COMPASSIONATE COMMUNITIES IN ACTION

Compassionate Communities in Action: Global Stories of Care, Loss and Connection brings together practical examples of compassionate cities and communities from around the world. Together they provide a practical road map, highlighting what has worked and what has been challenging, alongside reflections from the communities profiled.

Over the past 20 years, hundreds of areas globally have worked to develop compassionate cities and communities, in order to improve death, dying, loss, and caregiving for their residents. This book, designed to support those beginning their journey and those who want to continue to develop existing initiatives, highlights:

- Different models of organisation or structure for a Compassionate Community.
- How projects have engaged with wider civic society, including schools, workplaces, and the arts.
- Suggestions for reorientating health and care services towards community and well-being.
- The role of individual leaders in shaping grassroots activities.

Demonstrating public health palliative care in practice, this guide is an essential read for people working in the field of palliative and end-of-life care, as well as academics, students, and policymakers with an interest in the area.

Emma Hodges is the founder of Public Health Palliative Care UK and runs a management consultancy. This follows over 15 years' experience in public health palliative care including at Compassionate Communities UK and several years at a charitable hospice including as CEO. With 25 years' experience in healthcare with a focus on workforce and service redesign, she is driven by issues related to health and social inequity. Her doctoral research focused on UK hospices and dementia. She is Treasurer and an executive board member for Public Health Palliative Care International and a trustee of E-Hospice.

Manjula Patel is CEO of Murray Hall Community Trust, a community anchor hub, an organisation working to improve people's health and well-being through a social model of health from early years to end of life. Her doctoral research subject was about the development of compassionate communities, and she is a published author on the subject. She is also a Trustee of Locality and a member of the International Federation of Settlements.

COMPASSIONATE COMMUNITIES IN ACTION

Global Stories of Care, Loss and Connection

Edited by
Emma Hodges and Manjula Patel

Routledge
Taylor & Francis Group
LONDON AND NEW YORK

Designed cover image: Getty Images

First published 2026
by Routledge
4 Park Square, Milton Park, Abingdon, Oxon OX14 4RN

and by Routledge
605 Third Avenue, New York, NY 10158

Routledge is an imprint of the Taylor & Francis Group, an informa business

British Library Cataloguing-in-Publication Data
A catalogue record for this book is available from the British Library

ISBN: 978-1-041-02902-1 (hbk)
ISBN: 978-1-041-02901-4 (pbk)
ISBN: 978-1-003-62134-8 (ebk)

DOI: 10.4324/9781003621348

Typeset in Times New Roman
by codeMantra

CONTENTS

CONTRIBUTORS

Julian Abel is a retired palliative care physician, Director of Compassionate Communities UK, and Visiting Professor at the University of Northumbria, Newcastle.

Lacey Ahern, MPH, is the Executive Director of Global Partners in Care and Adjunct Associate Professor of the Practice in Global Health at the University of Notre Dame, Indiana, USA. She teaches on compassion and global health, and much of her work focuses on building partnerships to advance palliative care development globally.

Saphrah Amumpaire is an English and Literature teacher at Taibah International School in Uganda. She serves as the Patron of the Palliative Care Club at the school and has guided students in various community acts of kindness: caring for the suffering, easing pain, and making their days meaningful.

Samar Aoun, AM, is Perron Institute Research Chair in Palliative Care, University of Western Australia, Chair of Compassionate Communities Australia and the South West Compassionate Communities Network, and council member of Public Health Palliative Care International.

Julia Martínez Barbero is Project Manager at the *Agirre Lehendakaria Center for Social and Political Studies (ALC)* and a PhD candidate researching how experimentation portfolios that integrate cultural dynamics can support socio-ecological transitions. Her work ranges from the community-based redesign of drug policies in several Latin American countries to the facilitation of collaborative processes aimed at rethinking community-based care models in the Basque Country.

Rachael Basak is Head of Community Involvement and Support at Princess Alice Hospice in Surrey, UK. She leads work to build compassionate communities, supporting people to care for one another through illness, dying and bereavement. Rachael is passionate about partnership, inclusion and the role of local communities in shaping more compassionate responses to end of life.

Mary Ann Boe, an affiliate of Compassionate Communities UK and Healthcare Sector co-lead with the Charter for Compassion, is a grief companion and community weaver who fosters kindness, compassion, and belonging across sectors. As co-founder of the Journey Guide Project, she works to embed the science of narrative, connection, and mind-body integration into clinical care – addressing the gaps traditional medical models leave behind.

Georg Bollig, MD, PhD, MAS, is Associate Professor in Palliative Medicine in the Department of Palliative Medicine, University of Cologne, Germany and leader of Last Aid International. His scientific work focuses on Public Palliative Care Education, Telepalliative Care, and Ethics.

Alison Bunce, CEO, is a Queen's nurse, founder, leader, and guiding force of Compassionate Inverclyde, an award-winning community-led initiative that revolves around "ordinary people helping ordinary people" when confronted with crisis, illness, suffering, and other difficulties.

Katie Burbridge, MSc, PGCE, is Clinical Director at Acorns Children's Hospice after spending a little over a decade at an adult's hospice. She is driven by providing a high quality of care to patients and their loved ones.

James Byron lives in Bath and has worked for Dorothy House for the past six years and in the charity sector for more than two decades, spanning a range of causes. His passion for hospice care was inspired by personal experiences, not least the short life of his first son, Arthur.

Louise D'Eer, PhD, is postdoctoral researcher at the End-of-Life Care Research Group, Ghent University, Belgium. Her research is centred around the evaluation of civic engagement programmes around serious illness, death, and dying. She is a member of the Public Health Palliative Care International (PHPCI) and the Compassionate Communities Centre of Expertise (CoCo).

Erin Das, MN, RN, is a Canadian advanced practice nurse specializing in palliative care with 17 years of clinical and leadership experience across paediatric, cancer, and community-based care. She currently serves as practice lead at the Global Treehouse Foundation, Kidney Supportive Care Lead at AHN, and technical advisor for Oasis of Hope in Kenya, advancing access to holistic and integrated care models globally.

Elham Day, BA, MA, Grad Dip Couns. Grief&Loss, most recently was the Manager of the Family and Community Support Team at Hummingbird House, Queensland's only children's hospice. His work is focused on resourcing community-centred responses to (and involvement in) end-of-life, after-death care, and grief support for families.

Julen Larrañaga Martinez de Agirre is Project Manager at the "Agirre Lehendakaria Center for Social and Political Studies". He coordinates the social services area, with a particular focus on developmental evaluation in collaboration with Plena Inclusión, Matia Institute, and Agintzari. He also supports the work for the Deep Demonstration of the Diputación de Gipuzkoa. Before joining the ALC team, he worked on project coordination at the organisation Garabide and supported ethnographic work in countries such as Ecuador and Colombia.

Cara Doherty, BSocSc/BA, GradDipTAP, most recently was a community development worker at Hummingbird House children's hospice. She works alongside families, local communities, and stakeholders to strengthen community-held supports for families caring for, and grieving the death of, a child.

Leigh Donovan, BSW, PhD, Churchill Fellow, is a consultant in Thanatology with Collaboraide. Her work spans the clinical, programme, policy, and research domains within paediatric palliative care and bereavement care.

Sabine Eichberg, PhD, is Head of the Department for Health Planning and Health Promotion at the Cologne Public Health Office, Germany.

Constanza González is a clinical psychologist specialised in mindfulness and compassion training. She has led initiatives around end of life care and building communities of care in Colombia for the last 10 years.

Naomi Hasson is a palliative care nurse and compassionate communities coordinator, Getxo Zurekin – Fundación Doble Sonrisa and also President of the Basque Society for Palliative Care. Having worked for over 30 years in palliative care settings, she firmly believes in working alongside with the local communities in creating safe spaces for living and dying well.

Mark A. Hazelwood is CEO of the Scottish Partnership for Palliative Care (SPPC). Spanning policy, service improvement, and public health approaches, SPPC works collaboratively to improve all aspects of living with serious illness, dying, and bereavement.

Anne Hendry, Honorary Professor UWS and Director IFIC Scotland, is a geriatrician who held national clinical lead roles in Scotland for Long Term Conditions, Healthcare Quality, Reshaping Care for Older People, and integrated health and social care. Through IFIC's Academy and Solutions teams, she supports integrated care education and system coaching across the globe. She is the Chair of Kilbryde Hospice and Trustee of Compassionate Inverclyde.

Julieanne Hilbers, PhD, is the Compassionate Communities Project Lead for the Perron Institute and Deputy Chair of the South West Compassionate Communities Network.

Sheng-Jean Huang, MD, is a Taiwanese neurosurgeon and a leading advocate for palliative and community-based care. Former Superintendent of Taipei City Hospital and Director of NTU Hospital Jinshan Branch, he pioneered Taiwan's "aging and dying in place" model, integrating hospice and community health services. He played a key role in advancing Taiwan's Patient Autonomy Act. Recipient of the 2020 Presidential Innovation Award, he continues to promote compassionate, person-centred healthcare through education and writing, emphasizing dignity and quality of life over life prolongation.

Sumiko Kanegae, MD, MPH, PhD, is the Director of Compassionate Communities Japan and Hiramatsu Home Care Clinic. She has been involved in the development of compassionate communities in rural areas in Japan.

Allan Kellehear, OBE, is the academic founder and international lead for the public health approach to palliative and end-of-life care. He established and led the Palliative Care Unit at La Trobe University in Melbourne, Australia – the first non-clinical, public health practice-based, palliative care unit in the world. His foundational books on the topic – Health *Promoting Palliative Care* (1999) and *Compassionate Cities* (2005) – are widely cited in the international academic and policy literature. He has published some 25 books and over 120 articles on death, dying, and end-of-life care and has held numerous professorships in Australia, Japan, England, and the USA. Allan is currently Professor of End-of-Life Care at Northumbria University in Newcastle-upon-Tyne and elected Fellow of the Academy of Social Sciences. Allan was awarded an OBE in the King's Birthday Honours, in June 2025 for his exceptions contributions to palliative care

Leonard Kiprono, KRCHN, HDPC, BPsych, BTh, MPsych, MDivE, is a Kenyan Palliative Care nurse and trainer specialised in palliative care and counselling psychology as a practitioner as well as a trainer. He is also a licensed Christian Chaplain in Kenya and a programs coordinator for Oasis of Hope community-based organisation in Kericho County, Kenya.

Rosemary Kiwanuka is the first palliative care nurse in Uganda and has held several leadership positions. She was the founding Country Director of the Palliative Care Association of Uganda, where she retired and established the Lweza Community

Health Program. She continues to offer support and guidance for palliative care initiatives in Uganda across all levels of the healthcare system.

Anne Kreische works at the Division of Health Planning and Promotion in the Public Health Department, Cologne, Germany. Her work focuses on health promotion for elderly people.

Kerstin Kremeike is a trained physiotherapist, and social and health scientist. Her health services research focuses on dealing with the desire to die, dying in hospital, and death and grief literacy in the society. She is a spokesperson for the specialist group "Last Year of Life" at the German Network for Health Services Research (DNVF) and a board member of the German Association of Palliative Medicine (DGP).

Chia-Jen Liu holds a PhD in Business Administration (Health Care Management) from Fu Jen Catholic University and an EMBA in Business Administration from Tamkang University. His academic and professional background combines healthcare administration, business management, and social welfare, shaping his focus on integrating management innovation into community health and welfare systems.

Teresa Majkut is a recent graduate from the University of Notre Dame and interned at Global Partners in Care in her final year of studies. She is passionate about advancing global health equity and improving access to care for vulnerable populations worldwide.

Jenny Marshall is Executive Director at Mid & East Antrim Agewell Partnership, a charity which supports older people in Northern Ireland. She champions older adults' well-being through community-led, inclusive approaches and asset-based development, with a personal interest in death literacy and helping people plan and make informed choices around end of life.

Hugh McElhinney has been the lead for Compassionate Communities at St Elizabeth Hospice since 2022. Previously, he was the volunteer manager at East Anglia's Children's Hospice and has worked in the charity sector since 2012. His ongoing work focuses on improving underrepresented communities' knowledge of and access to palliative care, as well as helping people across different sectors of society gain the tolls and confidence to support those they live, socialise, and work with.

Sue Merriman is an experienced youth worker through founding and leading Vysions Youth Services, a youth-led organisation supporting children, young people, and families across Staffordshire, over the last decade. Her work through Brereton Million developed a deep understanding of trauma-informed care, emotional well-being, and creating safe, inclusive spaces for residents to thrive.

Saif Mohammed is a consultant and faculty member at the WHO Collaborating Centre, Institute of Palliative Medicine, and Membership Secretary of Public Health Palliative Care International. His work focuses on integrating palliative care into public health systems, building capacity in low- and middle-income countries, and advancing community-led bereavement support through the Bereavement Companionship Programme.

Paul Mwambi hold a BA degree in Education and an MA degree in IRD. He is a senior teacher at Taibah International School and the founding Patron of the School Compassionate Community Club/Program. He is passionate about empowering the youth for community action, and his work also focuses on eliminating barriers to education for young people.

Mark Mwesiga is the Executive Director of the Palliative Care Association of Uganda and part of the Lions Club of Entebbe Road. He is dedicated to community service, social justice, and spearheading grassroots initiatives aimed at transformation, particularly for vulnerable and humanitarian communities.

Jim Nininger, Co-Founder of Compassionate Ottawa, was President and CEO of the Conference Board of Canada from 1976 to 2001. He has served on private sector boards and has been active in a variety of community organisations.

Kerrie Noonan is Adjunct Associate Professor at the Public Health Palliative Care Unit, La Trobe University and Director of the Death Literacy Institute. Her research spans public health approaches to palliative care and bereavement, death literacy, compassionate communities and the development of the death literacy index.

Karin Ohler a trained communication scientist with several years of experience in the start-up sector, including in digital interaction. Since 2022, she has been leading the Caring Community Cologne project together with its steering group, overseeing the development, ongoing refinement, and implementation of local Caring Community structures and initiatives.

Monica Patten, former President and CEO of Community Foundations of Canada, is well known for her leadership in Canada's voluntary sector. She has been actively involved in the development of community philanthropy around the world and has received numerous awards for her work. She is a member of the Order of Canada.

Rebecca M. Patterson is Director of Good Life, Good Death, Good Grief, an initiative of the Scottish Partnership for Palliative Care. Guided by a community development approach, her work aims to increase death literacy and grief literacy across Scotland by taking actions in the five key domains outlined in the Ottawa Charter for Health Promotion.

Bert Quintiens works as a project coordinator at the End-of-Life Care Research Group and the Compassionate Communities Centre of Expertise (Vrije Universiteit Brussel & Ghent University). He obtained a PhD in Social Health Sciences by studying the development and evaluation of two Belgian Compassionate City projects. He has a background in nursing and clinical trials.

Niki Read is the Healthy End of Life Program Impact and Engagement Coordinator in the Public Health Palliative Care Unit at La Trobe University and Program Manager with the Death Literacy Institute. Her work is grounded in creative-, practice-based, and knowledge translation approaches.

Edward Roberts is a scientist turned public health professional, working at Birmingham Public Health. His work areas and interests are dementia, compassionate cities, the built environment, and issues of social justice.

Camila Ronderos is the Executive Director for Fundación Keralty and Keralty Compassionate Communities. Her work focuses on building capacity both in communities and healthcare institutions to connect social and community needs with community-based solutions that improve health and well-being outcomes.

Maider Grajales Saenz is specialist in Family and Community Medicine, with a Master's degree in Palliative Care She is at the Doble Sonrisa Foundation since 2017. Since 2016, she has been working in the community field, promoting awareness and visibility of palliative care.

Joseph Sawyer is a consultant in palliative care at St Elizabeth Hospice. He graduated from Imperial College in 2011 and holds a PhD in public health approaches to palliative care in dementia. His ongoing work focuses on supporting any given communities' capacity to provide care at the end of life.

Bee Hia Sim, Executive Director of the Singapore Hospice Council, leads national efforts in public education and community engagement of palliative care and builds compassionate communities across Singapore. She champions cross-sector partnerships that make end-of-life care "everyone's business".

Julia Strupp is senior researcher and coordinator in the Department of Palliative Medicine, University Hospital of Cologne, Germany. Her work focuses on health services and palliative care research, particularly the last year of life, patient and family experiences, and value-based healthcare. She leads and contributes to several national and international projects aimed at improving end-of-life care and promoting patient-centred and equitable health and social care systems.

Hirobumi Takenouchi is Professor of Philosophy and Death Studies at Shizuoka University and Representative Director of Compassionate Communities Japan. His research and social practice cover the themes of life and death as well as dialogue and compassion.

Raymond Voltz has held the Chair of Palliative Medicine at Cologne University Hospital since 2004 and is Director of the Department of Palliative Medicine. His scientific work focuses on the further development and evaluation of palliative care structures, the wish to die and the dying phase, Caring Communities, palliative care in neurological diseases, and neurological symptoms in palliative care.

Samuel Shih-Chih Wang, PhD, is Professor and Head of the Department of Health and Welfare at the University of Taipei. He holds a doctoral degree in Sociology from the University of Essex. His work spans interdisciplinary collaboration, volunteerism research, and integrated care. He is now focusing on social work practice research and social prescribing.

Birgit Weihrauch, MD, is former State Secretary and member of the Managing Board of the Caring Community Cologne Association.

FOREWORD

The public health approach is now a major policy and practice approach in hospice and palliative care. Known by numerous names as "public health palliative care", "health promoting palliative care", or the "compassionate communities movement", this social model of hospice and palliative care now sits alongside the more established public health approaches in all major areas of healthcare – from emergency medicine, disability public health, and sexual and reproductive health to public health work in drug and alcohol, school health, and heart and dementia healthcare.

Compassionate communities emphasise a number of key practices to support people at the end-of-life, their caregivers, and those living with grief and loss: community development, social ecology, death and grief literacy, health promotion, and services redesign. Key to all these practices are two central assumptions: (1) health and well-being are necessary and achievable goals for the end of life and (2) community action and participation are crucial to the achievement of those goals.

Community action and participation are vital elements to personal support because the lives of people living with life-limiting conditions, caregiving, and grief and loss are NOT confined to professional settings and institutions. Most of the time spent by these people occur in places and contexts of work, learning, play, shopping, and prayer, and this time is spent alone, or with friends, family, neighbours, or animal companions – occurring in the world, or online. These places and people are our compassionate communities of support and love. It is equally true that the promotion or preservation of health and well-being at the end-of-life balances and tempers our physical deterioration, sorrow, and difficulties of long-term care. Love, friendship, practical support and listening, companionship, shared reflection, and many other examples of the gifts of human support and accompaniment remain essential to the quality and continuity of care for one another in life as they do at the very end of it. These relationships are crucial to the steady supply – and maintenance – of hope, connection, and meaning. These gifts are the bold promise and vision of all compassionate communities.

This book showcases different models of organisation for these compassionate communities by helping readers to understand that there is no single model, no single best path to civic support at the end-of-life. The different chapters provide a practical insight into how community models have worked for compassionate community activists in their work with schools, workplaces, or in the arts. The different authors come from many different parts of the world and exemplify different roles of involvement – from healthcare to business to temples. This book demonstrates, through practical examples, the true value of reorienting our health and social care services by showing how these services can successfully move from our usual role of *providers-of-care* to a more promising future one as *partners-in-care*.

Professor Allan Kellehear OBE
Northumbria University

INTRODUCTION

Manjula Patel and Emma Hodges

Abstract

This chapter outlines the inspiration behind this book and the previous texts that it builds upon. It describes the current context, particularly as we move to super aged communities and why, amid changing demographics and social challenges it is timely. The chapter provides some of the background to compassionate cities and public health palliative and end of life care and the aspiration to normalise in the design of civic life key elements that improve the experiences of death, dying, loss and caregiving for all people. It goes on to provide an overview of the structure of the book and the appreciation of all the authors who have contributed to make this publication happen.

I.1 Introduction

2025 was the 20-year anniversary of the publication of *Compassionate Cities: Public Health and End of Life Care* [1]. Since then, hundreds of places have engaged in compassionate communities and cities activities aiming to improve death, dying, loss, and caregiving. This book brings together examples from around the world and provides a practical road map; what has worked well, what has worked less well with common themes and challenges. It also showcases the aspiration and dedication of the people behind the cities and communities featured.

This book builds on earlier texts, including *International Perspectives on Public Health and Palliative Care* [2] and *Compassionate Communities: Case Studies from Britain and Europe* [3] and it is hoped that this practice-based book will support anyone engaging in public health palliative care, compassionate city, or compassionate community initiatives.

DOI: 10.4324/9781003621348-1

Much of the literature on compassionate cities and compassionate communities is from a research perspective rather than practice with many more community examples than cities [4]. Discussions with some of the contributors to this book highlighted difficulties in translating theory into practice. This is particularly challenging where the word "compassion" does not have a direct translation. It is these discussions, the anniversary of the original text, and the knowledge that there are some wonderful examples from which everyone can learn, that inspired the idea for this book.

I.2 Why now

In addition to the anniversary of the original text [1], the global population is ageing [5], and this will put increased pressure on healthcare systems that have professionalised dying and on communities that are under resourced. It is essential, given the changing demographics, that public health palliative care approaches are developed alongside primary and secondary care.

Compassionate city and compassionate community initiatives provide practical approaches to building capacity within communities and civic structures. The aim is to reduce the taboo around death, dying, loss, and caregiving that can create barriers to support, for example within communities and workplaces. On average, 95% of the time that someone is seriously ill is spent amongst their own social networks, whatever that means for them, e.g. work, school playground, walking the dog or being alone [6]. It is this 95% of the time that offers the greatest opportunity to improve the experiences of people affected by death, dying, loss, and caregiving. Social morbidities such as time off school, time off work, depression, isolation, suicide, drug and alcohol usage, youth offending are all issues that can be addressed, at least in part, by public health palliative care.

Kellehear uses the comparison of health and safety, also a public health issue. It is taken for granted that our civic structures such as schools, workplaces, places of worship, and open spaces have been designed to incorporate health and safety and that there are sufficient policies and education in place to ensure there is no harm [7]. Similar tools, policies, education and design can be used to create compassionate cities and communities where all people can take it for granted, that when facing issues relating to death, dying, loss and caregiving they will be met with compassion and understanding by their employers, formal and informal services, family, friends, colleagues, their hairdresser or café owner, or wherever they spend their time.

No one has yet lived in a super-aged society, with the numbers of older people with multiple health conditions that will be visible across many communities globally. This is a whole population issue. For dementia alone, 82 billion hours of informal care is provided to people at home, women contributing 71% of these hours [8]. Wong [8] states that "changing family structures, coupled with changes to migration trends continue to weaken informal support systems, shifting the burden of care towards an (unprepared) wider society" [8, p. 58].

This is not just an issue for adults; our children have not previously, grown up amongst so many older people with the implications for them seeing the declining health and increased number of people dying. The ageing population may result in increasing numbers of young caregivers and the impact this has on their life chances. In addition, more young people with life-limiting illnesses are moving into adulthood with often inadequate planning from children's services to adult provision.

Many programmes separate out groups in society such as healthy ageing, dementia action planning, children, and young people. Death, dying, loss, and caregiving are universal experiences and need to be embedded across all health policy development and civic life, a whole population approach.

The challenge is not easy; however, the areas highlighted in this book show that change is possible and that there are many creative and practical ways to make a difference at all levels including grass roots communities, service providers, and policymakers.

I.3 Background

The history of compassionate cities and compassionate communities emerged from applying public health principles to palliative care. In public health palliative care, there is a focus on health policy and management, environmental health science, social and behavioural science as key strands. The field of public health palliative care practice includes elements of health promotion, including civic engagement, community development, public education, social ecology, and policy development [9].

The World Health Organisation's (WHO) Healthy Cities programme, founded on the principles of the Ottawa Charter for Health Promotion, did not adequately make provision for issues relating to death, dying and loss [1, 10]. The Compassionate City movement was "created as a policy and practice corrective" to the Healthy City Programme [11, p. 118]. In developing healthy cities, WHO decided that the "city" was "the lowest administrative level which can marshal the resources and has the political mandate and authority to develop and implemented intersectional approaches to health" [12].

The Healthy City programme focuses action on, "forging necessary connections in political, economic, and social arenas" [13]. These arenas include statutory health organisations, nursing homes, schools, workplaces, voluntary organisations, and places of worship and are key areas of action within the compassion city charter [14].

Whilst the narrative has a focus on "city" as the place of change, in practice where there is a different administrative level e.g. town, village, or county, that makes sense, then the compassionate city charter or a localised version is applied.

Professor Allan Kellehear's book [1] recommended nine policy visions and associated operating policies [1]; this later became the compassionate city charter [14]. Many people assume that the charter statements are standards to achieve and measure. Kellehear [5] is clear that they are purely guidance and areas of focus across civic life with many places writing their own charter that is relevant to their geographical, cultural, and social context [7].

Kellehear suggests that the way how to make compassionate city policies "real" is through "community development," "community capacity building," and "community work or community action" [1, p. 117], in other words, as compassionate communities.

I.4 Definitions

The terms compassionate city and compassionate community are used interchangeably in practice and in some of the chapters that form this book. We have not corrected these definitions and discuss this issue further in the conclusion chapter. However, for clarity, the following explanation is provided:

> Compassionate communities is a practice method of community development that forms part of the toolkit of public health palliative care [1]. A compassionate community is a naturally occurring community that might be place based or online.
>
> A Compassionate City, which would include compassionate communities, is a level of administrative authority that can also focus on policy change and structural redesign across several areas of civic life.

I.5 Structure of this book

The first part of this book has examples from 20 different communities around the world. These chapters have been organised alphabetically by place. These chapters provide insight into the many similar and dissimilar approaches and challenges when involved in a compassionate city or compassionate community initiative.

These place based chapters are followed by four chapters outlining common tools that are utilised in the practice of compassionate cities and compassionate communities. These include the death literacy index, community connectors, and community-focused service redesign.

Finally, there is a conclusion that brings together many of the themes from this book, the critical ingredients of practice, including partnerships, diversity, social capital, death, and grief literacy and many of the shared challenges such as definitions, resources, and size.

I.6 Contributions

In selecting contributions to this book, the editors wanted to ensure that the practice examples were diverse and truly global. There are 20 communities represented, including from Africa, Asia, Australia, Europe, North America, and South America. The chapters include countries that would be considered as resource rich and resource poor. The examples include diverse cultural settings and range from a village community, a large city, to a whole country in terms of size and structure of compassionate city and compassionate community examples. For people familiar with the field, there are some chapters from places that have been leading the way for some time, and there are also some from less well-known examples of compassionate city and compassionate community work.

The contributors to this book include many leaders in the field of public health palliative care, compassionate cities, and communities and, as this is a practice-based book, there are also community leaders doing amazing work, who would not count themselves as being at the forefront of this international movement. The editors are incredibly grateful to all the authors who have contributed to this book. By sharing their experiences, they are inspiring and enabling others around the world in the practicalities of developing compassionate cities and communities. Thank you.

References

1. A. Kellehear, *Compassionate Cities: Public Health and End of Life Care*, Oxfordshire: Routledge, 2005.
2. L. Sallnow, S. Kumar and A. Kellehear, *International Perspectives on Public Health and Palliative Care*, London: Routledge, 2013.
3. K. Wegleitner, K. Heimerl and A. Kellehear, *Compassionate Communities: Case Studies from Britain and Europe*, Oxon: Routledge, 2016.
4. S. Librada-Flores, M. Nabal-Vicuna, D. Forero-Vega, I. Munoz-Mayorga and M. D. Guerra-Martin, "Implementation Models of Compassionate Communities and Compassionate Cities at the End of Life: A Systematic Review," *International Journal of Environmental Research Public Health*, 2020, Vol 17, pp. 1–15 [Online]. Available: https://www.mdpi.com/1660-4601/17/17/6271 [Accessed 22 July 2025].
5. World Health Organisation, "Ageing: Global Population," 21 February 2025. [Online]. Available: https://www.who.int/news-room/questions-and-answers/item/population-ageing. [Accessed 27 October 2025].
6. A. Kellehear, "Workshop: Igniting CommUnity," [Powerpoint slldes]. *Compassionate Communities UK* Conference, Rugeley. 2024. [Online]. Available: https://compassionate-communitiesuk.com/wp-content/uploads/2025/04/About-CC-UK-Igniting-CommUnity-1-1.pdf. [Accessed 22 July 2025].
7. A. Kellehear, "*Discussions in Singapore*." [Interview] *Singapore Hospice Council*, Singapore. 2025. [Online]. Available: https://www.singaporehospice.org.sg/an-interview-with-professor-allan-kellehear/#. [Accessed 18 August 2025].
8. D. Wong, "Women and dementia: from caregiving disparities to economic opportunities," in *Dementia in the Commonwealth",* CommonAge, 2024. [Online]. Available: https://commonage.net/wp-content/uploads/2024/09/Dementia-in-the-Commonwealth-full-report-2024.pdf. [Accessed 18 August 2025].
9. J. Abel and A. Kellehear (Eds.), *Oxford Textbook of Public Health Palliative Care*, Oxford: Oxford University Press, 2022.
10. World Health Organisation, *Ottawa Charter for Health Promotion*, Ottawa Canada: World Health Organisation, 1987.
11. G. Wilson, E. Herrera Molina, L. F. Silvia Librada and A. Kellehear, "Compassionate Cities: A Social Ecology at the End of Life," in Abel and A. Kellehear (Eds.), *Oxford Textbook of Public Health Palliative Care*, Oxford: Oxford University Press, 2022, pp. 117–125.
12. J. Ashton, P. Grey and K. Barnard, "Healthy Cities – WHO's New Public Health Initiative," *Health Promotion*, vol. 1, no. 3, pp. 319–324, 1986.
13. World Health Organisation, "Creating Healthy Cities," [Online]. Available: https://www.who.int/activities/creating-healthy-cities. [Accessed 18 August 2025].
14. A. Kellehear, "Compassionate City Charter," 2020. [Online]. Available: https://compassionate-communitiesuk.com/the-compassionate-city-charter-3/. [Accessed 18 August 2025].

1

COMPASSIONATE BIRMINGHAM – CREATING, CARING, CONNECTED AND SUPPORTIVE COMMUNITIES IN BIRMINGHAM AND BEYOND

Edward Roberts and Emma Hodges

Abstract

Birmingham is a large, diverse city in the centre of England and became the first city to be endorsed as a compassionate city by Compassionate Communities UK in 2021. This chapter describes the complexity of navigating the different levels of action in developing a compassionate city (i) grassroots, (ii) organisations and services and (iii) city government and policy.

This is a story of learning by experience as the team involved in Compassionate Birmingham worked together to understand the structure, the approach and issues relating to monitoring and outcomes.

The learning is an ongoing process with new opportunities taking shape as this chapter is written. The Compassionate Birmingham Network acknowledges and thanks everyone who has been part of this journey so far.

1.1 Introduction

Birmingham is the second largest city in England. It is a city of 1.15 million people with complex demographics, and although considered a young city with an average age of 34 (compared to 40 for England), that does not mean there are not many older residents living in the city. The city's ethnic composition is diverse with 48.6% describing themselves at White, 31.0% as Asian, Asian British or Asian Welsh, and 11.0% as Black, Black British, Black Welsh, Caribbean or African [1,2]. Mixed, multiple or other ethnic groups make up the remaining population. In terms of ethnicity, this has earned the city the title: super diverse. However, the city also has diversity in terms of its LGBTQ+ population, people with disability, Birmingham's faith centres and more.

DOI: 10.4324/9781003621348-2

In the UK, we conceptualise deprivation through a decile-based system: every 10% is a decile, where decile 1 is the most deprived 10% and decile 10 is the least deprived 10%. Birmingham is a highly deprived city, with 41% of the city living in decile 1, and 60% of the city living in deciles 1–3. This leads to greater health and social challenges for residents. These deciles take account of the following factors:

- Income deprivation (22.5%)
- Employment deprivation (22.5%)
- Education, skills and training deprivation (13.5%)
- Health deprivation and disability (13.5%)
- Crime (9.3%)
- Barriers to housing and services (9.3%)
- Living environment deprivation (9.3%)

Birmingham's mortality data is significantly worse than the England average, which is a function of the high deprivation in the city. The city's mortality rates are in the worst 25th percentile for 61 of the 70 metrics used [3]. The remaining nine metrics are all below the England average. These metrics are split across the following categories:

- All causes
- Cancer
- Cardiovascular disease
- COVID-19
- Dementia and Alzheimer's disease
- Liver disease
- Respiratory disease

This data is, however, nuanced by ethnicity. For example, cancer rates are higher in the White population, but infant deaths are highest in the Black population (7.4 per 1,000 live births), S. Asian (7.0 per 1,000 live births), and then White (4.1 per 1,000 live births). Furthermore, data from 2011 to 2014 shows that people from White and Mixed-Ethnic groups had lower life expectancy than people from the Black African group. This may have changed in the intervening years, but there is no data to categorise it.

Place of death is captured in the system with 48% of people dying in hospital, 28% dying at home, 17% in a care home and 5% in a hospice. The remaining people die elsewhere. The most common causes of death are 45% frailty, 19% cancer, and 18% organ failure.

There is limited data regarding where people seek support around death, dying, loss and caregiving or the cultural appropriateness of the support available.

The communities of the city are bounded by certain government structures. Birmingham is divided into five localities, ten constituencies and 69 wards. The boundaries of these areas do change, which adds complexity, and they are not recognised in the same way by all organisations. For example, the police and National Health Service (NHS) recognise slightly different boundaries than the local government. For the police, this is due to the operational efficiency of the policing district and neighbourhoods. However, how the various large-scale organisations understand the city is invariably different to how the citizens recognise their neighbourhoods and communities.

One of the many community tools implemented by Birmingham City Council are Neighbourhood Network Schemes (NNS) [4]. These are funded by Adult Social Care (ASC) and Public Health (PH) departments within local government. They aim to provide support for people to live happy, healthy and independent lives in their own homes and communities. They do this by funding, supporting, and linking up local community groups and setting priorities for their areas. This offer was initially for older adults, but it was such a success that it was extended to all adults.

Birmingham is formed of many smaller communities that exist under one umbrella. Some of the better-known neighbourhoods in the city are Digbeth, known as a creative quarter with many music venues – also, the Jewellery Quarter with its rich heritage of craftsmanship. Then there is Mosely with many independent shops and Mosely Bog, which inspired J.R.R Tolkien's vision of the Old Forest in the Lord of the Rings. There are also many other communities both famous and invisible.

Birmingham is rich in its diverse culture with many museum, arts events and festivals. Birmingham has a calendar of events happening throughout the year. To date, the city has 18 annual events [5]. The yearly event that fits most clearly into the compassionate city objectives is the A Matter of Life and Death (AMOLAD) festival, organised by Brum YODO (you only die once), a CIC that aims to create a society that talks openly and honestly about death and dying [6]. However, there are additional festival and events that bring people together as communities in the city: Birmingham Pride, Birmingham Jazz and Blues Festival, Simmer Down Festival and Mosely Folk and Arts Festival, amongst others.

The characteristics of Birmingham make it challenging to work in because it cannot be approached as one area, but instead, it must be approached as many smaller communities. This hyper-local approach must then be connected at an organisational and service level where organisations are often working in several communities or city wide, and at local government level to influence policy and change.

1.2 Background to Compassionate Birmingham

Organisations working in Birmingham were some of the first in the country to actively engage in compassionate communities. Murray Hall Community Trust had been exploring and developing practice in compassionate communities since 2008 after hearing Allan Kellehear speak at a conference at Teesside University [7].

In 2009, the West Midlands Strategic Health Authority chose four sites and funded compassionate communities pilot projects one of these was Murray Hall Community Trust and the other Birmingham-based pilot was Birmingham St Mary's Hospice (now known as Birmingham Hospice) [7].

These pioneering organisations continued the dialogue about a compassionate communities' approach being key as part of a wider palliative and end-of-life care strategy. However, it was difficult to gain traction. Other local hospices also started to advocate for and build PH approaches. The focus remained on clinical pathways and the many challenges associated with reducing deaths in hospital, early identification of people who would benefit from palliative care and advance care planning. There was little interest in compassionate communities becoming a key strategy or policy driver across the city.

However, the impact of COVID created the necessary political and organisational will to move forward on this initiative. Key people from health, hospice and ASC started to reshape compassionate communities as a whole population approach that did not reside within just hospice or palliative care services.

Working with CCUK, funded by the ASC Department, two teams of people from across different sectors participated in compassionate communities' foundation training programme. This helped form a team and momentum to achieve Compassionate Birmingham status.

Because of the earlier work and the activities of Brum YODO [6] and others, there were already many examples of compassionate communities' activities that would demonstrate progress towards the compassionate city charter [8] and CCUK's endorsement process.

The endorsement is not awarded to the "perfect compassionate city" but is awarded to those who have shown significant progress and commitment across a range of the areas of action in the charter [8], senior sign up and a clear plan on what to focus on next. This is not about new projects but building on what is already in place.

This first team worked together gaining support from the Informal Cabinet of Birmingham and the City's Health and Wellbeing Board along with many other senior key stakeholders. The city was awarded compassionate city status in February 2022.

1.3 Maintaining momentum

After the achievement of the endorsement, it would be fair to say that there were some challenging times ahead. Some key people changed roles; there were more changes within the health and care policy landscape and trying to move the programme forward was difficult and lacked clarity.

In April 2022, the city's PH Department took a lead role and formed a partnership with CCUK to create some additional capacity for the Compassionate Birmingham programme.

One of the key aims was to understand all the activities across the city that contributed to Compassionate Birmingham and there were lots of examples, many of which came out of the public response to COVID.

During COVID, many people organised to support those in their community's needing assistance, and this was done at a grassroots level. For example, Northfield Community Partnership (NCP), which was a small community group at the time, coordinated a stakeholder network consisting of numerous organisations and people. They organised through Zoom and would have 100–200 people on a Zoom call at its height. They organised support for vulnerable people in their community by actions such as delivering food parcels and collecting medications. Different groups were able to bring different contributions to the initiative, such as vans (Bournville Village Trust) or faith centres, who knew who needed what.

One of the elements that created confusion was the interchangeability of the terms "compassionate city" and "compassionate community". The Compassionate Birmingham Network define these as follows:

- Compassionate city is a civic society that recognises that care for one another at times of crisis and loss is everyone's responsibility. It amplifies, supports, and celebrates compassionate communities.

- Compassionate communities are naturally occurring communities that support each other using their skills and assets. Making the most of associational life, reducing social isolation and creating a resilience that reduces the reliance on services for challenges that do not need a formal intervention.

Of course, having an agreed definition does not stop the terms still being used interchangeably! The aim of Compassionate Birmingham is to bring together the wonderful compassionate communities in the city, with clear policy support across civic society and a recognition and action regarding inequity relating to death, dying, loss and caregiving. When the term compassionate city is used, it is recognised that compassionate communities are a vital part of its success.

The concern around momentum has been a continual theme as the team learned together and better understood the PH approach. Another cohort of local people has been involved in the compassionate city foundation programme training which has also helped engage new stakeholders in understanding this work.

There have been several changes to the structure and governance of the programme as part of trying to find the right fit that supports all three levels of activity and forward momentum.

1.3.1 Structure

The Compassionate Birmingham programme sits with the PH Team. Originally, the aim had been to have no single lead organisation to enable the co-leadership and to prevent the model becoming embedded in a service mindset. However, it was clear that there did need to be a lead body, and this needed to be carefully considered. The PH Team, for Birmingham, is the ideal home for the city-wide strategy as they are not a service provider and there is a desire to consider how the Ottawa charter principles [9] relate to palliative and end-of-life care.

Initially, there was a plan to have a subgroup for each of the standards in the charter [8]; however, this seemed to create a focus on new projects rather than connecting with everything that was already happening.

The second iteration was that someone who sat on any other overlapping meeting, e.g. the bereavement forum and homelessness forum should be a member of the Compassionate Birmingham Network and update at the meetings. The only subgroups would be for those areas where there was not an existing group.

This also did not work very well as the other groups were not meeting regularly or were not talking about relevant topics to the network which made the meetings rather dull.

The third iteration was a Compassionate Birmingham Network that meets monthly. Anyone can join the network. There have been many meetings, however, discussing structure and strategy which is not particularly appealing for community leaders and activists.

The latest iteration is that the network will meet every other month, and a new group has been created focusing on public participation in Compassionate Birmingham and network members can choose to attend that meeting as well as, or instead of the more formal meeting. In addition, a group focusing on the charter domain of children and young people has also been established. Our model is now more fluid, setting up groups as needed for the programme, but keeping a strong core of people engaged via the network meetings and the contract between PH and CCUK.

As part of the endorsement, there was a document that listed all the activities there were already in place in Birmingham and what the next steps would be for each of the areas in the city charter [8]. This was helpful and is updated annually.

As part of the aim is to capture existing activities that contribute to Compassionate Birmingham, the PH lead for compassionate cities goes out to the networks to collect as many examples as possible. Only a fraction of true resident-led activity is being collected; the examples tend to be at that middle level of organisations' activities. The hope is that the new public participation group will start to better understand the existing strengths and challenges in the many communities that make up Birmingham.

Birmingham is also involved in Ageing Well and Dementia-Friendly programmes and along with other key policies such as frailty and falls prevention understands the connection between these complimentary policies.

Both Compassionate Cities and Age-Friendly Cities have been named as key drivers for Birmingham's emerging Ageing Well strategy and a compassionate cities focus is being adopted including:

1 Use the values of compassionate cities to inform the vision and approach to Ageing Well
2 Compassion as one of three principles alongside independence and choice

3 The emerging Ageing Well Strategy has four themes:

   a Dying well
   b Brain health
   c Planning for retirement
   d Falls and frailty

4 These themes are nuanced, through the use of the eight pillars of Age-Friendly Cities:

   a Community and health services
   b Transportation
   c Housing
   d Social participation
   e Outdoor spaces and buildings
   f Respect and social inclusion
   g Civic participation and employment
   h Communication and information [10]

This progress reinforces the need to focus on all three levels (i.e. city (i) grassroots, (ii) organisations and services and (iii) city government and policy). If the programme was all grassroots, this sort of embedding of strategy into cross-civic society policies would not be happening. However, without a focus on grassroots any policy-led initiative will not achieve the outcomes that are important to the people of Birmingham.

1.4 Activities

1.4.1 A Matter of Life and Death Festival

Annually, during Dying Matters Week, Brum YODO holds the city's A Matter of Life and Death Festival (AMOLAD) [6]. This is a festival that focuses on arts and creativity to convey its message, and they have been organising this since 2015. The members of Brum YODO, who were initially involved in the death economy, have delivered this festival both with and without funding. The events that make up this festival are held in different parts of the city, though there are areas that are more involved, which leads to a greater concentration of events in those parts of the city. Each year, there are about 20 events that happen over an approximate two-week period in early May. Although it has been possible to organise this festival without funding, doing so requires the goodwill of numerous organisations and is logistically challenging, taking up significant time for the volunteer organisers.

1.4.2 Northfield Community Partnership (NCP)

In 2023, NCP, a local charity working in the Northfield area of Birmingham, received funding from the PH Department to establish a compassionate city project.

NCP were commissioned to deliver this project as a pilot within the Northfield Constituency using their NNS (Neighbourhood Network) team. This project led to numerous events and training opportunities within the local area.

Northfield NNS used the funding to upskill community groups in their area and launch their own events. They set out to do some research on what compassionate cities are by attending as many events as they could during the 2023 AMOLAD festival run by Brum YODO. The very next month, they organised a compassionate communities launch event for their community organisations, at which various speakers linked to the compassionate city ethos gave talks and hosted discussions – essentially, raising awareness of the topic. Additionally, at the annual NCP Beach event in August 2023, which attracted over 23,000 people over five days, Northfield NNS hosted a specific compassionate communities' marquee. They had Birmingham Hospice, A Natural Undertaking, Coffin Club, Methodist Housing Association, Brum YODO and Cruse Bereavement, all attending at different points. They also had an art installation by local artist Jemma Mellor, to which people were able to add their memories. This art installation was turned into a travelling art installation and continued to grow. Lastly, they organised bereavement training for local community organisations and set up three new, local bereavement groups: Weaving and Grieving, Golden Threads at the Scrap store and a bereavement church group.

1.4.3 Bereavement and prisons

Birmingham Hospice worked with the prison in the city to deliver palliative care when required. However, during this time, it was realised that there was a lack of bereavement support for inmates who were coping with loss. This was an important piece of work because it is recognised that grief and bereavement are experienced at higher rates by prisoners and their situations are more complex, and due to their context, dealing with this is often extremely isolating. This piece of work developed a training toolkit to:

1. Enable prisons to establish their own bereavement group.
2. Improve the understanding for imprisoned people of the impacts of grief and how to support peers within the prison facility affected by it.
3. Develop suitable resources and tools to help support people in prison to deal with loss and grief more effectively.

For the project to start, support was needed from the prison governor. This led to the hospice community-development workers co-designing a grief awareness programme with the inmate volunteer health and well-being coordinators in the prison.

Training of inmates showed a significant improvement in their ability to recognise the symptoms of grief and support fellow inmates within the prison. It also gave inmates another place to receive support other than the chaplaincy. From this, several key themes emerged:

1 Tools to help with hopelessness
2 What to say and not to say
3 Bereavement and suicide
4 Resources for peers and families
5 Grieving for loss of a child
6 Culture and diversity

There were some key learning from the project. First, poor prison staffing levels hindered the setup of the project. Also, prison security meant that hospice staff could not bring their own laptops or training materials to the prison, and sessions had to fit into 90-minute segments to align with prison procedures. Importantly, not only did publicity of the project have to be handled carefully, but some hospice staff questioned why hospices were working with prisoners, demonstrating the stigma associated with this group of people. Lastly, the project primarily hinged upon the goodwill of one member of prison staff.

1.4.4 Increasing death and grief literacy in communities

Evolve and Flourish, a local community interest company specialising in compassionate communities, was funded by the Birmingham Voluntary Service Council to run a project to increase death and grief literacy in five of the city's ten constituencies.

The topics of death, dying and grief were received differently in various areas of the city. Some of the constituencies had large ethnically diverse populations, and these, compared to those constituencies with less diversity had less take up of the project. This is further nuanced by each NNS (we have one for each constituency) having their own set of priorities, of which some would map more closely to this project than others. Lastly, the relationships of voluntary, community, and social enterprise organisations present in each constituency with the NNS team also influenced engagement.

The project delivered bereavement awareness training to 122 staff and volunteers from local assets and 46 members of the public, hosted 15 death literacy events and helped assets deliver a range of compassion cafes using creativity to help facilitate conversations and bonding over grief.

Birmingham LGBT offers a well-being support service to LGBTQ+ people aged 50 and over. The service includes one-to-one well-being support sessions, combined with a range of group activities, open to anyone from this age group.

From March to June 2024, Birmingham LGBT ran a series of workshops under the banner "Living Your Best Life", which concluded with "Planning Your Fab Funeral – Planning the End of Your Life". This workshop encouraged participants to set up their own end-of-life folder, with sections on lasting power of attorney, advance directives, insurance and payments, my funeral, my will, important documents and contracts (passwords, etc.). We used good practice guidance from Age

UK, Independent Age, Bereavement Advice Centre, a local undertaker: A Natural Undertaking, and "Making Informed Choices When Planning a Funeral – a guide for queer people" by Ash Hayhurst [11].

Whilst many heterosexuals and/or cisgender people have family who are involved in their end-of-life decisions, LGBTQ+ people, especially of this generation, may be estranged from family, even their own children. They often build a "family of choice", and the workshops emphasised the importance of involving their chosen family members in their plans, especially where there was the risk of "blood" family being hostile to the LGBTQ+ person's plans. We know about trans people whose family have buried them under their birth, "dead", name and excluded their family of choice, for instance. So, having the tools to be able to live their later life and end-of-life in an affirmative way and having made plans for their death, funeral and will is very important for the LGBTQ+ community.

1.4.5 Death literacy index

In addition to a range of local activities, some of which are described in this section. At a city-wide level, the Compassionate Birmingham Network decided to test the death literacy index, which was developed by Noonan et al. [12], and is validated for use in the UK [13].

The aim was to try to get a representative sample and to see whether the index would provide useful information as part of the compassionate city programme. There were known limitations in the methodology of testing the index, the main one, being that links to the survey, were going out via existing networks and social media. This would impact the types of people completing the survey. However, this risk was accepted as a "broad test" rather than a deep dive into any specific community.

Statistical significance for Birmingham was calculated at 386 survey responses, and the network were relieved to hit 391 with some last-minute pleas for completion. However, statistical significance does not mean the sample is representative; this is covered in Chapter 24.

The result of the test provided useful feedback on the index itself as well as some indication for future actions. Most people who completed the survey were White women and therefore whilst the number for statistical significance was reached, because demographic data was collected, the results are not representative of the diversity of the city.

The other feedback that was key to next steps was that for some members of the community who reviewed the survey, the language was complex. The survey has been adjusted to comply with Plain English standards to address those concerns [14].

Whilst the death literacy index is being used in many countries internationally, a key concern is the acceptability of the survey title and questions to some of the diverse communities in Birmingham. This is being taken forward as part of a future project.

More information on the results of the death literacy survey is in Chapter 24.

1.4.6 Evaluation

Much of the work mentioned above was evaluated and a conference in 2023 brought together stakeholders across Birmingham to hear and learn about compassionate city activities.

The death literacy index is being used as a community development tool as one of the methods of capturing change in addition to surveys and conversations to demonstrate the impact of the various programmes.

These evaluations often say the same thing; people feel uncomfortable talking about death, dying, bereavement or sharing their grief. Once they have been through a training session and talked about their experiences and feelings, it becomes much easier to discuss the topics and offer support to people around them. People are often grateful for information on creating wills and powers of attorneys, and sessions are, for some people, a trigger for conversations at home about these matters. This message has come through repeatedly.

However, the size of Birmingham is challenging. The work that is happening does not have the funding to operate at the scale of the entire city. This means that there are pockets in which change happens, but it is not reaching everyone.

The hope is that by growing public participation in Compassionate Birmingham, we can develop programmes such as community connectors, bereavement awareness and palliative care for non-healthcare professionals via cascade models at scale.

1.5 New programmes in 2025

Whilst the Compassionate Birmingham Network aims to collect and connect with many of the grassroots existing activities, the network can also work to co-create city-wide solutions to some of the common challenges.

1.5.1 A city wide approach to bereavement

The aim of this work is to help people in Birmingham feel better able to support their family, friends, neighbours and colleagues who are impacted by grief. The project will create free resources, including films, that will be available to everyone and everywhere across the city. The resources will include films of local people sharing their experience of grieving, what helped, what did not and what they wish others had understood. People often feel isolated when grieving because either no one knows what to say or people say things that may be well meaning but make things worse. People's attitudes towards us when we are grieving are key to us feeling understood and less isolated.

The films will also show different experiences based on diversity and types of deaths. This recognises that family, friends and colleagues may feel more able to provide informal support to some types of deaths than others. Therefore, the aim is to have films that talk about different religious and cultural backgrounds, parents who have had a child die including those who have experience a long illness and those who have experienced miscarriage or a still birth, people from the LGBTQIA+ community, people widowed at different ages, people who are neurodivergent and people who are bereaved following a long illness and sudden death. The project is also considering other experiences including violent crime resulting in death.

The catalyst for this work was when the Birmingham Bereavement Forum flagged to the Compassionate Birmingham Network that there is an increased demand for support alongside competition for charitable funding. The statutory funding challenges for the NHS are considerable and therefore a different approach was needed.

Research shows that the most effective form of bereavement support is family, friends and colleagues rather than formal services [15,16]. Therefore, a PH approach to bereavement as part of Compassionate Birmingham is a far more effective solution than investing in more formal services.

Through consultation and collaboration, a paper has been created called a City-wide Approach to Bereavement. Many of the key stakeholders, including national and local bereavement charities, have been engaged in the development of the paper and have endorsed a compassionate community approach.

Key to the success of this project, in addition to finding local people willing to be filmed, is the wide dissemination of the films across employers' networks, community groups and faith networks along with a communications strategy.

1.5.2 Befriending

The next city-wide focus is on befriending. There are many organisations and groups across the city that have "befriending" programmes of one sort or another. There are new programmes being considered and the city also has other roles locally such as end-of-life care doulas and soul midwives who are not widely known.

The aim of the project is to engage with this wide befriending community to understand their experiences and challenges, to explore local grassroots solutions to loneliness and isolation and to find out about levels of death literacy.

1.5.3 Fairer futures

Compassionate Birmingham is engaged in a project with the city's South Asian community. The project is operating across 12 community centres for this community, which is primarily formed of Bangladeshi, Pakistani and Indian groups. The project comprises four goals.

The project's goals are the development of Communities of Practice (CoP), which are facilitated groups that co-produce interventions to local problems with the aim of becoming self-sufficient. Then, there is the Talk Listen Connect initiative, which aims to make support easier to find in communities when people need it. Finally, the project will deliver work on social ecology mapping and health systems mapping, completed by partners at Birmingham University, to gain a deeper understanding of South Asian needs in Birmingham.

Due to the co-produced nature of the CoP element of the project, the way the project will be evaluated needs to be adaptable given the unknown (at time of writing) nature of the interventions that local groups will deem important. As such, there will be several potential evaluation measures used, though the aims and objectives of each CoP will be captured together with the potential impact for mental health and well-being of each intervention as well as what will be finally realised.

As with many projects, it became apparent that organising work like this takes more time than initially estimated. Additionally, it helped significantly that our community development workers were primarily South Asian and multi-lingual. This made a significant difference in gaining community trust. Lastly, we are beginning to find (at time of writing) that working with faith organisation may be the best way to yield results because they are extant social and community structures, which makes a difference to the delivery timeline of the projects.

1.6 Size and tiers

Every place is different, and from hearing stories from other areas, it feels that it may be easier to see change at a smaller scale e.g. village size. Understanding the cause and effect of activities, grassroots involvement and ownership all seem easier in a smaller geographical area.

However, a village programme may not be able to influence some of the city- or county-wide policies they have no control over. Many relevant policies, strategies and funding operate across larger populations and are not devolved to town and parish councils.

Working at a larger scale can be problematic because though it brings together organisations that operate at the city level in a strategic manner. This can create a space that is unwelcoming for smaller organisations working at a community level. Working at scale can make it harder to see change and to capture all the amazing activities that are taking place, particularly at grassroots level.

Attempting to link together various strands of civic life and the broad opportunities of a compassionate city programme against an increasingly fraught funding environment is challenging. Organisations do not have the capacity to champion the goals of a myriad of initiatives.

In Birmingham, the NNS deliver a significant amount of work that would be classified as compassionate community, whilst also funding support for people who are dying, bereaved, grieving or have caring responsibilities. However, the NNS was set up prior to the compassionate city work, and due to challenges such as capacity and oversight, the links between the compassionate city network and the NNS have historically been variable. This is an example of one of the issues of trying to capture the great work happening in Birmingham given the size and complexity of the system. There are no incentives for all organisations to use compassionate cities as a central repository of knowledge for what is happening in the city and a lack of capacity to make it so.

Understanding how to operate at multiple tiers has been a key reflection and recognising that not everyone can work across all three levels e.g. grassroots, organisations and service providers and local government and city strategy. This is an ongoing challenge for Birmingham.

The hope is that the funding for a marketing and communication campaign will be secured for the bereavement project and that this, acts as a catalyst for Compassionate Birmingham.

1.7 Inclusivity

There have been some really great examples of work with many of the diverse communities in Birmingham. However, again these are restricted by capacity and are often subject to short-term project money.

Death rites vary greatly by heritage and religion. We, on the Compassionate City steering group, do not currently have the diversity to represent the 18 primary ethnic groups and 31 documented languages spoken in the city [2]. This is further complicated by the strength or weakness or absence of links to these different communities, of which some are spread across the city, and this does not account for our LGBTQ+ population, Gypsy, Roma and traveller communities or migrants and refugees.

The aim is that programmes such as the City-wide Approach to Bereavement and Fairer Futures can help connect further with some of our diverse communities.

Learning from other international examples, Compassionate Birmingham is fortunate to have links with an inter-faith network and there is more that can be explored in this area.

In the context of inclusivity, Compassionate Birmingham is aware that there needs to be a greater focus on understanding the experiences of such a diverse city. The focus of the new subgroup focusing on public participation in Compassionate Birmingham must lean into this challenge.

A sustainable model of really exploring the experiences of death, dying, loss and caregiving in diverse communities requires a real shift from a service mindset to one where the experts, the residents, are leading this agenda. There is optimism that some of the changes made to the structure of the network along with current programmes will start to evidence change and improved inclusivity and social justice.

1.8 Messaging and communications

If there was one element of the charter that should have taken a more prominent role (with funding), it is communications [8].

Greater clarity about the overall purpose of Compassionate Birmingham would have helped increase engagement in some of the work to date. There has not been any funding to invest in a marketing and communications campaign. There is now a logo for Compassionate Birmingham co-designed by network members and a "strapline" "creating caring, connected & supportive communities in Birmingham and beyond". There is some funding to start to develop a Compassionate Birmingham website.

Funding to support Brum YODO's AMOLAD festival which is doing an amazing job in highlighting issues relating to death, dying, loss and caregiving in such a creative way would help with public engagement.

1.9 Conclusion

The journey from the compassionate city programme being launched in mid-2021 to writing this chapter, feels like a lot longer than four years!

Much of this chapter is about lessons learnt along the way and challenges. However, there are some real positives to celebrate.

1. The concept of the compassionate city is increasingly embedded in city strategy for relevant health and care agendas.
2. The network of individuals who have been on the journey have all been learning and in doing so advocating for the 95% of the time that people who are seriously ill and grieving are in their community.
3. There have been incredible annual events and festivals promoting a shift in how society relates to death, dying and loss.
4. There have been hundreds of events, workshops and conversations all with the shared aim of making death, dying, loss and caregiving better for the people of Birmingham.
5. There has been investment to support new ways of working and thinking.
6. There are new, potentially transformative PH palliative and end-of-life care initiatives being signed up to by key stakeholders across the city.

Compassionate Birmingham continues to develop with more people becoming involved as awareness grows.

References

1. Office for National Statistics, "How Life Has Changed in Birmingham: Census 2021," 19 January 2023. [Online]. Available: https://www.ons.gov.uk/visualisations/censusareachanges/E08000025/.

2. Birmingham City Council, “Population Overview,” [Online]. Available: https://www.birmingham.gov.uk/info/50265/supporting_healthier_communities/2438/ethnic_communities/2. [Accessed 19 September 2025].
3. Department of Health and Social Care, “Mortality Data,” [Online]. Available: https://fingertips.phe.org.uk/profile/mortality-profile/data#page/1/gid/1938133009/ati/501/iid/93823/age/1/sex/4/cat/-1/ctp/-1/yrr/1/cid/4/tbm/1. [Accessed 21 September 2025].
4. Birmingham Connect to Support, “Neighbourhood Network Schemes,” 7 September 2021. [Online]. Available: https://birmingham.connecttosupport.org/prevention-and-communities/neighbourhood-network-schemes-nns/. [Accessed 19 September 2025].
5. Visit Birmingham, “Annual Festival,” [Online]. Available: https://visitbirmingham.com/whats-on/annual-festivals/. [Accessed 18 September 2025].
6. Brum YODO, “A Matter of Life and Death,” [Online]. Available: https://brumyodo.org.uk/. [Accessed 19 September 2025].
7. *National Council for Palliative Care: Dying Matters Coalition, “An Overview of Compassionate Communities in England,”* London, NCPC, 2013.
8. A. Kellehear, “Compassionate City Charter,” 2020. [Online]. Available: https://compassionate-communitiesuk.com/the-compassionate-city-charter-3/. [Accessed 18 August 2025].
9. World Health Organisation, *Ottawa Charter for Health Promotion*, Washington Dc, World Health Organisation, 1987.
10. Birmingham City Council, “Ageing Well Strategy Partnership (draft),” in B. Yakoob (Ed.), *Compassionate City Network Meeting*, Birmingham, 2025.
11. Ash Hayhurst, “Making Informed Choices When Planning a Funeral: A Guide for Queer People,” Ash Hayhurst, 2019.
12. Death Literacy Institute, “Death Literacy Institute,” [Online]. Available: https://www.deathliteracy.institute/.
13. L., Graham-Wisener, P., Toner, R., Leonard, and Groarke, J. M., “Validation of the Death Literacy Index and Benchmarking of Death Literacy Level in a Representative UK Population Sample,” *BMC Palliative Care. Preprint, 10*, 2022.
14. Plain English Campaign, “Plain English Campaign,” [Online]. Available: https://www.plainenglish.co.uk/. [Accessed 19 September 2025].
15. J. Abel, S. Aoun and A. Kellehear, “Bereavement Care Reimagined,” *Annals of Palliative Medicine*, Vol. 12, No. 4, pp. 816–825, 2023.
16. S. Aoun and B. Rumbold, “Public Health Approaches to Bereavement Support,” in J. Abel and A. Kellehear (Eds.), *Oxford Textbook of Public Health Palliative Care*, Oxford, Oxford University Press, pp. 187–196, 2022.

2

RESIDENT LED – BRERETON, A COMPASSIONATE VILLAGE

Sue Merriman

Abstract

Compassionate Brereton and Ravenhill (known locally as Brereton) tells the story of a village in Staffordshire, England. The journey to becoming a compassionate community does not start with a focus on palliative and end-of-life care, although, of course, naturally residents were supported with these issues. The need to respond to the community amid the COVID-19 pandemic resulted in a support network that was built on existing community strength. The flexibility and adaptation of Brereton Million, now called Vysions, has been key, as has responding to the changing needs within the community and building knowledge, skills and capacity to focus on the best solutions for residents. This chapter is a story about local people, not systems and services.

2.1 Introduction

The community of Brereton has a population of 7,000 in c. 3,000 households. It is in central England, about 40 minutes north of Birmingham in the county of Staffordshire. Based on 2023 data, 22.8% of children under 16 live in low-income families and 15.7% of people aged over 60 live in income-deprived households [1]. The village is on the edge of Cannock Chase, an area of outstanding natural beauty and has its own large park in the middle of the village.

Brereton was a large, close-knit, coal mining village, and whilst the mines have closed, the community spirit remains. The village has its own Parish Council which is now run by local residents. Parish councils are the lowest tier of government in England and are responsible for representing the local community, delivering local services and managing local facilities as well as working to improve quality of life.

DOI: 10.4324/9781003621348-3

Central to the village is a large grass area, a children's play park and paddling pool. The community has always had the traditional range of community activities, for example, a grassroots football club, girl guiding and scout clubs, a local school, library, pubs, church and parish hall.

2.2 The Brereton Million community

The National Lottery, which raises money via the sale of lottery tickets across the country, invests into local charities and community projects. The lottery funded a programme called Local Trust, working with Big Local (a lottery programme) [2], the project was to fund 150 areas around the UK to try and get communities to start working together again. Each community selected would be given ten years to spend one million pounds to achieve a range of outcomes, designed by local people.

The Big Local looked for areas where there used to be a good working industry that had gone away and areas that had not had much investment. Brereton was one of these areas and was awarded £1m in 2015. This investment created the organisation Brereton Millon [3].

Brereton Million is made up of a board of 12 members from the local community. This board oversees the budget and is the decision-maker in prioritising projects and managing investment. The board is also responsible for ensuring local consultation to make sure all the residents have their say, making sure that the projects match what the residents want and feel is needed. The board are local volunteers who have other responsibilities such as full-time employment and caring responsibilities.

Big Local recognised during the first year of the programme that a community development and coordination post was essential in delivering the benefits for local people from the investment. Sue Merriman was employed in this role, and this is her story.

2.3 Building Brereton Million

I have lived in Brereton all my life and know the history of the community. I was already well-connected helping at the local school, the football club and running a Brownie Guiding group. When I was approached to fulfil the role of Community Development Worker for Brereton Million, it was something I knew I had to say yes to.

Within the next 12 months, with a team of volunteers we posted leaflets across the whole of the village, we did lots of little events, we went to every community group, ran meetings, talked to businesses and went to schools. We wanted to ensure that everyone had the opportunity to say what they thought the £1m should be spent on.

A lot of the residents told us that the park was the heart of our community, and they loved it. We have a 1950s-type play park and are one of only a few areas that still have a paddling pool. Whilst this was important to the community, by the time, children were six they were bored. Lots of residents wanted the park upgraded.

Another priority was our war memorial. It was starting to look worn and untidy. Our older residents were keen that this be properly looked after.

The common theme was that everyone wanted the community spirit back. It was still there in pockets but not across the whole community.

Whilst Brereton Million was just starting, discussions were also taking place about reinstating our local carnival. Some of our older residents remember the old carnival and the difference it made to the village therefore a committee was formed to bring this back. The carnival is now the biggest event in Brereton, and it's really brought the village back together. The carnival includes a walking event around the village, with people and vehicles decorated and then events in the park. Local charities and groups can have tents up in the park to talk to local people about how they can support a wide range of issues including joining local groups, caring for older people, local wildlife charities and promoting the youth programmes and clubs. We also have local businesses and food vendors all getting involved and lots of singing and dancing.

As we identified priorities, we engaged with people on the design; for example, we have three primary schools in our area. Once we'd created two designs with all their images, we then let the rest of the residents in Brereton vote, but we only let the adults do that once the kids had chosen.

The play park was truly designed by the kids. We had a running track in our play park; it was absolutely overgrown with weeds and grass. We dug that out and we've relayed it. So, it's back to being a running track now.

We put in an open-air gym that is free for anyone to use. We've put in a woodland walk, an edible forest, mud kitchens, a fairy trail and since COVID-19 a memorial area. We are really maximising the use of our outside space for the benefit of residents.

Brereton Million purchased a community centre, known as 'the hub'. It was a social club that was going to get knocked down. Residents petitioned to save it, which created a centre for our work. There are lots of activities that run from the 'hub' such as craft groups, woodworking groups and lunch clubs, things are starting to come together since opening back up after COVID-19.

One of our projects is called Brereton Grows. We've put planters all around our village, so we get streets working together by having a planter in their street, where they all work together to grow things. We're in the process of creating a map, so we can get people to go on a healthy walk and collect fruit and veg from the planters as they go.

Funding had been withdrawn so we had lost our youth services here in Staffordshire. Brereton Million took over our youth group, which is named Vysions, and we've been running that since 2014. That's going from strength to strength providing opportunities for children and young people.

Our youth group is a bit different to your traditional youth groups where you just go along and play. They are a volunteer youth group. They go out into the community and do volunteering projects. And then they earn reward points for every hour that they do in the community.

2.4 Brereton Million, COVID and compassionate communities

The pandemic brought a whole new series of challenges for the community. We spotted an elderly resident who should have been shielding on her way to the shop, her son had COVID and was locked in his room whilst she was sitting at home watching the news telling her she needed to stay indoors. It turned out she hadn't eaten for four days, and she was absolutely petrified. We sent her back home and went to the local grocery store, the Co-op, for her. That's when we got talking about how there must be lots of residents like this. The Co-op said they could provide surplus bread, and with our Brereton Million volunteers, we started knocking on all the doors.

We knocked on every door in the village, all 3,000 of them. Every time we knocked on a door, we found a new problem. Kids with no pens or supplies for school, families struggling for food and disabled people whose support services had stopped. Mental health was at an all-time low. As the weeks went by, we'd got residents who were so low and lonely because they'd not spoken to anyone for weeks.

As we went through the village, we kept appealing for people to help us and we got a volunteer co-ordinator who really jumped on board and started organising a mass of volunteers. Then we got a phone buddies co-ordinator who would get people to ring those lonely residents who didn't have anyone to speak to.

We had a food co-ordinator who would do brilliant appeals. That led to supermarket lorries turning up at my house with trucks loading up my living room.

We created a craft group who made personal protective equipment because we couldn't get any in the shops. There was a book and jigsaw group set up for residents who were used to going to community groups that had shut down so that they could enjoy books and jigsaws at home. The Brereton Grows group encouraged the sharing of equipment and plants, anything that would keep people busy.

It just kept growing and growing, we had over 150 residents volunteering in any way they could across the village.

The same volunteers were also there for people when someone died, whether it was a listening ear or offering help with all the paperwork associated with dying.

Despite all the community support bringing people together, there were tough times. There were times when the phone didn't stop ringing with the different challenges people were facing.

We'll never forget one man who was too proud to tell his family he couldn't afford to feed them so I arranged to meet him round the corner from his house so they would think he'd gone shopping.

During the first round of door knocking, we stopped a man from killing himself.

We had so much food donated, it helped when we were knocking on the door, it broke the ice to be able to hand over a gift of food, along with my number and an offer of help.

2.5 'The heart of a compassionate community is simple: no one should face loneliness, death, or grief alone'.

Of all the problems we encountered, loneliness and isolation were number one. So many people just hadn't got anyone to talk to. It was like people were not speaking to each other anymore as they hadn't got anything positive to say and didn't want to drag their friends and family down when everyone was trying to stay positive. Hence, the phone buddy system to try and resolve this.

We were getting calls from around the country phoning us and saying, my mum lives in Brereton and she hasn't answered the phone. We're worried. Can you go and check? And, from that, we ended up making relationships with these families and being the go-between for them.

We had elderly people who didn't understand, who had serious illnesses, and their carers had been cut from four times a day to one, but when you've got no family and your four-day carers only come once, we knew something wasn't right.

We had a lady ask us to go shopping and a couple of days later, she rang again and asked for the same things. She'd asked for grapes and milk, and that kind of thing was flagged up that it wasn't quite right. When the volunteer dropped off her shopping, her clothes were back to front, and she was not in a very good hygienic way. So, I went around to see what was going on, and her stair lift was broken. And there was no downstairs toilet. We started to try and sort this out with her, and it was clear she had the early stages of dementia and no support had been put into place; however, she decided to go to the shops by herself and had a fall, so we sorted out an ambulance, we were able to share what we had learned and she is now in residential care.

Twice, we had to break into people's houses when they were sick with COVID and wait for ambulances. We couldn't help people by standing at the door and telling the ambulance service or GP what we could see, so we had to break the isolation rules to go into their homes and explain what we were seeing to get emergency care.

People were still ill through other illnesses such as cancer during COVID, those deaths didn't stop happening. The lockdown massively reduced the support available, carers weren't working at full capacity, some services had shut down, friends and family were doing what they could but couldn't fill the gap on their own. Plus, lots of people were shielding.

For us, it wasn't so much about COVID during the pandemic; people were getting ill from cancer and other illnesses. It was because of the COVID lockdowns that people couldn't be supported in the way they would have been. We started to have calls from people asking us to support their family. Not necessarily themselves, but their family. They didn't know who to go to or what they needed to do, and of course people didn't want to go to hospital due to the fear of COVID.

We started to work out which services were still running and were able to liaise with the hospice nurses, try and help identify carers, link in with the GP. In some instances, we'd got a wife who was poorly, but they were the main carer for their husband creating a crisis.

Some of the regular tests that some residents needed were being done at home rather than in the doctor's surgery. We needed to get involved in that as people couldn't manage on their own.

With services absent or reduced, partners were exhausted trying to provide 24/7 care for their loved ones.

2.6 'Compassionate communities are built by residents, not services – neighbours supporting each other through life, death, and everything in between'.

I, and a few volunteers, started to step in and sit with people who were seriously ill and dying to allow their partners to sleep. We could provide the support and reassurance the family needed.

Most of the time it would just be sitting them up, giving them a drink, putting their blankets on, then they want their blankets off, brushing teeth and hair, and listening to them when they want to talk. And most of the time, it was just reassuring them that you were there. They just needed to know they weren't on their own.

There was no training, and there were plenty of times where I was petrified. There was no choice, and we just had to get up the next day and keep going.

Even now, after the pandemic, there is still a lot of support needed around death, dying and loss. There is the funeral to organise, and some people don't have support to do that and there is a lot of paperwork to deal with. We've supported all of that too. Luckily, one of our residents has experience in this and has been able to help.

We still check in on residents who had a loved one die during COVID and since. We're still doing jobs for them, the youth group have just been to one of our gentlemen and painted his shed, his wife's favourite place was the garden, so we're making sure that that's kept on top of for him.

2.7 Life after COVID

Writing this in 2025 as our £1m-funded programme comes to an end and five years after the pandemic is quite timely.

Whilst the intensity of support is different after the pandemic, the issues remain. Loneliness and isolation are also big problems across all age groups, our youth work and developing new intergenerational activities are key. In many ways, it is an ongoing process of listening and understanding the issues residents have and matching skills within the community to help resolve these issues.

There are challenges in Brereton's social issues that play out nationally and impact the village too, e.g. government funding cuts, lack of capacity in the NHS, lack of capacity in mental health services and issues relating to social cohesion and immigration. Taking over the Parish Council has enabled a greater input for residents on how we can tackle these issues locally.

The village has experienced a lot of death, including suicide. The support around death, dying, loss and caregiving remains essential for us as a community organisation.

We were awarded compassionate community status in September 2021, the first area endorsed in the UK. This award recognised not only the community we were going into the pandemic and how we came together dealing with the crisis we were facing regarding death, dying, loss and caregiving but also how we recognised the work we now needed to continue to do because of what we'd learnt.

The process of being endorsed allowed us to step back from the work and see it from the perspective of the compassionate community's movement. We were able to see that we'd been working with schools, businesses, healthcare partners and the church, all neighbourhoods, considered memorials, communication plans, used arts and crafts and considered which residents might be missing from our work.

It also helped us consider what else we needed to do in this area of work.

We have run some awareness events encouraging people to 'get their affairs in order'. Members of the team have had training in bereavement support, so that we can feel more confident when residents talk about their loss.

The impact of COVID is still felt today. I will never forget the community spirit we experienced and feel that the Brereton Million, having been established prior to the pandemic, gave us some infrastructure and connectedness that enabled us to mobilise and get organised quickly.

2.8 How do we know the difference we make

We haven't started this programme to create an evidence base or be part of a research project. We have been providing updates and reports to Big Local as part of the funding arrangements. So, we can evidence what programmes have been run and how the money has been spent.

The partnership board, our youth leaders' group and our volunteers all know the community and see day to day either the difference we've made or what else we need to do.

When we travel around the village, we can see that the play park is full, we can see whether our events are busy. We can see that the war memorial is being properly cared for. We can see the planting boxes growing, the dog walkers in the forest. We know how many young people access youth programmes. We know which groups are popular and which aren't. We can see all the knitted crafts around the village such as on remembrance Sunday, royal events and just for fun.

We see and hear the stories of individuals like the two young people going back to mainstream schooling having been part of our youth programme and home-schooling support. We have quotes that we can use to demonstrate impact.

> When I lost my wife, I joined the buddy system because I really needed help. It was really helpful to put something in the diary to say I was going to have a phone call on a particular day because it's so easy to descend into the rough of

> despair. It's made a huge difference to my life, and I honestly don't know how I would have coped without it.
>
> —*Brereton Resident*

We don't have the capacity to focus on counting what we do rather than just getting on with trying to make a difference. However, we know that some people want to see more measurable, numerical-type outcomes and some tools are useful in developing community approaches.

For example, with regard to death, dying, loss and caregiving, we did undertake an exercise using the Death Literacy Index and in comparison to others, our results seem to indicate that what we are doing is working. The death literacy index helped us identify areas we can focus on going forward, for example, community training.

2.9 What has been learnt along the way?

Creating a compassionate community takes time and capacity. It became apparent during year one that relying on busy volunteers, often juggling jobs and families, was insufficient for the programme outcomes. Current discussions about another round of Big Local funding have recognised, particularly from Brereton's experience, that there needs to be a small dedicated, employed team working in the community.

Events, bringing the community together, are far more effective than formal consultation methods. Consultation meetings might have 50 people attending, whereas events were starting to bring together 3,000 residents.

For Brereton Million, we were responding to residents with a simple goal of 'bringing the community back together'. We didn't have a specific agenda or area of focus e.g. older people or mental health. This means that for the team they can hear about so many things that they may have no experience of including death, dying, loss and caregiving.

We could not have anticipated a pandemic and all that this brought. However, with training and support, we could possibly have felt better equipped in supporting residents on issues relating to death, dying, loss and caregiving.

It is fair to say that at times the role and the work have been overwhelming and heartbreaking. Community development staff and volunteers need time to debrief, reflect and recuperate.

There is something about the balance of being supported by service organisations, without losing the ethos of a resident-led community.

2.10 Next steps

Brereton Million will be known as Vysions (the current name of the youth programme). This new charity will combine all community activities across all ages.

Bordering areas such as neighbouring towns and surrounding villages also want to be involved and we need to consider how to scale up or create new resident-led community programmes. Some activities can lend themselves to a wider population, others need to be focused on smaller numbers.

We have no shortage of ideas. We need to continue to grow the number of volunteers and ensure the new charity is financially sustainable. We also want to ensure that there is appropriate support and training in place for our volunteers.

Specifically with regard to death, dying, loss and caregiving, we are taking part in two programmes with Compassionate Communities UK.

The first is piloting the use of Pallilearn, which was developed in Australia. This is a series of workshops designed to raise the awareness and skills of residents on palliative and end-of-life care.

The second is a programme from Japan called Lessons of Life. This is a workshop aimed at helping young people be better able to support each other during life's tougher times.

We have been talking about a Day of the Dead festival or other events that encourage people to think about putting things like funeral plans, wills and lasting power of attorney documents in place.

> Brereton's story shows that when people face loss together, they don't just survive - they grow stronger, more connected, and more compassionate.
>
> *[4]*

2.11 Summary

This chapter shows that organised, well-resourced community development makes a real difference. It highlights the value of programmes led by trusted local residents, not outside organisations. Brereton's story also reminds us that death, dying, loss and caregiving affect everyone, and when communities face these together, they build resilience and reduce loneliness. Finally, it reinforces that those doing the work, staff and volunteers must be supported with training, partnerships and time to reflect, so they can continue making change without burning out.

References

1. Cannock Chase Council, "Brereton and Ravenhill, 2023," 2023. [Online]. Available: https://www.cannockchasedc.gov.uk/sites/default/files/site-old/brereton_and_ravenhill_2023.pdf. [Accessed 2 September 2025].
2. Local Trust, "Big Local," [Online]. Available: https://localtrust.org.uk/big-local/. [Accessed 17 September 2025].
3. Brereton Million, "Brereton Million," [Online]. Available: https://www.breretonmillion.co.uk/. [Accessed 17 September 2025].
4. J. Abel, *Survival of the Kindest – We Need to Do Something*, [Online] Available https://podcast24.co.uk/episodes/survival-of-the-kindest/survival-of-the-kindest-sue-merriman-we-need-to-do-something-TAONTX1AN. [Accessed 26 January 2026].

3

COMPASSIONATE COMMUNITIES IN FLANDERS

An account of the development and implementation of Compassionate Bruges and Compassionate Herzele

Louise D'Eer and Bert Quintiens

Abstract

This chapter describes the development and implementation of Compassionate Bruges and Compassionate Herzele, the first compassionate cities in Flanders, Belgium. Combining city-wide strategies with neighbourhood-level initiatives, both cities aimed to foster supportive environments around serious illness, caregiving, dying, and loss. Using a co-creative approach with diverse stakeholders, each city developed unique programmes, entailing activities such as compassionate schools in Herzele and the Node City Festival in Bruges. This chapter describes key activities, impacts and facilitators and barriers. The latter including resource limitations, the influence of COVID-19, and strategies for sustaining engagement. It highlights how locally sensitive, participatory processes can promote civic responses to end-of-life experiences and contribute to long-term social change.

3.1 Introduction

The cities of Bruges and Herzele were the first in Flanders to develop a compassionate cities programme, with a city-wide focus, as well as a neighbourhood-specific programme around the topics of serious illness, caregiving, dying, and loss.

The development of the two compassionate cities in Flanders was initiated in 2019 under the impulse of a group of researchers from the End-of-Life Care Research Group at the Vrije Universiteit Brussel and Ghent University. With funding from the Flemish Research Foundation, the research project aimed to explore how cities and neighbourhoods could foster more supportive environments around serious illness, caregiving, dying, death, and bereavement. Candidate compassionate cities

DOI: 10.4324/9781003621348-4

were cross-checked against a priori developed criteria, such as having support and commitment from the city council, cities having prior experience with social change projects, cities providing access to existing stakeholder coalitions, and the willingness to focus both on a city-wide and a neighbourhood-level programme [1]. Bruges and Herzele were then selected based on their responses to these criteria.

Bruges, a highly urbanised city with a population of around 120,000, is known for its historical city centre [2]. Herzele, by contrast, is a semi-urban municipality with approximately 18,500 residents [3]. The compassionate neighbourhoods were located in a sub-municipality of the city of Bruges and in the city centre of Herzele, each comprising around 10,000 inhabitants.

Both cities share common demographic characteristics, including a high proportion of older residents and a growing number of individuals living alone [3]. Survey studies conducted by the researchers at the start of the compassionate cities programmes revealed that many residents were dealing with recent or ongoing experiences related to serious illness, caregiving, dying, and loss [4,5]. This convergence of experiences with these topics, alongside heightened risks of social isolation, highlighted the pressing need to foster more compassionate environments concerning serious illness, caregiving, dying, and loss in the two cities.

3.1.1 Compassionate cities and communities: what's in the name?

Although the terms compassionate communities and compassionate cities are often used interchangeably, there is a semantic difference between the two concepts. Compassionate communities represent a broader implementation of the compassionate cities concept, extending its principles to encompass entire local communities, rather than geographically fixed urban areas [6]. While compassionate cities are often equated with a top-down approach, this characterisation is not always accurate. Initiatives within compassionate cities can also be driven by grassroots efforts within communities, even within the context of a city-wide program [6,7]. However, the aspect of bottom-up approaches is more pronounced for compassionate communities since they focus on initiatives that originate from within the communities themselves, driven by the efforts of local residents, organisations, and community groups.

In both Bruges and Herzele, the compassionate cities programmes were developed by combining a city-wide strategy with a neighbourhood-level initiative focused on serious illness, caregiving, dying, and loss. These neighbourhood initiatives represent the local character of the compassionate communities approach, integrated within the broader compassionate cities framework.

3.1.2 A co-creative development process involving multiple, local stakeholders

From the outset, the project was grounded in the philosophy that it should neither be a top-down initiative directed by municipal authorities, nor solely an academic endeavour. Rather, it was conceived as a collaborative effort aimed at integrating research, policy, and grassroots action. Central to this approach was the development of the programme in co-creation with local stakeholders. The term *stakeholders* is understood here in a broad sense, encompassing all interested parties in the cities and neighbourhoods, including healthcare and well-being providers, teachers, and representatives from cultural organisations and volunteer organisations.

Each city appointed a project leader who was responsible for coordinating the local compassionate city and neighbourhood programme and for facilitating the development process with the local stakeholders. In both cities, the project leaders were guided and supervised by city aldermen. The selection of aldermen was based on their mandate in relevant policy domains as well as their willingness to provide support for the initiative, for instance, through access to networks and local resources. Additionally, in Bruges, a designated neighbourhood worker was appointed to facilitate the development of the neighbourhood programme. In contrast, in Herzele, this role was fulfilled by the project leader, as no dedicated neighbourhood worker was assigned.

In addition to these appointed project leaders, the university hired an external change manager to support the development process and to serve as a liaison between the cities' interests and the research objectives.

The researchers' role in the compassionate cities and the neighbourhoods programmes shifted from mainly observing to becoming more actively involved, as they offered input and recommendations based on insights from stakeholder meetings and preliminary research findings.

3.1.3 Bruges

In Bruges, the compassionate city programme was launched with the formation of a steering group composed of stakeholders from a range of sectors, including healthcare, education, religion, and culture. This cross-sectoral coalition collaboratively identified key areas for action, which led to the creation of seven dedicated working groups: Compassionate Schools, Comforting Care, Care After Death, Lonely Deaths, Compassionate Employers, Public Places of Mourning, and the Compassionate neighbourhood programme.

Initially, all seven groups were active, but over time, many became less engaged. In response, the organisational structure shifted from a steering group to a more flexible learning network structure. This network allowed for independent working group activities and informal exchanges among stakeholders, aligning better with participants' availability and preferences.

Due to limited resources and the project leader's constrained capacity, the neighbourhood programme began to develop separately from the city-wide programme. After the neighbourhood programme received additional funding from the Flemish Government in 2021, a dedicated neighbourhood worker was appointed, and a local stakeholder group was formed, comprising representatives from health and social care organisations, the volunteer centre, the library, etc.

3.1.4 *Herzele*

In Herzele, the compassionate city programme was launched with a deliberate focus on the educational sector. The city council identified schools as a strategic entry point and initiated a compassionate schools programme. Nine schools took part, each establishing a working group to design context-specific activities. Teachers had access to ongoing guidance from experts on cultivating compassion among both students and staff.

Parallel to the school-based compassionate city programme, the neighbourhood programme in Herzele was developed and built on an existing caregiver peer support group. The caregiver peer support group enabled participants to define and shape their own areas of focus. This process was facilitated by the project leader from Compassionate Herzele.

3.2 Co-creatively developed initiatives and activities

Since the compassionate city and neighbourhood programmes were developed through co-creation with stakeholders, only a few aspects were predefined regarding their direction, activities, or outcomes. This open approach made the development process less predictable, with the direction of the activities and their results depending on the specific local context.

3.2.1 *Bruges*

In Compassionate Bruges, a series of city-wide activities were developed, among which the Node City Festival stood out as a key highlight. This week-long thematic festival, held in 2022 and repeated in 2024, was initiated by the stakeholders from the Compassionate Bruges learning network. The festival adopted a diverse and inclusive programme, ranging from information sessions and city walks to theatre performances and exhibitions, all around the topics of serious illness, caregiving, dying, and loss. A wide array of stakeholders in Bruges were involved in the development and implementation of the festival, including museums, sociocultural organisations like senior advocacy groups, schools, self-employed professionals including undertakers, and civil servants from varying municipal departments such as diversity and inclusion. All events were open to the public.

One of the key activities within the Node City Festival was The Healing Museum, which featured an exhibition by Otobong Nkanga, an artist whose work explores themes of separation, death, and loss with emotional depth and nuance [8]. Complementing the exhibition, a series of events and performances took place in and around the museum site. One such event was the Soul Repair Café, where visitors could voluntarily share a loss experience. In response, an artist would translate each story into a personalised creation, a poem, a song, an illustration, or a letter, offering a meaningful and creative act of remembrance [8].

On the neighbourhood level, a community conversation event called Soup with Chats was organised to engage in dialogue with local residents. Held in a public meeting space next to the library, with soup provided by a local initiative, the event aimed to spark conversations about serious illness, caregiving, dying, and loss, and to identify the neighbourhood's needs around these themes. Through these discussions, three key themes emerged: the need to bring loss and bereavement more visibly into public spaces, the importance of encouraging "small help" in the neighbourhood – everyday acts of kindness and support between neighbours - and the need for stronger collaboration between healthcare providers and social services and informal or grassroots initiatives such as volunteer groups or community associations. These themes formed the foundation for the neighbourhood programme's future activities and priorities.

The Consolation Walk, an activity resulting from the neighbourhood programme, connected six public spaces of solace. The walk provided a moment for personal reflection while also nurturing a shared sense of community around the experience of mourning. Another initiative, Coffee with Your Neighbour(hood), involved a mobile coffee cart that visited a different street in the neighbourhood each month. The gatherings created an informal setting for residents to connect and engage in conversations about loneliness, serious illness, caregiving, dying, and loss.

3.2.2 Herzele

In Herzele, where the development of Compassionate Schools was a central focus, a wide range of activities were initiated within the nine participating schools. These activities aligned with four key areas: education and awareness, resource mobilisation, help, support, and care in the school context, and building partnerships and collaborations [9]. Examples of activities included a mailbox where students could anonymously share personal experiences about serious illness, dying, caregiving, or bereavement, and a dedicated guide that was created to support teachers in responding to loss within the school community. To encourage conversations about death among younger children, the local library curated a selection of age-appropriate books around the topic. Additional supportive measures included the installation of a "grieving bench" as a visible symbol of remembrance and care.

In conducting these activities, professional support was provided to the schools: an expert on death and loss delivered a lecture to teachers, and another training was organised to help teachers respond with greater compassion. Students participated in a parallel training to build their own "compassionate skills".

In the caregiver peer support group, the neighbourhood programme in Herzele, two participatory sessions enabled family carers to express their needs and priorities. From these conversations, three key themes emerged: the importance of self-care and allowing external support, the need for practical and financial information, and clarity on where to turn with caregiving-related questions and needs. In response, nine monthly sessions were organised, alternating between interactive workshops and informational meetings. The interactive sessions encouraged family carers to reflect on how accepting external support could improve their caregiving situation while challenging the notion that seeking help implies failure as a caregiver.

3.3 Outcomes and impact within Compassionate Bruges and Herzele

The development of the compassionate cities and their neighbourhood programmes was context-specific, influenced by factors such as local politics, economic factors, and the quality of social relations between local stakeholders and residents [10]. Because of this complexity, using before-and-after measurements to capture impact was not feasible, nor desirable. Instead, we found that ethnographically based methods like interviews, observations, and group discussions gave us a better understanding of people's experiences and of how the local context shaped the programmes [10].

3.3.1 Bruges

In Bruges, the Node City Festival enabled various stakeholders to collaborate and inform the public. Such collaborations not only within the city, but also across administrative city departments, were innovative and a first step towards integrating serious illness, caregiving, dying, and loss beyond the healthcare domain into the cultural and educational domain.

Additionally, stakeholders involved in the project reported on their increased skills and confidence in facilitating initiatives around serious illness, caregiving, dying, and loss; topics they had initially perceived as highly sensitive to stigma and community resistance. At the start, the project leaders felt unsure about how to create meaningful activities in their neighbourhoods or cities. To address this, they received targeted coaching from the change manager. A key focus of this coaching was to help them shift their role, from designing activities themselves to facilitating a process in which the initiatives were developed co-creatively.

At the neighbourhood level, a preliminary impact was reported in the form of strengthened social cohesion around the themes of serious illness, caregiving, dying, and loss. While this did not yet amount to the broad cultural shift that was initially hoped for, the stakeholders acknowledged that this increased sense of connection and mutual support was a valuable first step towards achieving that broader, cultural change.

3.3.2 Herzele

In Herzele, the compassionate schools initiative contributed to building new skills and capacities among teachers, which helped them support both each other and students when confronted with serious illness, caregiving, dying, and loss. Teachers received training focused on fostering compassion within the school environment, both towards students and among colleagues [11]. This training equipped them to better handle sensitive situations related to serious illness, caregiving, dying, and loss. Importantly, the trainer remained available after the initial sessions to offer advice and support in specific end-of-life situations that arose in the school context. This continued access to expert guidance was highly valued by the teachers, who felt more confident and supported in navigating these emotionally complex topics [11].

At the neighbourhood level, a specific method was used to identify meaningful changes resulting from the family carer peer support group. This method, known as the Most Significant Change Technique, involved participants sharing stories about the change they experienced through their involvement [12]. Using this method, family carers reported a wide range of meaningful changes, from learning from peers and feeling more confident in facing future challenges, to experiencing relief in their caregiving roles and considering the local service centre as a more accessible and trusted place for support [13].

Through reflection and discussion, the most significant change that was selected at the policy-level of the compassionate city programme [12], centred on the emergence of peer learning. For policymakers, this change reflected a shift from relying on outside experts to provide information to becoming a self-sustaining, community-based source of support and knowledge.

3.4 Facilitators and barriers to the development process

The development and implementation of the compassionate cities and the neighbourhood programmes were shaped by several facilitators and barriers, which can be grouped into four main themes. The first theme centres around the role of the city officials who held the decision-making power within the programme, influencing how priorities within the city were set. The second theme was the COVID-19 pandemic, having both a limiting and reshaping impact on the initiatives' development and implementation. The third theme was the stakeholders' prior experiences with serious illness, caregiving, death, or loss, shaping their engagement and perspective towards the programme. The last theme focuses on the continuation of the developed initiatives through embedding them into the city policy.

The findings presented here are based on observations, interviews, and group discussions conducted by the two researchers (LD and BQ) over the four years of development of the compassionate cities and neighbourhood programmes, 2020–2024 [11,14]. Data were collected from residents, local stakeholders, the city aldermen, the city project leaders, and the change manager who facilitated the programme.

3.5 The key role of the cities in the development process

The compassionate cities and the neighbourhood programmes being initiated and facilitated by the local government of the cities, influenced how the projects took shape and how stakeholders experienced the development process.

3.5.1 The available resources

A key facilitating factor to the development process was the stakeholders' newfound access, or lack thereof, to city resources that had previously been difficult, or even impossible, to mobilise. These resources included not only financial and logistical support but also the use of established communication channels and opportunities for policy integration. However, several stakeholders found that accessing these resources was often hampered by slow and bureaucratic processes. While this initially discouraged some from making use of the available support, many described gradually adapting to these bureaucratic constraints.

However, the resources provided by the cities were limited, and financial constraints became apparent in both cities studied. In one city, funding that had originally been allocated to the compassionate city programme was redirected to another social welfare initiative. Furthermore, financial limitations were not confined to the municipal level; participating stakeholder organisations also reported similar challenges from within their organisations, as one project leader explained.

> I hear nothing else but the social partners saying they're doing core exercises. A core exercise is a disguised exercise to see what can be cut [in the budget], and what can still be done with limited staff to maintain quality.

3.5.2 The prioritisation of the actions developed

Due to limited financial resources, and consequently, the limited time that project coordinators could devote to developing both the compassionate city and the neighbourhood programme, activities at the neighbourhood level were delayed and prioritisation was given to the compassionate city. As a result, the neighbourhood programme evolved separately from the broader city-wide programme. This division was further reinforced by the project leader, who viewed the city and neighbourhood programme as distinct and had no intention of integrating them:

> The neighbourhood project and compassionate city programme? No, I don't even have to think about it. No, the neighbourhood work will continue with [name of the neighbourhood worker], and the compassionate city,… No, that shouldn't coincide.

Nevertheless, the Node City Festival in Compassionate Bruges effectively illustrated how city-level activities could also serve as a catalyst for initiating and strengthening neighbourhood-level programmes, as one of the local stakeholders explained.

> It was a positive experience. There were a lot of people. I found that very good, it was [name project leader] who organised a networking and introductory moment online, and then there were breakout rooms where you could get to know each other and find points of connection. For me, it stimulates ideas for the neighbourhood.

3.5.3 *The decision-making power within the programme*

The development and implementation of the compassionate cities and the neighbourhood programmes within a city-led structure also impacted the partnership between the stakeholders and the project coordinators from the city.

A notable barrier related to the cities' profound role in the decision-making process, which diminished local stakeholders' sense of ownership over the project. For example, in one neighbourhood, stakeholders advocated for leveraging existing mobile neighbourhood teams to build local connections. However, the municipality instead opted to create a new neighbourhood worker position, which was ultimately implemented. This was experienced by the local stakeholder as follows:

> I think... in my opinion, we as [name organisation] have been involved, but it was the way how... The city had in mind that they were going to appoint a neighbourhood worker, and then we indicated that, as we are already in the neighbourhood, we could contribute there. We already have those teams in the neighbourhoods, mobile ambulatory teams. But for the city that wasn't a possibility, and neighbourhood work was set up there.

Over time, more trust was built between the city and the stakeholders, which led to a change in dynamic wherein stakeholders began to assume greater responsibility and develop a stronger sense of ownership over the initiative.

3.5.4 *A responsibility on the shoulders of a few stakeholders*

In the development of the city and neighbourhood programmes, the city officials deliberately chose to work with professional stakeholders from organisations, rather than involving local residents. This decision had several implications.

First, many of these professionals struggled to find the time to contribute to the project on top of their regular responsibilities, as one of them explained:

> I also have my assignments and can't afford to invest a lot of my time in extra activities. That's why, when I was asked to take on a leading role, I made it clear that the request should be directed to my employer. They decide whether I can take on additional responsibilities. Once I received the green light, I had a clear mandate within specific boundaries, and that made it manageable for me.

Additionally, by choosing to work with a select group of partners and not extending the development process to a broader audience, a high degree of responsibility rested on the shoulders of a few individuals, who in return had to carry much of the workload. This was explained by the change manager as follows:

> Looking back, I think [name of the project coordinator] already had too much on her plate to take this on as well. That ultimately became the biggest issue—too

> much all at once. I think we underestimated at the beginning just how much work would still be needed.

Furthermore, this organisational setup also created a vulnerability: when key figures dropped out, the entire programme was affected. This became evident when the neighbourhood worker unexpectedly left the project after seven months, which initially led to a delay in the project. However, it also created an opportunity by allowing space for other stakeholders to step forward and take on greater responsibility within the project. One of the city aldermen reflected on this shift in responsibility.

> I've understood that the person leading the neighbourhood steering group has stepped down. But what's remarkable in that group is that someone spontaneously stood up to organise something. This Saturday, September 23rd, there's an action with 'BankContact'. That kind of initiative just emerged from the group itself, and I think that's beautiful. There's a form of self-direction coming from the network, so to speak.

3.5.5 COVID-19

Both compassionate cities programmes were initiated during the COVID-19 pandemic, which simultaneously created opportunities and posed challenges for their development.

First, the COVID-19 pandemic facilitated the importance of working around serious illness, caregiving, dying, and loss, as these topics gained greater societal visibility and urgency. Additionally, it contributed to a shift in public consciousness, emphasising the importance of social connection and collective support in facing experiences around these topics. One of the stakeholders explained this as follows:

> The pandemic made people more open to talking about death and loss; it was suddenly part of everyday life. That created space for us to connect and support each other in ways that didn't seem possible before.

Conversely, the COVID-19 pandemic hindered the development of a shared vision and the establishment of interpersonal connections. Nevertheless, once in-person meetings were allowed, these relationships gradually took shape, strengthening further collaboration. A stakeholder explained this as follows:

> The initial setup we had was all digital. That was a loss in terms of building those personal relationships. Now, when I meet with my partners, I meet in person again. I take the time to say, "Are you coming here, or should I come to you?" It's a double-time investment, but the gain you get from physically seeing someone, that makes such a huge difference compared to a digital chat, especially in building trust.

3.5.6 Contributing to cultural change through action and shared vision

Stakeholders involved in compassionate cities programmes participated with a long-term aim of fostering cultural change around serious illness, death, and bereavement. However, translating these ambitions into practical action proved challenging. Many stakeholders, particularly those involved in the compassionate schools initiative, found it difficult to engage with abstract, long-term planning without visible outcomes. Their professional cultures often prioritised action and concrete results. As one teacher involved in a compassionate schools project explained:

> It was a bit confusing. In education, we are 'doers'. We want to do something, grasp it, and see immediate results. That was the difficulty at first; we kept mapping things out, but we wanted something concrete, something finished. That was my struggle: Is something concrete coming now?

This tension between broad cultural change and practical actions also affected the development of a shared vision among stakeholders, which was especially the case at the neighbourhood level. Neighbourhood residents prioritised grassroots concerns, such as helping neighbours, improving communication between formal and informal networks, and acknowledging grief in public spaces. Stakeholders from local organisations, on the other hand, attributed more importance to understanding the local landscape of organisations, aligning services, and exploring opportunities for collaboration, as one of them explained:

> I mainly want to see the bigger picture… Who are the other partners, and what are they already doing? There are many initiatives in the neighbourhood that could be useful to know about.

Over time, the repeated organisation of concrete, tangible activities, such as the Node City Festival or the local consolation walks, played a pivotal role in bridging these gaps and providing a common ground for stakeholders both at the resident-level and at the organisational level:

> By organising a consolation walk, we started from the need in our city and from our need to connect our initiatives, and that's why it's working now.

3.5.7 Death and loss experiences and perceptions

Most participating stakeholders had prior personal or professional experiences with serious illness, caregiving, dying, or loss. These experiences shaped their willingness to engage around these topics in two different ways: for some, it made them more susceptible to participating, while for others, these experiences created hesitation or emotional distance. Both responses were reported among stakeholders.

> I have to say, I'm an emotional person, when I bring those books into the classroom [laughs], then I also get, well… I find it difficult to work with that, because, well, that emotional aspect, that's also present in me. I lost my dad four years ago, so when it comes to sorrow, I find it difficult to deal with the children.

> Compassionate cities and I, that was a good match. I've had a personal journey with a lot of experiences of loss, but I've also followed a training as a grief and loss counsellor. That's a common thread running through my life.

3.6 Ensuring the continuation of the developed initiatives

Challenges in continuing the compassionate cities and the neighbourhood programmes stemmed in the first place from resource constraints. In one of the cities, the project leader expressed concerns that over time, there would not be sufficient staffing to continue the initiative.

> The biggest pitfall is that I can't imagine us having the staff to carry out this project within five years. So, we will have to find ways to make the network self-sustaining.

One proposed strategy for ensuring the programme's continuity was to expand its reach to include local residents, rather than relying solely on stakeholders from professional organisations who had been the primary participants during its development and implementation.

> I think that up until today, we still lack the active participation of local residents in this entire story. There have been discussions here and there, but there hasn't been a specific request for participation, for providing input into what is currently on the table. I think that these are definitely missed opportunities.

Additionally, there was a realisation that sustaining stakeholder motivation required careful attention to pacing, with an emphasis on setting realistic and manageable goals rather than pursuing overly ambitious objectives, as the project coordinator explained:

> Yeah, I think that's our biggest challenge. Keeping the project alive. And it…I always say that you shouldn't run before you can walk. You first have to take small steps before you can run. How can I explain that? Sometimes people want to achieve very big things within the project. But sometimes it is better to accomplish some small things, maintain them, and only then work towards expansion.

3.7 The Future of Compassionate Bruges and Herzele

Both Compassionate Bruges and Herzele are currently still active. In Bruges, a second edition of the Node City Festival took place in November 2024, and the learning network continues to meet bimonthly. The network is steadily expanding, organising, and sharing activities within the wider group. Examples of such activities include an inspiration session on the theme of loneliness for first-line professional carers, and an aftercare initiative for bereaved individuals, including workshops for children on the topic of loss.

Even after the project funding ended, the neighbourhood programme continued joint activities, such as "Coffee with Your Neighbour(hood)". Stakeholders report closer collaboration, ongoing exchanges, and expanded involvement of new partners and local residents, exemplified in a networking event they organised in May 2025.

The continued presence of both the compassionate city learning network and the neighbourhood programme demonstrates a sustained commitment in Bruges.

In Compassionate Herzele, participating schools aim to continue to operate as compassionate schools, integrating themes of serious illness, caregiving, death, and loss into their educational practices. At the neighbourhood level, the caregiver support group remains active, providing family carers with a space to share experiences and learn from each other.

References

1. B. Quintiens, T. Smets, K. Chambaere, L. Van Den Block, L. Deliens and J. Cohen, "Researching two Compassionate Cities: study protocol for a mixed-methods process and outcome evaluation," *Palliative Care and Social Practice*, vol. 16, no. 26323524221137601, pp. 1–13, 2022.
2. Stad Brugge Team, "Brugge in cifers - Stedenbeleid Interprovinciale werking Data & Analyse," [Online]. Available: https://brugge.incijfers.be/dashboard/dashboard/bevolking-3. [Accessed 3 April 2024].
3. A. Bestuur, "Gemeente-Stadsmonitor," [Online]. Available: https://www.herzele.be/gemeentemonitor-cijfers-en-statistieken-over-herzele. [Accessed 4 April 2024].
4. L. D'Eer, K. Chambaere, L. Van den Block, S. Dury, L. Sallnow, L. Deliens, T. Smets and J. Cohen, "How compassionate is your neighborhood? Results of a cross-sectional survey on neighborhood participation regarding serious illness, death, and loss," *Death Studies*, vol. 48, no. 8, pp. 810–819, 2024.
5. B. Quintiens, T. Smets, K. Chambaere, L. Van den Block, L. Deliens, L. Sallnow and J. Cohen, "Discomfort with suffering and dying, a cross-sectional survey of the general public," *Journal of Pain and Symptom Management*, vol. 66, no. 5, pp. 529–540, 2023.
6. A. Kellehear, "Compassionate cities: global significance and meaning for palliative care," *Progress in Palliative Care*, vol. 28, no. 2, pp. 1–15, 2019. doi: 10.1080/09699260.2019.1701835.
7. A. Kellehear, *Compassionate Cities: Public Health and End of Life Care*, Oxfordshire: Routledge, 2005.
8. M. Brugge, *Persdossier: The Healing Museum*, [online]. Available: https://www.museabrugge.be/objects/production/general/persdossier_TheHealingMuseum_web.pdf. [Accessed 4 April 2024].

9. K. Dumont, I. Marcoux, E. Warren, F. Alem, B. Alvar, G. Ballu, A. Bostock, S. R. Cohen, S. Daneault, V. Dube, J. Houle, A. Minyaoui, G. Rouly, D. Weil, A. Kelleahear and A. Boivin, “How compassionate communities are implemented and evaluated in practice: a scoping review,” *BMC Palliative Care*, vol. 21, no. 1, p. 131, 2022.
10. H. Bakelants, S. Vanderstichelen, K. Chambaere, F. Van Droogenbroeck, L. De Donder, L. Deliens, S. Dury and J. Cohen, ““Researching compassionate communities: identifying theoretical frameworks to evaluate the complex processes behind public health palliative care initiatives,” *Palliative Medicine*, vol. 32, no. 2, pp. 291–301, 2023.
11. R. Davies and J. Dart, The most significant change (MSC) technique: a guide to its use, Melbourne: MandE. Available: https://ahi.sub.jp/eng/wp-content/uploads/2022/02/MSCGuide-1.pdf. [Accessed 4 April 2024].

4

BUILDING AN ECOSYSTEM OF COMPASSIONATE CARE

Connecting healthcare and communities

Camila Ronderos and Constanza González

Abstract

This chapter describes the development and implementation of Keralty's ecosystem of care in Colombia, a community-centred model that integrates health care delivery with social, community, and educational strategies to improve health and well-being. Rooted in a fully integrated health system, Keralty's approach is structured around three interconnected components: (1) building a community network of health assets, (2) incorporating a community approach within clinical care, and (3) fostering compassionate neighbourhoods through locally led communities of care. The model emphasises the identification and activation of formal, informal, and community-based resources, supported by community health workers and an open-access health asset platform. Within health care settings, social connection and loneliness are systematically assessed using validated tools, enabling social prescribing pathways tailored to patients' levels of readiness and need. At the community level, Fundación Keralty leads the creation of compassionate neighbourhoods, empowering residents to map care needs, develop local leadership, and co-design practical solutions to support caregiving, connection, and well-being. Early results demonstrate high uptake of social prescriptions, improved patient experiences, strengthened social networks, and preliminary evidence of reduced health care utilization and avoided costs. The chapter illustrates how integrating community assets, social connection, and local leadership into health systems can contribute to more person-centred, sustainable, and effective approaches to health and well-being, positioning communities as the smallest and most fundamental unit of health.

DOI: 10.4324/9781003621348-5

4.1 Introduction

Keralty is a global healthcare organisation that started in Colombia over 30 years ago and that has, in Colombia, a fully integrated healthcare system including primary care centres, high complexity hospitals, insurance both premium and basic as well as a university and a nonprofit, Fundación Keralty.

At the core of Keralty's mission is the will to care for every one of their patients, and to do so, they have set out a four-axis model of care that not only encompasses having excellent clinical services but also includes the social and community realities of each one as well as having innovation and education at its core.

This is what is understood as an ecosystem of care by Keralty. There is a need to build a healthcare system that puts communities at the centre and connects with their reality, but communities themselves must also become empowered around their well-being and their needs and assets to truly transform health and well-being overall.

This chapter will present the strategy that Keralty has implemented in Colombia for building that ecosystem, which has three components. This strategy involves the participation of the primary care centres and the nonprofit, Fundación Keralty, to reach all levels.

The first component is building a network of organisations, community-based strategies and informal services (i.e., people that consistently meet at a park) and making it available to everyone. The second one is around incorporating a community approach to healthcare and making them aware of the importance of incorporating assessments around the real needs of people like care, connections and support. The healthcare setting identifies the needs of patients and their families and connects them to resources in their own community, using the resource directory amongst other available. The third strategy is around building local communities of care, working directly at the neighbourhood level, which identify their needs and assets and build community plans to transform their own realities.

4.2 Building a network of support

As presented above, the first strategy is building a network of resources in each community. Every community is rich in resources, or health assets, that can transform realities; they, however, are often not known by everyone. The resources that exist from the public and private sector are usually more known, but there are also many resources that are community-based, and many times informally run and therefore harder to identify.

To build that network, Keralty has included the role of a community promoter or community health worker (CHW) both within the primary care centres and from the nonprofit side (Fundación Keralty). Their role is to identify the health assets that are in each of the communities that can help build better well-being. Health assets are not just about health resources, it is about identifying all the elements in a community that could help everyone become healthier, happier and thrive; this includes, for instance, book clubs, painting classes, walking clubs and many more of that sort.

The community promoters are in charge of connecting to the different levels and key players to map all of them and make them available.

They connect with the public sector in each locality to identify what they have to offer, for instance public libraries, schools, sports and recreation offices amongst others. They also reach out to private organisations working in the area to understand what they bring to the community, private universities or schools, shopping malls, stores, businesses or large corporations. And finally, they walk around the community to see what informal things are happening, is there a group that meets at the park to walk together, is there a group of people who play dominos regularly, how is the community centre used, where do children gather to play, where do mothers meet up; and they identify how they can connect these informal activities to people that might need them.

All this information is inputted into an open database that anyone can access, using filters for location, gender, age and topic, so that they can also start using those resources. This platform, called Activos de salud Keralty [1], is available to all the other organisations that are part of the network so they also see what new connections they can make, how can they join forces and create new strategies together.

The asset database is the basis to connect people to people, bridge gaps of information and build truly connected communities. It is a resource that can be used by anyone both for uploading resources identified in the communities and for finding out possible connections. Community leaders are encouraged to become familiar with the resource database and help other use it and signpost people to all the resources available.

4.3 Community approach to healthcare

The second strategy is around building a community approach to healthcare, how to change the way clinical settings connect to their patients, having a more salutogenic approach to their conditions, understanding the need for connection, of having resources, connecting their social determinants of health to the recommendations that they made and having a truly person-centred approach.

Having strong social connections and a support system is key to achieving health outcomes. As the report of the World Health Organisation "From Loneliness to Social Connection" [2] outlined, about one in six people in the world feels lonely. This report also highlighted the impacts of social isolation and loneliness, emphasizing that people who have stronger connections are healthier, for one having support from others lowers inflammation and reduces the risk of heart disease and stroke. Data also shows that loneliness and isolation increase the risk of serious health problems and can even lead to death, according to the report "over 871,000 deaths around the world were linked to loneliness annually (2014–2019) [2]."

It can also impact mental health outcomes, leading to depression and anxiety. Taking all of this into account, healthcare organisations have no choice but to address loneliness and social isolation as much as they address hypertension, obesity or any other condition; however, it is not often done. Keralty, however, designed a strategy that could allow providers in different settings to address this as a key component of healthcare.

This strategy started within Fundación Keralty´s implementation of the compassionate cities strategy, from the Todos Contigo Methodology of The New Health Foundation [3]. The Foundation started working with different healthcare settings to integrate circles of care assessments or loneliness scales, initially with patients from palliative care programmes. The invitation was for the teams in palliative care to understand who was part of the caring process for each patient, was there a risk of loneliness, was there a primary caregiver with high burnout, who else could be part of that network of care and what would they need to participate in it.

This presented a challenge at the beginning since healthcare professionals are not trained traditionally to address these issues, even in palliative care where this conversation is a little more common. However, many institutions were willing to try it and include these assessments, and as they did, they discovered that this was an issue for many of their patients and their caretakers and that increasing the network actually improved quality of care and outcomes and that with the right information from the health assets platform, they were able to recommend other resources that were already canvassed. Furthermore, conversations started happening with family members, friends and neighbours amongst others of how they could participate in that process of caring.

Two major things were identified in the process of inviting other members to this process; one was that many identified caring as doing things considered complicated or too personal, like helping them take a bath or cleaning them. The second was that many feared being there; on one hand, most people did not know how to address the fact that the person was dying and did not know how to support them or how to help. Identifying this allowed the team to develop sensibilization and training strategies around those issues to increase their willingness to participate in the care process. Workshops around bereavement, talking about death and more instrumental ones like caring for a person that is bedridden and how to feed them according to different conditions were offered to all those who wanted to be part of the network of care.

As the numbers from the compassionate communities' strategies started to increase and show the impact it was having on the patients and their families as well as the impact of the network, Fundacion Keralty and the primary care medical centres decided to do a pilot at that level to widen the reach of the intervention.

The strategy in the primary care centres needed to be simpler and faster, given that the average consult is 20 minutes with the primary care provider (PCP) and needs to cover all the basics of a traditional visit. To achieve a wider reach, we decided to use the abbreviated Lubben scale as an assessment for network support for the patients, allowing the PCP to have a simple one-number assessment that they could easily understand and then address the issue if they were identified as having a low support system.

Currently, in 25 of Keralty´s primary care centres in Colombia, patients with a diagnosis of mild mental health, diabetes and hypertension are now being assessed with the Lubben scale by their medical teams. This is a cohort of around one million five hundred people.

The patient journey is as follows, the PCP or one of the members of the healthcare team applies the Lubben scale on the patient while they do the traditional assessment of any visit. If the Lubben scale comes out as positive for lack of a support network, meaning 12 and under, the team member who applied the scale addresses the issue with the patient the same way they would address a high blood pressure number or a high haemoglobin diagnosis. This makes both the healthcare team member aware of the importance of addressing this issue as well as the patient. If the patient tests positive for loneliness, there are three possible pathways to address it by doing a social prescription to local resources.

The first one is for those patients who are more empowered and willing to connect directly to the possible resources identified both in the resource database and the activities that are offered through volunteers directly within the medical centres. As the team member talks to the patient about their loneliness or lack of support system and offer the possibility of connecting them to resources in their community, they assess how likely it is that they will do it by themselves; this is usually associated with the type of loneliness and personal character, people that are more shy might not be as willing to connect directly.

The second path is identified as an assisted social prescription, where the patient does not seem willing to connect directly to the resource and support is needed. The patient is therefore referred to the community promoter who will do a telephone encounter with the patient to get to know him or her better and help them identify the best resource for them and offer to help in the first connection to it.

The third path is for those patients that are identified as not willing or able to connect with the resources or identified as having the biggest challenges in meeting their health and well-being goals. This group participates in a strategy called "Communities of Well-being," which takes the participants on a seven-week support group with other patients. The support group addresses each week one of the jewels of health, mind, nutrition, movement, community, environment and relationships through questions that allow them to share their struggles in each one, strategies that have helped them overcome them and build relationships with the other members of the group. In each session, resources associated with the specific topic are also shared so that they have them available for when they feel ready to use them. The first session is designed so that the members of the community can choose in what order they want to address the different jewels so that they feel they have ownership of the strategy and that it is for them to support each other based on what they feel they need more support in.

Furthermore, the Colsanitas Medical Centres have become a hub for the community where activities are held to connect patients and their communities in a place where they feel safe to do so. Community promoters lead and organise activities that are of interest to them mainly with volunteers from the community, for instance knitting classes, book clubs and arts and crafts.

Lubben scales are reapplied every six months for those patients who tested positive for loneliness or social disconnection and every year for those who did not, understanding that situations can change. Members of the Communities of Well-being also get a Warwick Well-being assessment done at the beginning and the end of the seven-week strategy.

In 2024, around 230,000 social prescriptions were done to different resources; 60% of them were level 1, meaning they were sent directly to the resource, 30% to level 2 and 10% to the communities of well-being. Most of the referrals were done to public resources in the community, followed by resources offered by the private sector. Health is impacted by having stronger connections; therefore, analysis regarding the impact on health outcomes is also being done, especially around hospitalizations, ER visits and medication usage. The economic impact analysis is showing in preliminary outcomes that for those patients who have received a social prescription, regardless of the level or path, there are avoided costs around hospitalization of around USD600,000 for the cohorts analysed.

Furthermore, qualitative interviews have also been done with the patients participating, which has allowed us to identify that they are very grateful to be able to be connected to resources in their communities and to other members of the community, that they feel better cared for now that they are seen as a whole person and not just a list of symptoms and that they feel better, healthier and happier in the process.

Therefore, implementing a strategy that allows medical facilities to address key issues such as loneliness and isolation and not just disease-related conversations is not just good for the patient, it is also good for the healthcare system. Having better cared for patients who are healthier reduces costs both now and in the long run by having avoided costs associated to conditions that are not well taken care of. This also improves company recognition and fidelity of clients since they feel that they are truly cared for.

4.4 Communities of care – building compassionate neighbourhoods

The third strategy led directly by Fundación Keralty is the promotion of Communities of care to achieve compassionate neighbourhoods.

Caring should happen in your community, staying connected, feeling cared for, having support and well-being are built into your everyday life and environments. Caring for your health when you need it must have not just the clinical aspect but a crucial component from your own community, your family, friends, neighbours, coworkers, amongst others.

However, how can you have that support when social capital has decreased worldwide, Colombia not being the exception, loneliness and isolation are happening in every community, neighbours do not know each other anymore and therefore cannot build strategies together.

As the WHO report also stated, "Communities are where connection happens. They are where people live, work, learn, play, and age. That's why community-level strategies are important for helping people feel more connected and less lonely [2]."

The compassionate neighbourhood strategy seeks to connect communities at the micro level to build strategies to address care needs for everyone involved, understanding care in a wider definition not just around healthcare but care in terms of support for caring for yourself, for others and your community in general. Currently, the strategy is being implemented in 30 communities in 6 cities in Colombia, Bogotá, Ibagué, Manizales, Santa Marta, Cartagena and Villavicencio in partnership with other allies in each city.

To build compassionate neighbourhoods, CHWs work directly with local communities to build a community plan to address their care needs. The first step to achieving this is gaining trust in the community. CHWs start by identifying different members of the community that can help them begin conversations with different groups in the community to understand who they are, what their story as a community has been and where they see each other in the future as a community. This allows the community to start seeing a common goal, what unites them instead of what can bring them apart and how they can build on those things that they have in common. The CHW identifies in these activities' positive leaders in the community that are already leading activities for the community and its well-being and that could be the leaders of the compassionate community.

The second step includes two components, one around training the identified leaders and another around mapping the community. Fundación developed a training strategy of 100 hours called "Compassionate leadership for the building of caring communities" that trains the leaders on how to lead community building strategies, mapping assets, promoting collective solutions for care needs. At the same time, those leaders are mapping their community, house by house, to identify the caring needs; for instance, people who are home bound with a single primary caregiver, people who live alone, people who have a diagnosis that makes it harder for them to connect.

Once they have the map built, they come back to the drawing board with different members of the community that want to be part of the caring process to develop strategies that could support those in needs. Strategies are to be feasible and starting with solutions that can show quick results so that the community wants to continue participating. Examples of the solutions that the communities have come with are:

1 The Matedeagua Community in Manizales identified eight households with people who were home bound and that had one primary caregiver that was suffering burnout. The community developed two strategies, one around supporting instrumental care by creating a WhatsApp group where they could ask for

support when they needed to buy groceries, pick up medication and such. The community volunteers who joined the communication strategy could offer to either care for the person at home so that the caregiver goes out or run the errand for them. However, they also decided that the care takers also needed to be cared for and every two weeks a volunteer of the community would take over the caring and the care takers would go to a community centre were other volunteers would organise an activity to care for them.

2 The Bosa Community in Bogotá built an urban garden as a place of gathering in the community, of supporting mental health and connecting and providing healthier food for the members in the community to help them have better health and well-being.

The strategies implemented by the communities of care have connected the members of the community so that they can feel supported by others, develop strategies that achieve well-being for everyone and that make better use of all the treasures that are in each community.

As a conclusion, achieving true health and well-being is not possible without understanding that it all happens in the communities, that they can transform their reality, that by supporting their connections they can develop strategies to tackle the major health and well-being issues that can be more effective, efficient and sustainable. Healthcare must understand that and connect with their communities and their patients to truly care for them. As Wendell Berry said it, "I believe that the community, in the fullest sense: a place and all its creatures, is the smallest unit of health and that to speak of the health of an isolated individual is a contradiction in terms" [4].

References

1. Keralty, "Keralty," [Online]. Available: https://keralty.activosdesalud.com/.
2. World Health Organisation, "From loneliness to social connection: charting a path to healthier societies," World Health Organisation, 30 June 2025. [Online]. Available: https://www.who.int/publications/i/item/978240112360. [Accessed 23 October 2025].
3. New Health Foundation, "La Universidad de Huelva obtiene el reconocimiento como Universidad Compasiva," [Online]. Available: https://www.newhealthfoundation.org/. [Accessed 23 October 2025].
4. W. Berry. "Health is membership" delivered as a speech at the conference "Spirituality and Healing" on October 17, 1994. Louisville, KY.

5

GETXO ZUREKIN BASQUE REGION SPAIN COMPASSIONATE COMMUNITY

Naomi Hasson, Julen Larrañaga Martinez de Agirre, Julia Martinez Barbero and Maider Grajales Saenz

Abstract

Getxo Zurekin is conceived as a social awareness, training and research programme with the aim of transferring the importance of end-of-life care to the community. The project is intended to promote a new social movement in Getxo for the creation of a compassionate environment for people at the end of their lives through the involvement and participation of the community. Rather than replacing existing palliative services and health and social care, the aim is to contribute to the well-being and improvement of the quality of life of people in dependency and end-of-life situations, capitalizing on existing community strengths and networks.

This initiative, launched in 2017, also had the aim of gaining an in-depth understanding of the challenges related to advanced illness, end-of-life and the bereavement process, as well as the existing capacities, resources and opportunities for the design and implementation of innovative and well-being, generating actions from a community perspective. Throughout this process of listening, network management and collective interpretation, focused on carers, care workers and their immediate environment (from care home staff to the public sector, including pharmacists, undertakers, cemetery workers and hairdressers for cancer patients), the programme was able to determine a series of challenges and opportunities that can serve as a basis for work on compassionate environments.

Getxo Zurekin Basque Region Spain was endorsed as a compassionate community by Public Health Palliative Care International in October 2025.

DOI: 10.4324/9781003621348-6

5.1 Introduction

Located on the Biscay coast in the Basque Country, Getxo is often described as a vibrant and attractive municipality that combines the elegance of its seaside heritage with a strong sense of community and cultural vitality. Traditionally considered an affluent residential area within Greater Bilbao, its urban landscape blends stately homes, working-class neighbourhoods and lively coastal spaces that foster an active civic life. According to 2024 records from Eustat [1], Getxo has 75,306 inhabitants (53.3% women and 46.7% men), of whom 28.5% are aged 65 or older, confirming its status as one of the most ageing municipalities in the region. That same year, 417 births and 749 deaths were registered, reflecting a demographic trend of population decline and an increasing need for care and social support systems.

Beneath its appearance of prosperity lies a more complex reality defined by the significant presence of migrant residents, particularly women employed in domestic and care work, who sustain much of the local care system. Their contribution has transformed Getxo into an increasingly diverse and interdependent community, revealing both the solidarity and inequalities that underpin daily life. In recent years, initiatives such as *Getxo Zurekin* have sought to acknowledge this plural social fabric, promoting intercultural dialogue and a shared vision of care that reflects the municipality's evolving identity.

5.2 Why Getxo Zurekin

In 2017, the Doble Sonrisa Foundation, a local family foundation established with a mission committed to care and support, launched Getxo Zurekin to develop innovative approaches to end-of-life care, inspired by the Todos Contigo® methodology of the New Health Foundation [2].

The initiative began when a palliative care doctor from Álava connected with the compassionate community programme: Sevilla Contigo [3] discovering a new model of care that placed the community at its heart. In a field where healthcare professionals often feel overstretched and where in many cases people and their families face their final journey in isolation with immense suffering, the idea of engaging the wider community as active partners sparked the creation of Getxo Zurekin compassionate community.

This movement recognises Getxo's diverse social fabric and promotes intercultural dialogue and a shared vision of care that reflects how the municipality lives and dies together, especially in times of crisis.

Throughout its journey, Getxo Zurekin has worked alongside committed partners such as the Agirre Lehendakaria Center (ALC) [4], which promotes social innovation and cultural transformation, and Deusto Business School Health, which underscores the importance of evidence and measurement. These collaborations have helped identify community needs and key actors already working in palliative and social care, forming a network united by a single goal: building an integrated model of health, social and community care that enhances well-being and grief literacy.

Conceived as a programme of social awareness, training and research, Getxo Zurekin aims to embed end-of-life care as a shared community responsibility. Rather than replacing existing services, it strengthens them by mobilizing local capacities and networks to support people with advanced illness, dependency or at the end-of-life.

Since 2017, the initiative has carried out extensive research to understand the realities of advanced illness, end-of-life and bereavement, identifying challenges and opportunities to design meaningful, community-led actions. By listening to carers, healthcare workers and those in their immediate circles, from care home staff to pharmacists, undertakers, cemetery workers and hairdressers for cancer patients, the programme has laid the foundation for developing compassionate environments in the municipality and being able to support others in the creation of their own compassionate community wherever they may be.

5.3 The WHAT

Through the Getxo Zurekin project, stakeholders in Getxo and its surrounding areas are experimenting with a portfolio of socially innovative services designed to complement the existing care system from a *community-based and compassionate* perspective.

One of the distinctive features of Getxo Zurekin is the creation of community roles that connect, coordinate and energise the various agents in the ecosystem. These roles help develop initiatives that holistically address care-related challenges, enabling the construction of a comprehensive community care model that strengthens and complements formal services.

The active involvement of community members, including citizens, public institutions, the private sector and third-sector organisations, has fostered a strong and cohesive social fabric. This collaboration has given rise to what we now call the compassionate community of Getxo, a network of interconnected actors working together to promote the holistic well-being of the municipality's residents.

At the heart of this network is the figure of the Lokarria, one of the central community roles within Getxo Zurekin. Inspired by the social innovation approach of the ALC, and examples such as the health connector in Mendip compassionate community [5], the Lokarria acts as a connector and facilitator, linking existing efforts, coordinating listening processes to understand community needs and co-creating new initiatives with local agents. This role is also key to engaging community members and encouraging their active participation in shaping the care ecosystem.

Getxo Zurekin relies on a group of highly committed volunteers, many trained in care and bereavement, who work closely with the Lokarria in the project's steering group. These volunteers promote community initiatives and help connect residents with local resources. Within the project, they are known as community connectors.

In addition, the project's influence enables many of the community members who have been informed and trained in community connections. Getting to know the resources available to them, understanding that small actions, conversations can change people's lives. These people are not formal volunteers but become part of a community empowered to become agents of change in their environment; these people are weavers.

The self-organization of these participants, particularly the community connectors, led to the creation of the Getxo Bihozbera association in 2023. This collective emerged to consolidate community initiatives born from Getxo Zurekin and now supports projects such as Getxo ZUrt! [6], a community co-created initiative focused on suicide prevention, intervention and postvention. The association remains closely linked to Getxo Zurekin and other local partners.

Other relevant actors include social and healthcare professionals connected to the Getxo community, as well as third-sector organisations and palliative care specialists. The scale of the initiative is reflected not only in the number of people involved but also in the strength of the networks and partnerships built across the territory.

A crucial aspect of this work is the connection with public health and social services. Getxo Zurekin maintains close collaboration with local institutions, health centres, hospitals and social services, ensuring alignment and coordination across care systems.

Finally, Getxo Zurekin is deeply engaged in wider regional and national networks that promote collaboration and shared learning, such as Arinduz (Basque Country Palliative Care Society), the Basque Country compassionate communities network and Eraldatuz (Network of People for Social Change), as well as partnerships with other municipalities. The Lokarria also plays an active role in supporting neighbouring municipalities to develop their own compassionate community initiatives.

Getxo Zurekin has a series of scaled initiatives that work in an interconnected manner at different levels of intervention, responding to the shortcomings of the social and healthcare system in addressing care, complementing it. The main ones are:

1 Bereavement support groups and one-on-one support.
2 Talking cafes: Space to talk, to connect with resources and create new relationships and caring for those people who feel isolated in the community [7].
3 Death cafes: In the community and in the prison services [8].
4 Training for people at risk of social exclusion in particular migrant workers in collaboration with local NGO´s because they are in many cases the carer for this elderly population.
5 Workshops for volunteers in local NGOs.
6 Workshops for teachers in local schools.
7 Community weavers workshop. Two-hour training based on the Mendip Compassionate Community model [9].
8 Palliative care and support for people and their families who are approaching end-of-life.
9 Space of silence and meditation. A space for reflection and guided meditation for self-care, launched in 2023 in response to the need to create a place of meditation for people with advanced illness and their families.

10 Soul weavers group. A mutual support group for women who care for their partners, children or other family members, or carers who have lost a loved one. It is a self-help group based on friendship and connection.
11 Community theatre: In collaboration with a local theatre group, we have developed "Rumbo Desconocido" community performance to raise awareness of the end-of-life. Since its premiere, it has been performed in around 15 municipalities and 6 universities across the country [10].
12 Monthly talks open to the community. These talks aim to raise awareness and provide training on end-of-life care, advanced illness and grief.
13 Connection with local funeral parlours to normalise the spaces prior to death.
14 Formalization of the Advance Directive document in community.
15 Specific activities to raise awareness and sensitivity in the community. These are activities carried out on a more ad hoc basis with the aim of transforming the community's perceptions of the end-of-life, death, grief and unwanted loneliness. They aim to break the existing taboo and destigmatise these issues.
16 Les Elis Group: Mutual support group formed by people with motor neurone disease in the municipality.
17 Getxo ZUrt! [6] A series of initiatives aimed at the prevention, treatment and postvention of suicidal behaviour through community involvement.

5.4 Have we made a difference?

To understand the most significant changes in the Getxo community since 2017, an analysis of the evolution of narrative patterns has been carried out, with the aim of understanding the community's deep-rooted beliefs about the evolution of the care model, the driving forces behind its change, social values and the perception of death and the meaning of life. To this end, a comparative analysis was carried out of the perceptual patterns of 2017–2018 with those of 2024 [11]. This work has been done with the support of ALC, who have been possibly the most valuable partner we have had since the beginning of this journey. The most significant changes found in the four key areas are described below, where you will also find some excerpts from the testimonies that have been collected through the listening platform. These conversations, safe spaces and workshops have allowed us to listen, gather information in real time to understand the impact of the Getxo Zurekin project.

5.5 Care model

Between 2017 and 2018, the care model in Getxo was understood from a strongly medicalised perspective, focused almost exclusively on healthcare and with little consideration for the emotional, social and spiritual dimensions of care. The supposed model of care focused on the curative sphere, mainly centred on treating the physical body and sometimes the mental body. In contrast, the emotional and spiritual spheres (and usually the mental sphere) were not considered by the care system; there was no comprehensive approach to care. A welfare-based approach prevailed, in which the public administration was solely responsible, and the community was not recognised as a participating agent.

> The protagonist is the doctor, the protagonists are those who treat you while you're lying on your back, exhausted, but your mind is still working, it's an insult to your intelligence, on top of being bedridden, they're abusing you, because if you're normal they don't abuse you, they don't say such nonsense to you, that way they treat you, from top to bottom, both them and her.
>
> *(Adult male with amyotrophic lateral sclerosis)*

> We need a trade coordinator, like when you do work on your house and someone organises the carpenter, painter, and bricklayer for you. This is the same thing. We need someone to accompany us and connect us because we are exhausted.
>
> *(Wife of a gentleman with Parkinsons)*

In 2024, the narrative shifted towards a comprehensive concept of care, recognizing the need to involve multiple actors, especially the community, in the construction of a shared model. Although structural deficiencies persist—such as a lack of end-of-life training or resources in the social and healthcare field—a cultural shift towards more humane, collaborative and sensitive relationships within the care system is evident.

> The community aspect is extremely important and must be very present, but it is true that we can provide support, we can be there, but I believe that public institutions also need to change their perspective and become part of the care system. If a migrant is unable to understand their appointments for the following week, it should not only be the community that ensures they have access to those appointments, but the public system should also provide that care. Community cannot sustain everything. From within the community, we can detect problems,
>
> *(Adult woman with a social and health care profile)*

5.6 Traction of the care model

In the 2017–2018 period, the transformation of the care model lacked a clear agent to drive change: neither public institutions nor the community felt responsible or capable of leading it. Care remained relegated to the family sphere, especially to women, and remained invisible in public debate.

> A nurse who doesn't know him very well says to me, "You leave him alone at night," and I say, "He's been in hospital for two months, I'm his nephew (…) you have no right to ask me to do anything at work or anything else."
>
> *(Adult male, primary carer for a dependent relative)*

> I can do it, I do it, I don't have to ask anyone for anything, but not because I'm arrogant, because I'm no better than anyone else, but it's my turn, he's my husband and it's my turn.
>
> *(Elderly woman, primary carer for a dependent family member)*

In 2024, the narrative is reversed: the community emerges as the main driver of transformation thanks to training processes, the creation of support networks and the development of meaningful links. The Getxo Zurekin project has facilitated this process, making care a topic of collective interest and positioning the community as an agent with real capacity for action and shared leadership alongside institutions. The impetus for community action stems from the fact that the people who have become involved in the process have wanted to give back what the community has offered them, and that the creation of bonds and a community care network has generated a sense of belonging that encourages the involvement of the municipality's residents in care.

> You talk to them, and you can tell they're well trained. People with the same experiences, it's like a meeting point for all of us who have been through the same thing, you feel understood, but I would say that in the only one I've been to so far, I haven't found anywhere else like it.
>
> *(Lady who attends the bereavement group)*

> It is true that society is often ahead of institutions in terms of many initiatives.
>
> *(Mature adult male, associative profile)*

5.7 Social values

In the early years of the analysis, an individualistic metanarrative prevailed, limiting the possibility of community care. It was assumed that each person should take care of themselves or their immediate environment, while society had no reason to be involved in the well-being of others. There was a perception that individualistic values were so deeply rooted that community development was not a possibility. Community care requires a change in values to progress. From an individualistic perspective, care is a burden for which society should not be responsible, but rather each person is responsible for themselves (or at least for their closest relatives). Care provided by and within the community is not considered desirable.

> He had never come to my house to take him out, to take him anywhere. He only came to my house when I invited him to eat so that he could be with him. (…) And then he comes asking for money that his father has.
>
> *(Elderly woman, primary carer for a dependent relative)*

> They tell me that at 80 years old I have to go to a care home and live with an aunt I don't know at all and that I have to live there… come on.
>
> *(Adult woman, employed in a residential centre).*

By 2024, this framework had changed: community care is valued as a space for connection and meaning in life. People no longer see it as a burden, but as an opportunity to build bonds and mutual well-being. This change is accompanied by the recognition of the need for spaces and tools that facilitate community self-organization, consolidating an ethic of interdependence in the face of previous individualism. Although society is individualised, we need a push. In other words, we are not individualistic, but rather the current system individualises us, but this is not something immutable. On a deeper level, people connected to the compassionate community are aware that this is about giving and receiving, needing each other.

> Well, yes, I do have friends, I mean, now I get along very well. X and I don't talk much, but I get along very well. It's something that comes from the heart. (…) And well, friends, I've made quite a few friends here. You feel comfortable.
>
> *(Elderly woman, attends talking cafes)*

> I usually say that I have invented another life for myself, I have reinvented myself. Despite the pain and everything else, which is very hard, this situation has allowed me to meet some very valuable people, and the rapport we have motivates and helps you. Sometimes they help you and other times you help them.
>
> *(Elderly woman, community connector)*

> Creating a support network, collaborating with those people who need support, whether at home or in different areas, so they don't feel alone, knowing that there is someone there to support them at any time.
>
> *(Mature adult woman, community connector)*

5.8 Death and meaning of life

In 2017–2018, death was a taboo subject that led to social disconnection and a loss of meaning in life. Coping with death was restricted to the individual sphere, with no spaces or tools for processing it collectively, which led to loneliness and emotional distress. There were no spaces or tools that allowed for the normalization of death as part of the process of life. Death was limited to individual management, not even to the private sphere (family and/or other close support networks), making it difficult to deal with end-of-life processes and grief alone. The difficulty of socializing these issues led to the loss of pre-existing bonds in situations of illness and death, often resulting in unwanted loneliness. The shortcomings in addressing end-of-life and bereavement processes had negative impacts on the mental, emotional and spiritual well-being of people who felt their sense of purpose in life was being questioned.

> With dementia, your network disappears, everyone, even your friends from church, there is no one left. When I bump into a friend on the street and she says

> to me, 'I know I behaved badly towards your mother, but I feel so sorry for her that I'd rather not go,' lifelong friends.
>
> *(Adult woman, primary carer for a dependent family member)*

> I am someone who likes to talk about my sister above all else (...) People don't want to talk about those who are no longer here, but the dead are part of life.
>
> *(Adult woman, social and health care profile)*

In 2024, thanks to initiatives such as ceath cafés, community spaces and the promotion of advance directives, the community is beginning to integrate death as part of the life cycle, generating a progressive openness to dialogue about the end-of-life. Although cultural change is still in its infancy, community networks are consolidating as spaces for support and reframing, where talking about death contributes to strengthening the meaning of life and social bonds. Destigmatizing death and associated processes (illness, end-of-life and unwanted loneliness) takes time as it is a profound cultural change.

Although some pre-existing bonds continue to disappear, community bonds are emerging as a resource. Meeting people in similar life situations allows them to be replaced and new support networks to be consolidated, thus alleviating potential situations of unwanted loneliness. Participants have reframed death as part of the life process, which prevents negative impacts on people's health and well-being, allowing them to accept death as a natural and inevitable process.

> I used to be afraid of death. But now, for example, with everything we usually talk about, the experiences that each person shares, testimonies and so on, I think that's very, very good. I'm not afraid of it anymore.
>
> *(Adult female migrant, Death cafe)*

> I talk to my daughters about it, and sometimes they say, "I don't want to talk about that," but I tell them that it's something that will happen sooner or later. And so this coffee thing helped me a lot.
>
> *(Adult female attends death café)*

> Personally, I am extremely grateful because I don't think I would have been able to say goodbye to X, me and my children (...) it was wonderful to be at home as we all were, with that serenity, that peace, love and that farewell, thanks to the support I had from the palliative care team and from the lokarria.
>
> *(Adult woman, primary carer for dependent family members)*

Many of these quotes and references can be found in the reports published by the fundacion doble sonirsa in collaboration with ALC.

5.9 Reflections/challenges

The compassionate community of Getxo meets the criteria to be considered an example of community development and more recently tremendously grateful to have been given an endorsement by Public Health Palliative Care International in October 2025. Meaningfully connecting people in the community fosters participation and collaboration among the various community stakeholders, strengthens internal assets and resources, promotes collective well-being, encourages civic participation and local leadership, takes a holistic and sustainable approach, considers innovation and adaptation to the context and changing needs and promotes community resilience, diversity and inclusion.

Furthermore, considering the community-owned approach [12], the compassionate community of Getxo is mobilised and empowered in the development of its self-government, establishing priorities, implementing actions and developing sustainable mechanisms for health promotion with external allies and support by building networks. This network structure allows the complex challenge of care to be addressed through the development of personal skills, the strengthening of community action, the creation of supportive environments, the construction of healthy public policies and the reorientation of health systems.

Community training through the support of the Lokarria, and now through community connectors, as well as the development of specific initiatives such as the community weavers' workshop, have enabled the acquisition of specific skills, allowing people to consolidate themselves as assets to the community. In addition, community awareness-raising, education and training have indirectly generated natural links between community members, forming a daily support network that transcends the compassionate community process.

The process has also had a positive impact on public policies in the area. Examples include the establishment of a service in municipalities for drawing up advance directives [13,14] on the need for a community care system in end-of-life situations. All of this promotes the reorientation of the care system towards a comprehensive model in which the community plays a significant role.

The case of the compassionate community of Getxo confirms that community development enables systemic change, in this case addressing the issue of care through the implementation of a comprehensive care system with a community focus.

In addition to having a consolidated community approach, listening closely to community members through community leaders and other community agents allows the portfolio of initiatives to respond to the specific and changing needs and preferences of the municipality's residents. This is why we can talk about a people-centred approach, thus framing the Getxo compassionate community within the state strategy for a new model of care in the community [15] as an example of the deinstitutionalization of care, particularly in situations of end-of-life care, bereavement, unwanted loneliness and suicidal behaviour.

5.10 Conclusions and reflections for the future

The Getxo Zurekin project has successfully implemented the *figure of the Lokarria* through an evolutionary evaluation approach, positioning itself as a prototype for community development. Tested in the field of care, it contributes to building a comprehensive, community-based and people-centred care system that complements existing structures. This approach demonstrates how community development can drive systemic change, promoting collective well-being and health across the ecosystem.

In relation to the care model, the initiative has shown that a shift towards integrated social and healthcare is possible through community-driven transformation. Although limitations persist in the public sector, such as limited flexibility and a lack of incentives to reframe traditional care dynamics, community training and a strengthened sense of belonging have empowered residents to self-organise and act as agents of change. When the community takes ownership of the process, sustainability and growth become achievable. However, such transformation can only occur through alliances with other key actors in the care ecosystem.

To enable this, different community roles have been developed to coordinate and guide collective action. These roles facilitate the co-creation of initiatives through deep listening, connect diverse agents and resources, channel the community towards support systems and promote new initiatives, training and awareness-raising activities.

The evolving needs of the compassionate community of Getxo have inspired the team to learn from similar global experiences, such as health connectors, community weavers and connectors in other parts of the world. This process reaffirms that community action does not happen spontaneously; rather, it emerges through structured social innovation that fosters shared ownership and collective agency.

The implementation of the Lokarria figure, combined with an evolutionary evaluation approach, has proven effective as a flexible prototype capable of adapting to the unique challenges and opportunities of different territories. Furthermore, the network of multi-level community figures, supported by digital and collaborative management tools, has become essential for ensuring the sustainability and scalability of initiatives like Getxo Zurekin.

The compassionate community of Getxo stands as a methodological example of how to implement a comprehensive care system grounded in compassion, participation and systemic thinking.

We are deeply grateful to all those who have connected with us since 2017, those who have shared the understanding and desire to do things differently and who continue to demonstrate that change is both possible and necessary. As Allan Kellehear reminds us, *Death and dying is everyone's business.* [16]. Little by little, this understanding has taken root in Getxo, in its people, its organisations and its systems.

References

1. Eustat, "Getxo," [Online]. Available: https://en.eustat.eus/municipal/datos_estadisticos/getxo.html. [Accessed 22 October 2025].
2. New Health Foundation, "Un nuevo modelo de salud," [Online]. Available: https://www.newhealthfoundation.org/. [Accessed 22 October 2025].
3. New Health Foundation, "SEVILLA CONTIGO, ciudad compasiva," [Online]. Available: https://www.newhealthfoundation.org/sevilla-contigo/. [Accessed 22 October 2025].
4. Agirre Lehendakaria Center, "ALCK diseña Plataformas de Innovación para el abordaje de retos sociales complejos," [Online]. Available: https://www.agirrecenter.eus/. [Accessed 22 October 2025].
5. Health Connections, "Health Connections Mendip," [Online]. Available: https://healthconnectionsmendip.org/. [Accessed 22 October 2025].
6. Getxo Bihozbera, "Alerta Zurt," [Online]. Available: https://zurt.org/. [Accessed 22 October 2025].
7. Health Connections, "Talking cafes," [Online]. Available: https://healthconnectionsmendip.org/lets-connect/projects/talking-cafes/. [Accessed 22 October 2025].
8. Death Cafe, "Welcome to death cafe," [Online]. Available: https://deathcafe.com/. [Accessed 22 October 2025].
9. Health Connections, "Community connector training," [Online]. Available: https://healthconnectionsmendip.org/lets-connect/training/community-connectors/. [Accessed 22 October 2025].
10. *Teaser Rumbo Desconocido. Cia Utopian.* [Film]. Utopian Getxo.
11. N. Hasson, M. Grajales, I. Grajales and G. Espiau, "Building a narrative for compassionate communities: the case of Getxo Zurekin," *International Journal of Integrated Care,* 2018. Available: https://ijic.org/articles/10.5334/ijic.s2321.
12. World Health Organisation, *COMMUNITY ENGAGEMENT A health promotion guide for universal health coverage in the hands of the people*, WHO, 2020.
13. Department of Health, *Basque Country Palliative care plan 2023–2027*, Department of Health, 2023.
14. El Correo, "Living wills are growing in Bizkaia despite waits of more than a year to process them," 2 April 2024. [Online]. Available: https://www.elcorreo.com/bizkaia/testamento-vital-crece-bizkaia-pese-esperas-ano-20240402005225-nt.html?ref=https://www.elcorreo.com/bizkaia/testamento-vital-crece-bizkaia-pese-esperas-ano-20240402005225-nt.html#vtm_funnel=exito-login-gis&vtm_tipoProceso=. [Accessed 27 October 2025].
15. Ministerio de Derechos Sociales, "Estrategia estatal para un nuevo modelo de cuidados en la comunidad Un proceso de desinstitucionalización (2024–2030). Available: https://estrategiadesinstitucionalizacion.gob.es/wp-content/uploads/2024/06/Estrategia-para-nuevo-modelo-cuidados-en-la-comunidad.pdf.
16. Ashgate Hospice, "'We need an end of life care system worthy of our democracy' with Professor Allan Kellehear," 30 June 2025. Available: https://ashgatehospice.org.uk/2025/06/30/we-need-an-end-of-life-care-system-worthy-of-our-democracy-with-professor-allan-kellehear/.

6

COMPASSIONATE INVERCLYDE

Alison Bunce and Anne Hendry

Abstract

This chapter charts the journey of Compassionate Inverclyde from 2016 to date, evolving from an award-winning social movement to an independent community-led charitable organisation and the first compassionate community in Scotland. The authors describe the range of initiatives developed by Compassionate Inverclyde and the benefits realised for local citizens, communities and organisations, including an important contribution to individual, relational and community outcomes and social value. This chapter ends with insights and practical tips on creating the conditions for a compassionate community to flourish.

6.1 Introduction

Inverclyde is a mixed urban/coastal community of considerable scenic beauty in West Central Scotland. The population of around 80,000 is diverse. Some areas of high income sit alongside neighbourhoods with high levels of poverty, unemployment, disability and trauma. Life expectancy at birth is lower than the Scottish average but the population is ageing faster, and the dependency ratio is increasing. The area has a single district general hospital which is well integrated with local community health and social care services overseen by Inverclyde Health and Social Care Partnership (HSCP). Since 2015, following legislation to integrate health and social care in Scotland, Inverclyde HSCP has had statutory responsibility for planning, commissioning and delivering health and care services to meet the needs of the local population [1]. The HSCP team work closely with a wide range of public sector organisations, business, community and voluntary sector partners as a Community Planning Partnership, Inverclyde Alliance [2]. This integrated

DOI: 10.4324/9781003621348-7

context and the relatively compact size of Inverclyde foster positive relationships between the local leaders. This positive receptive context for a compassionate community is further supported by a strong cultural identity and pride, and the generosity and friendliness of its people.

6.2 Planting the seed

In 2016, inspired by Professor Allan Kellehear's work on compassionate communities [3], the Director of Care at Ardgowan Hospice began to explore the attitudes and behaviours of Inverclyde citizens around loneliness, isolation, death, dying and bereavement. Through community listening events, over 200 people identified what they valued most about living in Inverclyde. Uniting around values of kindness, helpfulness and neighbourliness, they pledged to make Inverclyde a more compassionate community. The initial aim was to begin to transform attitudes about death and dying in a natural, locally relevant way and to reduce suffering associated with life-limiting illness, survivorship, dying, death and bereavement.

6.3 Getting started

Ardgowan Hospice seconded their Director of Care to lead the programme and provided funding for part-time administrative support. The lead secured a Florence Nightingale Foundation scholarship to learn from global leaders of compassionate communities. The reflective report of this travel scholarship shares insights from visiting compassionate communities in England, Australia and the USA [4]. On her return, the lead established a programme board, co-chaired by a local councillor and by the HSCP Chief Officer. Members included local citizens and representatives from healthcare, social care, schools, college, voluntary sector organisations, police, prison service and local businesses. This diverse membership and a bottom-up community-led approach have enabled Compassionate Inverclyde to evolve organically and become a vibrant social movement of compassionate citizens who care for each other and work alongside local services. Over time, through listening to what matters to local people, Compassionate Inverclyde has expanded its focus to support people experiencing loneliness, social isolation or poor mental well-being as well as those experiencing crisis or loss.

6.4 Activities

The programme has tested and delivered a wide range of activities that are at varying stages of maturity. Some were seasonal and others time-limited responses to the COVID-19 pandemic. All activities apply a strength-based [5] and asset-based community development approach [6], recognising and nurturing the assets of individuals, families and neighbourhoods.

The first initiative was the most ambitious, introducing No One Dies Alone (NODA) Companions to support people in the last hours of life. NODA Companions are trained to understand the dying process and are supported through monthly peer supervision circles. NODA was initially introduced in hospital wards but gradually extended to the community, principally in care homes. The Comfort Care Bag carried by NODA Companions contains a CD player, a variety of genres of music, a NODA vigil journal, a notebook to record thoughts/experiences, NODA cards and envelopes to leave a note for the patient or family, a Bible or rosary if applicable, insightful readings and poems and evaluation forms that the Companion completes at the end of the vigil. Other related developments include Palliative Care Companions who may offer support or respite for carers, Back Home Visitors for people returning home from hospital who face loneliness or isolation, Dog Walking volunteers and Companions to support young mums who lack family support.

The second major initiative emerged from community awareness of the vulnerability of people returning home from hospital. Volunteers began to coordinate supply and delivery of Back Home Boxes to adults of all ages returning home from hospital alone. Citizens, businesses, organisations and groups across Inverclyde donate essential items such as tea, milk, bread and tinned food so recipients don't have to worry about shopping immediately on return home and can focus on their recovery. Boxes also contain a get-well card made by local children and a hand-knitted blanket from members of the local community. During lockdown as hospital activity decreased, Compassionate Inverclyde rapidly pivoted their Back Home Boxes support to provide Helping Hand Food Boxes for people isolating at home who did not have local family support. They also mobilised a volunteer prescription delivery service and distributed toiletries, clean nightwear and other essential items for patients isolating in hospital and unable to have visitors.

The third strand of activity supported well-being across the generations. Over 500 adults have completed Compassionate Inverclyde's High 5 well-being programme. This was developed from the 5 Ways to Wellbeing outlined in the New Economics Foundation 2008 report [7] and through pilots with local citizens, prisoners and college students. The High 5 programme has been further developed for primary school pupils in a fun and creative way, tailored to their age and learning style and to the mental, emotional, social and physical well-being experience and outcomes of the national Curriculum for Excellence. A version of High 5 has been developed for High School pupils and for staff working with the Homeless Centre. The High 5 approach inspired a Self-Care 360 project which includes mindfulness and a Capacitar healing workshop [8].

A bereavement café has evolved into a community friendship hub at a local church where around 45 people meet weekly offering networks of support for people who are lonely or isolated. Jolly Boxes are distributed every Christmas, a time when loneliness is often experienced more acutely. There is a strong sense of reciprocity among the 90 Compassionate Inverclyde volunteers who help in various roles. Volunteers formed a singing group in 2019. This continues to meet monthly.

Organisations from the third, public and private sectors who embrace Compassionate Inverclyde values have worked together to adopt Scotland's Bereavement Charter for Children and Adults [9]. The charter contains 13 statements which describe what we can do to support individuals and communities who struggle with the death of someone they know or someone in their community. An example of the collaboration is the Inverclyde Culture Collective work with local health and care organisations. The series of creative research events inspired a No One Grieves Alone event as part of the National Demystifying Death Week. An eight-week Tailz of Love programme was developed to help people who have lost a beloved pet to express their feelings of grief in a safe space accompanied by compassionate facilitators.

6.5 Estimating impact

In 2018, just two years after setting up the programme, an independent formative evaluation was commissioned. Around 100 people involved with Compassionate Inverclyde were interviewed to understand the individual, relational and community outcomes achieved. Three reports describe the many benefits for citizens, communities and organisations, and the contribution the programme makes to realising local and national health and well-being outcomes [10]. However, cause and effect relationships are not linear and there are many interdependencies in factors contributing to outcomes.

As the programme has continued to grow, the team have continued to gather information on benefits. For example, over 200 patients have now directly benefited from a NODA Companion at the end of their life. Their families also benefit, particularly if they are living at some distance or juggling other caring responsibilities. A sense of comfort and reassurance for families will have a positive impact on experience and recovery during the early stages of bereavement. Health and care professionals value the NODA offer too, not least as it avoids struggling to source additional staff to sit alongside a patient who would otherwise be alone. Monetary benefits in terms of costs avoided from compassionate companions releasing staff time are matched by the social value from a more positive bereavement experience and the intangible benefits experienced by volunteers who find purpose and well-being from their role.

Back Home Boxes directly benefit recipients and their family members and touch the lives of thousands of people of all ages across Inverclyde who knit blankets, make cards and donate goods for the boxes. The material value of 5,236 Back Home Boxes and countless other goods supplied to date is significant. However, the social value is considerably greater because of personal outcomes achieved: feeling less alone and better equipped to manage on return home from hospital, a sense of belonging and purpose, and a sense of significance, that you matter and people care. HSCP staff acknowledge the Back Home Boxes make a contribution to their strong performance in reducing delays to discharge and preventing early readmission to hospital. The Back Home Boxes may mitigate the need for an early post-discharge social care visit for a proportion of those returning home alone.

Compassionate Inverclyde's well-being activities and connections contribute to increased community cohesion and many positive outcomes across the life stages. These include enduring friendships, respect for diversity, networks of support and collaboration, community voice and pride, neighbourliness, resilience and active youth participation. Over 1,000 school pupils have completed the High 5 well-being programme and local high schools are now taking forward a Kindness challenge.

Bereavement-friendly workplaces support staff to return to productive work at the right time with less psychological morbidity, in turn benefiting the employing organisation. To date, more than 100 people in Inverclyde have participated in bereavement training and 14 Inverclyde-based organisations have achieved their Bereavement Charter Mark and so earned a Bronze Kindness Award. In total, 165 citizens have received an individual Kindness Award.

As public services strive to recover in the face of unprecedented economic and workforce challenges, investment in proactive care and prevention struggles to compete with the increasing demands for reactive care and support. The need to demonstrate impact from investment in prevention and community-led solutions is more pressing than ever. Social Return on Investment (SROI) methodology aims to identify wider socio-economic outcomes and a broader estimation of social value [11]. A high-level analysis of SROI for Compassionate Inverclyde in 2023 estimated at least a 3:1 SROI for people and communities through creating well-being, resilience and social capital in addition to the costs avoided for citizens and for statutory services [12]. This is almost certainly a conservative estimate as school pupil beneficiaries were not included in the analysis, and some supports had paused during the pandemic. More detailed analysis is required.

6.6 Reflections

Inverclyde's story has many lessons for other areas embarking on a similar journey. An important success factor is the empowerment at all levels: the Board, the lead and the network of local people, all bound together by shared values and mission described as "Ordinary people making a difference together." The Board governance enabled risk, knowing when to let go and leaving space for the lead and volunteers to be creative. The lead, a natural convenor and a positive role model for inclusion and co-creation, took care to build on the intrinsic values, strengths and ideas of local people. That required time to listen in an authentic way, uncovering, nurturing and appreciating the kindness that's already there. She strived to be inclusive, finding ways to make it easy for people of all ages and backgrounds to be involved and to contribute, ensuring they have a strong and equal voice. Building on local knowledge and established networks of support were essential. Understanding and affirming established relationships, community groups and the social and cultural heritage of the community were invaluable.

TABLE 6.1 Practical Tips

1	Start with community conversations about what matters most to local people
2	Invest in development support from a trusted, compassionate, authentic and humble leader
3	Develop collaborative leadership at all levels around a shared purpose and intrinsic values
4	Anchor the movement with a local community organisation that has a trusted brand
5	Establish a courageous guiding coalition that gives permission to act, purposefully avoids unnecessary bureaucracy and enables risk taking
6	Find creative ways to make it easy for local people to volunteer and for everyone to be kind, helpful and to have a can-do attitude
7	Value and empower all contributors and ensure they have a strong and equal voice
8	Nurture community volunteers through peer support, reflective practice and wholehearted facilitation
9	Use the power of social media as a practical communication and self-organising tool
10	Stay curious and keep learning from other compassionate communities
11	Continue to pay attention to what matters to people and share stories that touch hearts and inspire people to be kind
12	Plan for a sustainable model of leadership and governance that can exploit synergies with other developments and minimise unintended consequences

Compassionate Inverclyde is often described as a social movement or network. While largely self-organising, networks need to be managed and nurtured but in collaborative, non-hierarchical ways [13,14,15]. The programme lead functioned more as a systems convenor than a project manager. System convenors are often described as visionary and pragmatic and function as network weavers [16]. They open spaces for new kinds of conversations across traditional boundaries and silos to unleash unrealised potential [17].

Growth and spread were organic, enabled by making things easy, accessible and enjoyable to do, giving permission, restoring confidence, saying thank you with sincerity and remaining curious, continuously asking *how else can we help?* An active social media presence was invaluable – as were skills in the curation and telling of stories in ordinary language, touching people's hearts.

Based on the lessons learned, Table 6.1 offers tips for other communities embarking on this incredible journey. These tips must be viewed as a "compass" and not a prescriptive tool kit. How you develop your own compassionate community must make sense of the unique strengths, ideas and passions of your local people.

6.7 Moving forward

Early development capacity was provided by Ardgowan Hospice, later enhanced by financial support from the HSCP. As the community-driven movement matured and its scope broadened beyond end-of-life care, hosting by the Hospice became less critical. Following a period of transition planning, in 2024, Compassionate

Inverclyde became an independent Scottish Charitable Incorporated Organisation (SCIO). Inspired by the belief that everyone has a valuable role to play, the new SCIO brings together people from all walks of life to create positive change through being kind, brave and inclusive. This milestone coincided with the publication of a new strategic plan and partnership vision by the HSCP [18]. It is a testament to the influence and impact of Compassionate Inverclyde that the HSCP vision statement frames Inverclyde as a compassionate community, working together to ensure people live active, healthy and fulfilling lives.

Recent awards from the national Mental Health and Wellbeing Fund and from the National Lottery are supporting the new charity to continue its core work and to make progress on five new strategic objectives: to improve well-being; to promote and celebrate compassionate citizenship; to raise awareness about kindness through information and education; to recognise and foster compassionate organisations; and to build capacity, good governance and financial sustainability.

As Compassionate Inverclyde approaches its ten-year anniversary, all involved look back with gratitude and pride at which has been achieved. Moving forward as an SCIO offers a greater level of autonomy and opens new funding and development opportunities. These will be critical for succession planning and sustainability. We look forward with excitement to the many opportunities and challenges ahead.

References

1. Inverclyde HSCP Strategic Needs Assessment 2021/2022. Available at https://www.inverclyde.gov.uk/health-and-social-care
2. Inverclyde Community Planning Partnership. Available at https://www.inverclyde.gov.uk/council-and-government/community-planning-partnership
3. A. Kellehear. "Compassionate Communities: End-of-Life Care as Everyone's Responsibility." *Quarterly Journal of Medicine.* 2013 Dec;106(12):1071–1075. doi: 10.1093/qjmed/hct200. Epub 2013 Sep 30. PMID: 24082152.
4. A. Bunce. "Experiencing Compassionate Care in Practice: A Travel Scholarship." *British Journal of Nursing.* 2018 Jul 12;27(13):758–760. doi: 10.12968/bjon.2018.27.13.758. PMID: 29995503.
5. A. Morgan and E. Ziglio. "Revitalising the Evidence base for Public Health: An Assets Model." *Promotion and Education.* 2007;14(2 Suppl):17–22. doi: 10.1177/10253823070140020701x. PMID: 17685075.
6. I. Burkett. "Appreciating Assets: A New Report from the International Association for Community Development (IACD)." *Community Development Journal.* 201146(4):573–578. *JSTOR*, https://www.jstor.org/stable/44258309. Accessed 6 July 2025.
7. J. Aked, N. Marks, C. Cordon and S. Thompson. "Five Ways to Mental Wellbeing." *New Economics Foundation* (2008) Available online at: https://neweconomics.org/2008/10/five-ways-to-wellbeing
8. Capacitar UK. https://www.capacitaruk.org/
9. The Bereavement Charter for Adults and Children in Scotland. Available online https://www.goodlifedeathgrief.org.uk/about-charter/

10. A. Hendry, K. Barrie and E. Miller. "Compassionate Inverclyde Evaluation reports-Summary; Deeper Dive; Voices Narrative". 2018 Available at https://compassionateinverclyde.org/reports/
11. A.O. Banke-Thomas, B. Madaj, C.A. van den and N. Broek. "Social Return on Investment (SROI) Methodology to Account for Value for Money of Public Health Interventions: A Systematic Review." *BMC Public Health*. 2015;15:582. doi:10.1186/s12889-015-1935–7
12. A. Hendry. "Realising the Value of Kindness." 2023 Available online https://compassionateinverclyde.org/wp-content/uploads/2024/09/CI-Report-2023-_final.pdf
13. S. Hearn and E. Mendizabal. "Not Everything that Connects is a Network." *Overseas Development Institute*. 2011. Available online https://odi.org/en/publications/not-everything-that-connects-is-a-network/
14. R. Malby, K. Mervyn and L. Pirisi. "How Professionals Can Lead Networks in the NHS", *International Journal of Leadership in Public Services*. 2013;9(1/2):47–58. doi.org/10.1108/IJLPS-05-2013-0012
15. R. Arganoff R "Inside Collaborative Networks: Ten Lessons for Public Managers." *Public Administration Review*. 66(1) December 2006:56–65. doi.org/10.1111/j.1540-6210.2006.00666.x
16. Network weaver. A Space for Shared Knowledge on Network Weaving, Systems Change, and Transformation https://networkweaver.com/
17. Systems Convening. A Crucial form of Leadership for the 21stCentury. Available at https://www.wenger-trayner.com/systems-convening/
18. Inverclyde HSCP Strategic Commissioning Plan (2024–2027). Available at https://www.inverclyde.gov.uk/health-and-social-care

7

COMPASSIONATE COMMUNITIES GROWING IN JAPAN

Matsuzaki and Honaminosato

Hirobumi Takenouchi and Sumiko Kanegae

Abstract

The idea of compassionate cities and communities (abbreviated as CC) was recently introduced in Japan and fully-fledged activities are about to start. Some communities start from scratch, while others develop their practices with this 'new' idea. After sharing the attempt to create a nationwide network for compassionate communities, which overlaps with the short history of Compassionate Communities in Japan, this chapter approaches two cases. The first is a compassionate town, Matsuzaki in Shizuoka Prefecture with a population of 5,000, which officially announced in its comprehensive plan to aim to be the first compassionate city in Japan. The other is Honaminosato in Miyagi Prefecture with a history of 20 years, a compassionate community based on palliative care practices.

7.1 Introduction – Creating a nationwide network for compassionate communities

7.1.1 Outset

In October 2022, the Japanese edition of Allan Kellehear's *Compassionate Cities, Public Health and End-of-Life Care* (2005) was published, supervised by Prof. Hirobumi Takenouchi, Shizuoka University, and Prof. Satoko Hotta, Keio University [1]. In 2023, the Japanese Society for Hospice and Home Care organised a pre-conference and a main conference, thematising CC for the first time in Japan [2]. At the pre-conference in August, Dr. Julian Abel and Dr. Emma Hodges both from Compassionate Communities UK delivered online lectures. At the main conference in October, Kellehear delivered a keynote speech entitled 'Compassionate

DOI: 10.4324/9781003621348-8

Communities & Cities - Why do we need them? What are they? How to start them?' while Hodges led a workshop 'A practical approach to a Compassionate Community.'

Taking advantage of this opportunity, Takenouchi started monthly online meetings called 'CC Renrakukai' (CC liaison meetings) in November 2023. It is composed of three kinds of programmes:

1 Sharing various CC practices,
2 'Compassionate Café,' i.e. dialogical inquiries on themes such as compassion, community, and loss and death, and
3 Reading circle of *Compassionate Cities* and the Compassionate City Charter [1,3].

By March 2025, 15 meetings had been held, with a total of 400 participants (nurses, medical doctors, social workers, bereaved family members, and those concerned for loss and death).

7.2 Association's 'compassion and dialogue'

In January 2025, after a year of preparation, Takenouchi established an unincorporated association 'Compassion and Dialogue' to manage the programmes of 'Compassionate Communities Japan' with 15 other members including Ms. Michiko Uchimiya, Vice Representative Director, Dr. Sumiko Kanegae, coauthor of this chapter, Mr. Junya Fukazawa, mayor of Matsuzaki town, and Ms. Harumi Oishi, general manager of Honaminosato. The main programmes are:

1 A series of lectures on CC,
2 Online open lectures,
3 Dialogical cafes on loss and death in Shizuoka city, and
4 A summer school for dialogue and facilitation in Mishima city, Shizuoka Prefecture.

A series of courses on CC 2025–2026 started online on 4 July 2025 running until March 2026 [4].

1 Introduction (Hirobumi Takenouchi)
2 Sharing the experiences of loss and death and helping each other (Wakako Kaneko)
3 Cultural traditions of mutual support in loss and death (Susumu Shimazono)
4 Inclusive Community and Compassionate Cities and Communities (Satoko Hotta)
5 Palliative Care and Compassionate Cities and Communities (Shimon Tashiro)
6 Public Health and Compassionate Cities and Communities (Kenjiro Kawaguchi)
7 On Compassion (Hirobumi Takenouchi)

8 On Dialogue (Rei Nagai)
9 Compassionate Communities in Japan: Honaminosato and Matsuzaki Town (Harumi Oishi and Junya Fukazawa)
10 Compassionate Communities in Japan: Zensai Temple and CC Youth Group (Shunryo Yada and Asuka Ito)
11 Compassionate Communities in the UK (Emma Hodges)
12 Reflective dialogues with Allan Kellehear (Hirobumi Takenouchi)

Each lecture of 60 minutes is followed by 30 minutes of dialogue with participants. Hodges' lecture will be recorded in advance and watched with Japanese subtitles. Collecting questions from participants, Takenouchi will then have a dialogue with Kellehear, which will be recorded and watched with Japanese subtitles in the final session.

General course fee is 50,000 Japanese Yen (30,000 Yen for students). Calls for applications opened in April, and within a month all 45 places were filled. To meet this great demand, an on-demand course was established in parallel. The online open lecture course includes:

1 In June, two visit reports on the Institute of Palliative Medicine in Kerala, India, and Compassionate Communities in Hong Kong will be presented under the title 'Compassionate Communities in Asian countries'[5].
2 In August, there will be a lecture on Genshin's 985 year of work, Ojo Essential Collections (The Essentials of Rebirth in the Pure Land).
3 In October, there will be a symposium on 'community.'
4 In November, another symposium entitled 'Conceptual history of compassion, tracing back to the traditions of Ancient Greek and Primitive Buddhism' will take place.

In daily life, we relate to others both through verbal and non-verbal communications. Dialogue and compassion are complementary and go hand in hand. Based on this insight, 'Compassion and Dialogue' emphasises 'dialogue' as well as 'compassion.' Dialogical cafe on loss and death called 'Shiseigaku cafe' [6] (cafe for the mortals), launched by Takenouchi in Shizuoka in 2015, and was included as a programme of Compassionate Communities Japan. Every time, around 40 participants get together for dialogical inquiry. The summer school for dialogue and facilitation, launched by Takenouchi in Mishima in 2022, was also incorporated.

7.2.1 Next steps

'Compassion and Dialogue' will shortly make a transition to become a general incorporated association in August 2025. An annual CC Festival Japan will start in 2027, after pre-events are tested at a Buddhist temple in Kuwana City, Mie Prefecture. The leading concept of CC Festival Japan is to learn from each other's experiences and wisdom through dialogues and arts. Participants will share not only practices and ideas of CC but also their own lived experiences and enjoy together a story, tale, illustrated book, poem, music, and drama about loss and death.

A series of courses on CC will be modified. Three courses of Introductory, Practical, and Academic will be delivered in 2026–2027, responding to participants' various learning needs. Practical course graduates are expected to join in the nationwide CC network in Japan.

7.3 Compassionate town Matsuzaki

7.3.1 The town Matsuzaki

Matsuzaki town is in the western part of Izu Peninsula, in the southeast part of the main island. It has notable cultural traditions. In the days when shipping was thriving, this town flourished with its port 'waiting for the wind.' While at anchors, crews, and passengers from various parts of the country stayed and exchanged their diverse cultures. On the streets of the town namako (sea cucumber) walled structures, dating back to the premodern Edo period, are well preserved. It has a rich natural environment, surrounded by mountains and a varied coastline, recognised as a Geopark. The terraced rice fields of Ishibe overlook Mount Fuji and the Southern Alps over Suruga Bay. Salted cherry leaves, which account for 70% of the national market share, are a speciality product of the town.

7.3.2 Background

Since the late 1970s, Matsuzaki has promoted the community-building policies with a series of comprehensive town plans entitled 'creation of hometown with flowers and fascination.' A campaign to fill the town with flowers was run. Seven major festivals started, including 'Nakagawa Sansei festival' for commemorating the three pioneers of the town. Izunochohachi Museum opened as a hall of plaster trowel paintings [7]. Iwashina School, built with donations from residents in 1880, was registered as a national important cultural property. Matsuzaki became known as a tourist destination and welcomed many visitors. In the 1970s and 1980s, the town was full of vitality with economic growth.

However, the population began to decline in 1980, because of an exodus of young people. It decreased from 10,013 in 1980 to 6,250 in 2020. By August 2025, Matsuzaki is now the smallest municipality in Shizuoka Prefecture, with 5,589 inhabitants and 2,822 households. The ageing rate of the population is 50.8%. The number of elderly single-person and elderly-only households is 839 and 563, respectively. The population is projected to decline to 3,820 by 2045.

7.3.3 2030 Matsuzaki project

Against this background, '2030 Matsuzaki project' was launched in 2020 led by Junya Fukazawa, chief of Matsuzaki town hall, and Hirobumi Takenouchi, deputy director of the Organisation for Designing Future Society, Shizuoka University. Aiming for "building a town to live in with children" and "exploring new tourism possibilities", it started with intensive dialogical sessions with junior high and high school students. Including the diverse local populations, 13 goals to be achieved in 2030 were defined. Since then, residents, including junior high and high school students, have been working on a team basis, together with students and teaching staffs from Shizuoka University and other external partners to achieve the goals. In 2024, a team, consisting of university students, high school students, residents, and external cooperators, produced a short film entitled 'Benben,' which thematises spiritual legacy of the pioneer of the town, Benzo Yoda [8]. This film was shown at the 2025 Tokachi Little Film Festival in Obihiro, Hokkaido.

7.3.4 The comprehensive town plan for 2023–2032

In November 2021, Fukazawa was elected mayor of the town and nominated Takenouchi as a town development advisor. In January 2022, they started regular online meetings to develop the 6th comprehensive town plan for 2023–2032. In the two town meetings held in May, participants reflected on the earlier efforts including the town plan of 'creation of hometown with flowers and fascination' and the '2030 Matsuzaki project' and then presented ideas for community development. Making use of the feedback received, the draft was completed in October, after biweekly online meetings over for ten months.

The comprehensive town plan is called 'Compassionate Town Matsuzaki, in this place we can live proudly, peacefully and prosperously.' It is a town where people share difficult challenges and help each other, in cooperation with external partners. A rural municipality like Matsuzaki does not necessarily have to follow the manners of large cities. By cherishing the inherent richness of the land and human interaction, they can proudly, peacefully, and prosperously live in this place. Difficult challenges can be shared and dealt with in union. Let us extract some essence of the town plan.

7.3.4.1 Facing human vulnerability

Due to the spread of COVID-19 from early 2020 to early 2023, a state of emergency was declared, and preventive measures were introduced in Japan. This experience has exposed the fragility of human connection and community function in Japanese society. Prejudice and discrimination against infected individuals were outstanding. Understandings of 'ageing,' 'illness,' 'death,' and 'others' were questioned. People have become so accustomed to take for granted the care and services provided by government and professionals that they have shelved the effort of building a community that recognises and supports each other's vulnerabilities. Let us use these valuable lessons to build a sustainable town that supports each other, with a view to the well-being of each resident and the role of human connections and communities.

7.3.4.2 Dialogue and compassion

To share and realise the vision for the future of Matsuzaki, dialogue is essential. Even 'Matsuzaki town folks' have different family and work situations and environments. They may feel and think differently depending on their residential district, generation, gender, and beliefs. That is why it is important for each person to express his or her wishes and interests in words and to listen to each other through a process of dialogue.

In addition to 'dialogue,' 'compassion' is required to achieve the well-being of all residents so that 'no one is left behind.' Faced with suffering of others, we are moved and involuntarily extend helping hands. Compassion is a word that describes this kind of human response.

Compassion-based community building called 'Compassionate City and Community' has been positioned at the centre of social policies in many countries and regions around the world, including the United Kingdom, Australia, and Taiwan. In cooperation with these, Matsuzaki aims to become Japan's first 'Compassionate Town.' We will create a town where people share the challenges of life and death and help each other.

7.3.4.3 Partnership

How will community development be promoted over the next ten years? Who will be responsible for the town's development? There are many organisations and groups involved in community development in Matsuzaki. It is promoted in various ways, mainly by the residents of the town.

However, the town's residents are not the sole players in town development. For example, community development education programmes have been introduced at Matsuzaki Junior High and Matsuzaki High School, where many students commute to school from outside the town. Some workers commute from neighbouring towns and are involved in community development. Some others stay in Matsuzaki for longer periods of time to work. There are also people who repeatedly visit this town to attend such periodic events as rice planting and harvesting, festivals, and dialogue cafe 'waiting for the wind.' These people are so-called people of the wind attracted to the town. They are distinguished from mere consuming tourists ("exchange population"), though not "permanent residents." The people who are connected to Matsuzaki in various ways ('related population') will play an important role in town development.

With this outlook, we are working together with the '2030 Matsuzaki Project' to promote community development. This project has already brought together many people from inside and outside the town. In connection with this, the 'people of the soil' (residents) and the 'people of the wind' ('related population') will join forces to build a wider platform and a resilient and sustainable style of community development.

7.3.5 Five priority policies

The comprehensive plan has five priority policies as follows.

7.3.5.1 Disaster mitigation

We promote the development of a compassionate disaster-resistant community that incorporates preparedness for natural disasters (earthquakes and tsunamis) into daily life.

7.3.5.2 End-of-life accompanied by community members

The town is faced with a deficiency of healthcare services and resources. Expanding civil network and promoting collaboration between health services and medical and welfare professionals, we will construct the Matsuzaki style of the 'Integrated Community Care System' promoted by the Japanese government.

When someone has a difficulty or faces a challenge, community members can help and support that person, in some cases with new ideas and ingenuity. By sharing the challenges, our bond will be strengthened. By sharing the experiences of loss and death, each of us will learn about how to live our mortal lives.

7.3.5.3 Innovation and industrial promotion

We work for industrial development and sustainable tourism in response to changing social conditions. As part of this policy, we create new styles of succession and support the sustainability and continuity of establishments, as well as new businesses. We also build tourism that responds to new tourist values such as experience, learning, and human interaction.

7.3.5.4 Enjoyment and preservation of heritage in homeland

In appreciation of the bounty of nature and spiritual and cultural traditions, we build a restful town where residents can be proud to live. We inherit and hand over to future generations the beautiful landscape and culture, including plaster culture such as namako walls and trowel paintings of Chohachi, Sanyo Juku, terraced rice field, Mount Fuji over Suruga Bay, and the port of Kazemachi (waiting for wind).

7.3.5.5 Learning from one another and growing together

We restructure both school and social education so that everyone can draw up and realise each dream and continue to learn at any stage of life.

7.3.6 Learning programme for town connectors

In 2024, the town hall started the 'mutual learning programme for town connectors,' aiming at the following objectives.

1. Learn about 'compassion' and share the policies of 'Compassionate Town Matsuzaki' (the 6th comprehensive town plan).
2. Dig up treasures and challenges of the town with its historical backgrounds.
3. Find and train town connectors.
4. Shed light on the diverse activities of residents.
5. Create a major trend to realise the five priority policies by combining these activities.

The programme started in June with the keynote speech of Ms. Harumi Oishi, general manager of Honaminosato. As a leader of a preceding compassionate community, she shared the experiences and the ideas of compassion-based community building. Based on this practical learning, we focused on the idea of 'compassion' in July. In August, Dr. Eiji Matsubara, the former chief of Kitakyushu City Hall and the researcher in local governance, presented case studies of community building in Kitakyushu and other municipalities.

In September, three local speakers were invited as storytellers of Matsuzaki. The first speaker was a 92-year-old passionate leader of 'Kurara,' a workers' collective of the elderly. The second is chief priest of Shinto shrine 'Inashimo Jinja' located in town centre. The third contributed to the production of the previous comprehensive town plan's 'creation of hometown with flowers and fascination' as a former chief of Matsuzaki town hall. After learning about the lived history of Matsuzaki from different perspectives in this way, participants approached the basic ideas of current comprehensive town plan in October.

In November, participants were divided into five teams corresponding to the priority policies, according to their interests and activities. Each team then created and presented a map of the town's treasures and challenges from the perspectives of team members. In December, each team developed and presented an activity plan. In March 2025, after a group trial run of three months, achievements and challenges of the group activities were debriefed.

As the second step, 'mutual learning programme for town connectors 2025' started in May and runs until March 2026. In May, it started up with mayor's introduction, reflection on progress in the year 2024, and team meeting for planning the activities in 2025. A workshop entitled 'Practicing compassion in Matsuzaki' was held in July 2025. In September, five teams presented their interim activity report. Resident groups that had not yet joined up were also invited to present their activities. In October, a symposium was held with the title 'Compassionate town Matsuzaki, town of well-being walking together.' As a guest speaker, Shunryo Yada, practicing CC activities based in a Buddhist temple, was invited. In a workshop in December, participants will consider the treasures in Matsuzaki from the renewed perspectives. In March 2026, achievements and challenges of the group activities will be debriefed.

7.3.7 Other activities

Alongside the learning programme for town connectors, Fukazawa and Takenouchi organised the first council of religious leaders in Matsuzaki, inviting Shinto priest, Buddhist monk, and Church pastor. Participants exchanged their perspectives on the idea of 'compassion' and spiritual traditions of the town.

Attracted by the term 'Kazemachi' (waiting for wind), Takenouchi started dialogical cafe called 'Kazemachi cafe' in 2022. There are times in life, as well as sailing, when we must wait for the wind. In May and November every year, people waiting for wind in their lives come together from various parts of the country. The cafe is getting known to the local population and is expected to become a place for human interaction between the people of the wind and those of the soil.

7.3.8 Outcome

Every time around 50 people have attended the 'mutual learning programme for town connectors'. In the beginning, an odd feeling was expressed about the use of the English word 'compassion.' However, understanding the meaning of the term and learning other CC practices helped to resolve the discomfort. One participant stated, 'Like other words of foreign origin, in ten years, we will accept the word naturally.' Even in this short period of time, participants became more familiar with it.

Matsuzaki town consists of four districts. By engaging in mutual learning programmes and team activities across district boundaries, new relationships and trust are being forged. Several ideas were put forward, such as creating a third place for young people and community space where residents get information and interact with each other. Group members of 'enjoyment and preservation of heritage in homeland,' involved in maintaining historic and ancient roads, expressed a vision to establish a new town corporation in collaboration with tourist association.

Awareness of the 6th comprehensive town plan has been raised by the town newsletter, the website, social networking, by word of mouth, newspaper, and magazine coverage. Fukazawa is often asked about the town initiatives on various occasions, including at National Association of Chairpersons of Town and Village Assemblies. Many people contact Takenouchi with a vivid interest in Compassionate Town. An increasing number of people are keen to visit the Compassionate Town Matsuzaki. Banks, securities firms, and other companies are also beginning to participate in the town development. The unique challenges of Matsuzaki are becoming nationally recognised.

7.3.9 Reflections

Two years have passed since the introduction of the comprehensive town plan. In the year before that (2023), the first compassionate town meeting was organised, inviting a well-known home care physician who resonates with the idea of CC. In October 2023, Dr. Emma Hodges visited Matsuzaki after the conference of the Japanese Society for Hospice and Home Care in Sendai. She led a workshop with an introductory lecture 'Compassion-based community building' in the morning and delivered another lecture in the evening. Participants were delighted and encouraged to be able to learn from each other across borders and language barriers. In addition to the existing official website, a dedicated website for Compassionate Town Matsuzaki was created [9].

Prepared in this way, the 'mutual learning programme for town connectors' was launched in 2024. So far, the mutual learning programme is going well. The number of participants has been consistently secured, and the willingness and growth of the participants are also clear. Interest and understanding of residents in the comprehensive plan are steadily increasing. The fact that Takenouchi published the Japanese edition of Allan Kelleher's *Compassionate Cities* and represents the organisation 'Compassion and Dialogue' contributes to the great response outside of town. Above all, the success of the activity relies on Fukazawa's consistent leadership. He started the attempt with a determination to achieve the Compassionate Town Matsuzaki over the next ten years. One could say that the division of roles between the mayor and the community development advisor is working well.

7.3.10 Challenges

The number of participants, around 50 for each session, is not small. However, the population of Matsuzaki town is 5,589. Only a small percentage of residents participate in mutual learning courses. The number of residents participating in community development activities is also limited. To share the goals and the ideas in the entire town, more measures need to be taken.

Town newsletters are distributed to all households but are not well read. It is also difficult to share information online because it is not easy for the elderly to master the internet tools. New ideas are needed to develop to share information with all the residents. It is also challenging how to find more town connectors and expand platform functions. That is why it is planned to invite resident groups that have not yet participated to mutual learning programmes, by providing opportunities for presenting their activities. It is also important in this context to create a free-accessed community space where residents get information and interact with each other.

When visiting Brereton and Ravenhill, a compassionate community in the UK in 2024, the author learned the importance of such a common space. It has a community hub where anyone can visit and spend time in one's own way. According to their age and interests, residents enjoy themselves attending their clubs and they also see and talk with not only their club members but also other residents joining in other club activities. In this way, they come to know what activities are taking place. A sense of community is fostered beyond the club boundaries. There is a place where one can go to see one's friends. That seems to be the key to the development of compassionate communities. In a safe place where they can talk about anything, compassionate relationships grow. A platform for coping jointly with the challenges of loss and death will be built in this way.

As mentioned earlier, people tend to rely on the services provided by government and professionals. This hinders the development of compassionate communities. In the case of Matsuzaki, there is a high reliance on public services due to limited market services. Town hall employees are busy with too many jobs and are exhausted. Many have retired. A shift is inevitable from a service delivery to community development model. It is essential for Matsuzaki people to clarify the division of roles between town hall staff and residents and to work altogether for the development of the town. This awareness will lead to building a wider network of mutual help and support. A giant step forward towards a Compassion Town will be when they recognise themselves and all other inhabitants in Matsuzaki as mortal, vulnerable, and in need of mutual help.

7.3.11 Next steps

Discussions have started to create a third place for young people and community space for all the residents. The vision to establish a new town corporation will be elaborated. The council of religious leaders, started in 2024, will be developed. If residents work together across religious barriers, making the most of their differences, the spiritual traditions of the town will be inherited, and 'compassion' will be revived. A Buddhist monk Yada's visit and lecture will be a perfect opportunity for this. A partnership between Matsuzaki and Brereton in the UK will be strengthened and some exchange programmes will be launched.

7.4 A local palliative care hub, Honaminosato

The ground-breaking CC activities have been organised by a local community palliative care support centre which involves patients, bereaved families, friends, and neighbours and encourages social sectors to take part. They include person-tailored volunteer care, drama play, and intergenerational transmission of local traditions with an initial aim of building relationships for people at the end of their life. The support centre has been developing a compassionate community, fostering reciprocal support and autonomy for all people in the community for 20 years.

7.4.1 Compassionate community, Honaminosato

Compassionate community at Honaminosato (abbreviated as CC Honaminosato) is active in Osaki City, Miyagi Prefecture, in the north-east region of Japan. The population of the city is 120,053, with the ageing population ratio of 32.1%. Osaki Kodo (cultivated soil) is recognised as Globally Important Agricultural Heritage System for its rich traditional food culture. Osaki City is one of the areas severely affected by the Great East Japan Earthquake in 2011.

CC Honaminosato was started by staff members, patients, and their families of a home care clinic, Honaminosato Clinic [10]. It has then developed in cooperation with a local community palliative care support centre, 'Haruka,' which fosters community palliative care, involving bereaved families and residents as volunteers or neighbourhood supporters, and builds partnership with local communities and healthcare professionals.

7.4.2 Background

Honaminosato Clinic was launched by a physician, Dr. Masaetsu Miura, and a social worker, Ms. Harumi Oishi, in 2005, aiming to provide home visiting medical care to residents. Working for a public acute hospital in Osaki City before, they found that most citizens wanted to continue their lives at home, instead of hospitalisation. Clinic staff members carefully listened to their patients at the end-of-life stage and established a philosophy of CC Honaminosato as below.

1 Persistently support home care and connect people.
2 Foster bonds of empathy by sharing the process of palliative care with all concerned.
3 Value relations and spiritual home of life.
4 Respect all circumstances around the life, and the heart of homeland where life has been fostered.
5 Contribute to the local society through community care and creation of caring culture.

7.4.3 Main activities

CC Honaminosato provides a variety of activities, including members of volunteer clubs for those who are suffering such as the dying people and bereaved families, those with high care needs or isolated, and young families in need of childcare support. Activities are organised by two total healthcare planners at a palliative care support centre, Haruka. Catching voices of hopes and dreams from patients, caregivers, volunteers, healthcare professionals, and neighbours, they plan palliative care projects to meet individual needs. Members of the local community and healthcare professionals equally share important roles. There are three significant activities as follows.

7.4.3.1 A volunteer club, 'warm hearted home visiting club'

Most of the volunteers are senior former family carers. They take care of the multiple needs, hopes, and dreams of suffering people. They are also involved in educational programmes of community palliative care and end-of-life care for residents, school students, and caring professionals.

7.4.3.2 Kitchen lab

To empower all people involved, they provide lunches for participants of the palliative day care, staff, and volunteers, even for people in need of care at home. Meals are prepared under the direction of Mayumi Kakuta, a hairdresser, considering individual physical condition and seasonality and regionality of food.

7.4.3.3 Honami community theatre

Dramas are played at patients' homes and schools, as well as in Happy Farm, a small farm beside the palliative care support centre, where senior volunteers built Red Ogre House based on a popular Japanese fairy tale. To raise awareness for compassionate communities and community palliative care, fairy tales and stories related to life and death and fellow supports are played.

7.4.4 Outcomes

CC Honaminosato has actively collaborated with multi-generations, providing person-tailored reciprocal supports with mutual understanding, warm-hearted communication, and rich food culture. Here are some stories that show how the CC activities affected individual life stories in multi-generation.

7.4.4.1 Mutual understanding and person-tailored reciprocal supports

Two stories show how residents experience reciprocal support. Mr. and Mrs. T were engaged in their mother's end-of-life care at home, with the support of the Honaminosato Clinic home care team and volunteers of the CC several years ago. One day, Mr. T asked total health planners about home care for Mrs. T. Because of a brain tumour, she was staying at the nursing home, with high care needs and depression at that time.

Mrs. T wished to be back home. With her autonomy respected, she returned home. Empowered by the care team, he developed care skills for his wife. He then became involved in the CC through the opportunities of care, death, and bereavement of his wife. The CC members, including Warm Hearted Home Visiting Club's members and participants in the Life Improvement Club, helped with the harvest at Mr. T's farm, sharing the sufferings of Mr. and Mrs. T.

An end-of-life home care patient, 60-year-old Ms. Y, participated in palliative day care. However, she became unable to join it any longer. She told total health planners in December that she wanted to eat a slice of watermelon. Palliative care team discussed her wish with CC volunteer members. Mr. T willingly offered Ms. Y watermelons growing in his greenhouse. Two participants in palliative day care, both friends of Ms. Y, visited her with the watermelon supplied by Mr. T. They sang songs for her too. Ms. Y passed away peacefully in a few days.

7.4.4.2 Learning compassion through multi-generational exchange with traditional culture and agriculture

Based on the continuous relationship built, Mr. T presented pears to CC members when students from Shizuoka University started fieldwork in the summer. It was just before a typhoon. Total health planners suggested CC volunteers harvest potatoes in his field, to express appreciation for his kindness. A potato harvest team was organised, for community action, by the university students and senior volunteers. The senior volunteers showed university students how to dig potatoes with warm-hearted communication. The students learned reciprocity and togetherness by farming together in the potato field. They cooked lunch with the potatoes offered by Mr. T. and supplied to other CC members and some terminally ill patients at the Kitchen Lab. This story shows an example of multi-generational exchange in the CC.

7.4.4.3 Sharing the process of public health palliative care

Potato harvest for Mr. T enabled senior volunteer members and the university students to build a good partnership. They then participated in a Life Improvement Club together. Senior volunteers explained to the students how to play a card game regarding life, dying, death, loss, and care. They had meaningful dialogues during the card game, finding different recognitions about death and life between the generations. Senior members talked about their values about life, death, and loss to younger generations and found the recognition of uncertainties and anxieties surrounding life and death among younger generations. Such opportunities for multi-generational partnership building are essential, with a view to the sustainability of the CC. The total health planners and the students published Honaminosato daily newspaper in cooperation, not only reporting every activity but also the learning process on public health palliative care.

7.4.5 Reflections

7.4.5.1 The key factors

There are important factors that have contributed to the development of CC Honaminosato. First, the philosophy and activities are based on individual life stories, hopes, and the experience of natural disasters in the community. Second, most people involved respect their traditional culture, food, and agricultural practices, which play important roles in connecting people and providing reciprocal support in the community. Third, accessibility and openness of the CC as in the newspapers, their local cable TV station, outreach educational projects, and networks with other communities.

7.4.5.2 *The lessons learned*

1 Community palliative care projects based on individuals' 'dreams' and 'hopes' empower people and build community capacities and resilience around end-of-life.
2 This CC provides all people with multi-generational educational opportunities as in Life Improvement Club and Honami Community Theatre.
3 Within the CC, 'compassion' circulates, naturally practised every day and everywhere.

7.4.5.3 *A kaleidoscope of mutual caring*

The words express the characteristic of CC Honaminosato. In the case of Mr. T, he has not only received a lot of support from the CC, but he was also involved in the circle of supporting Ms. Y. This reminds us of the changeable patterns of a kaleidoscope. Compassion in action mirrors the beautiful image created by a kaleidoscope.

7.4.6 Next steps to extend CC to the whole city

CC Honaminosato has already built a good working partnership with the local government regarding health, educational programmes, and local tourism. As the next step, they are now working to extend CC to the whole city so that no one will be left behind. Their motto is 'You, I, and we all work together in Osaki City for human interaction, mutual respect, and reciprocal support.' The ongoing plans below will achieve respecting gratitude, enthusiasm, and deep emotions.

7.4.6.1 *School of life*

CC Honaminosato is planning to organise training camps, designed to nurture future community leaders, where teachers and students learn about life together.

7.4.6.2 *Compassionate communities nurses*

It has worked to develop a unique and original compassionate communities nurse training programme. Nurses from all over Japan join in the programme to empower all residents in their communities, with the values of respect, reciprocity, and human resource development. In the educational programme, they work together with volunteer members of 'Warm Hearted Home Visiting Club.'

7.4.6.3 *Caring for those who care*

CC Honaminosato takes care of those who care. An exhibition of photographs will be held to share some cases where people care for people.

References

1. A. Kellehear, *Compassionate Cities, Public Health and End of Life Care*, Keio University Press, 2022 ed., Oxfordshire: Routledge, 2005.
2. Japanese Society for Hospice and Home Care, "The 30th Japan Hospice and Home Care Study Group National Conference in Sendai," October 2023. [Online]. Available: https://jshh.jimdosite.com/. [Accessed 17 September 2025].
3. A. Kellehear, "Compassionate City Charter," 2020. [Online]. Available: https://compassionate-communitiesuk.com/the-compassionate-city-charter-3/. [Accessed 18 August 2025].
4. Compassionate Communities Japan, "Compassion and Dialogue," [Online]. Available: https://cc-jp.net/. [Accessed 17 September 2025].
5. The Hong Kong Council of Social Service, "The Hong Kong Council of Social Service," [Online]. Available: https://www.hkcss.org.hk/?lang=en. [Accessed 17 September 2025].
6. Shizuoka University, "Dialogue Cafe for the Mortals," [Online]. Available: https://wwp.shizuoka.ac.jp/shiseigakucafe/. [Accessed 17 September 2025].
7. Matsuzakicho public corporation, "Izunochohachi Museum," [Online]. Available: https://www.izu-matsuzaki.com/en/pages/69. [Accessed 17 September 2025].
8. Benben. [Film]. 2024. Available: https://www.youtube.com/watch?v=klGRlz_wYHQ. [Accessed 27 January 2026].
9. Compassionate Town Matsuzaki, "Compassion Town Matsuzaki," 2024. [Online]. Available: https://matsuzaki-compassion.jp/. [Accessed 17 September 2025].
10. Honaminosato Clinic, "Honaminosato Clinic," [Online]. Available: https://honamino-sato.studio.site/. [Accessed 17 September 2025].

8

FROM GRIEF TO BELONGING

The evaluation of a compassionate community movement

Mary Ann Boe

Abstract

This chapter traces the evolution, fracture, and renewal of a grassroots movement to build a compassionate community around grief, dying, and collective care. Sparked by the story of Déva Ram Dass Pollard, the initiative in Kato Towns (Mankato and North Mankato, Minnesota) led to the development of a Compassionate Charter, the training of end-of-life doulas, and the launch of NicBluCares, a compassionate community model rooted in belonging and public health.

As the movement grew, structural tensions emerged. The creation of the Compassionate Community Centre marked a milestone but revealed divergent visions. The doulas' departure raised questions about leadership, sustainability, and the balance between professional focus and community inclusion. Yet, this fracture became a clarifying moment, prompting reflection on shared purpose and relational infrastructure.

Guided by Ubuntu, this chapter demonstrates the adaptability and resilience of a community vision rooted in belonging and collective care. A community festival, co-created by diverse partners and inspired by global leaders, reignited the movement with new energy and expanded reach. Ultimately, this chapter affirms that movements evolve, and when grounded in compassion, they can adapt, deepen, and continue, making space for parallel paths that remain united in purpose.

DOI: 10.4324/9781003621348-9

8.1 Introduction – The hero within: grief and the path to meaning

8.1.1 How loss calls us to show up, for ourselves and each other

> Déva Ram Dass Pollard (figure 8.1) came to teach, and his lessons were many. Life is pain and great suffering. Life is joy. Life is also marbles in a dump truck, King Castle stories, a Lois Lane sister needing to be rescued, and hospital slumber parties. Who is Déva? A shining one whose light is ever guiding, ever brilliant. A child, like so many, who comes bearing special gifts that sometimes take all our strength to hold and all our lives to open. And the treasure inside? Perhaps a true healing, a greater understanding of life's meaning, or the longed-for embrace of a natural great peace.
>
> Excerpt from Déva's Story by Mary Ann Boe [1]

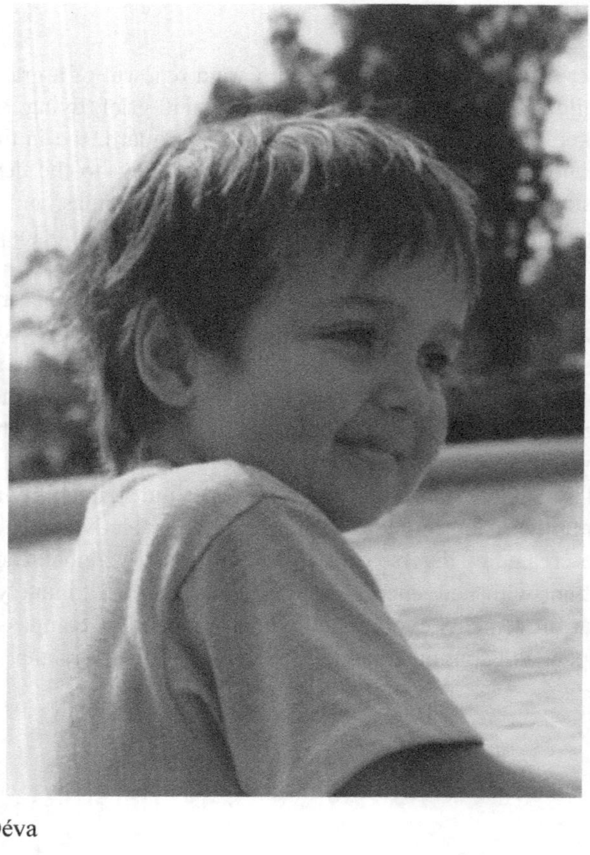

FIGURE 8.1 Déva

Source: Déva 1972–1986

The "why" of an initiative often begins with one person's quest to make sense of suffering. Déva spent his life surrounded by medical care with professionals who cared deeply. Yet, in his final eight months of hospitalization, the health system failed him. Death was never named, only the next surgery. His emotional needs were silenced by the frantic effort to keep his body alive. He died in intensive care, with everyone still fighting for his life.

After caring for her medically fragile son for 14 years and facing his difficult death, Mary Ann was driven to find meaning in the experience. She longed to make the journey through serious illness and dying less isolating, to support those facing fear, and to foster education and conversation that might bring peace at life's end.

Her personal journey, gifted by her son, became the spark that united the "whys" of an entire community. As others shared their stories and struggles, individual pain was woven into a collective purpose, reflecting the needs and experiences of many, not just her own.

8.2 Enter the compassionate community movement

8.2.1 Building a civic and public health framework for compassionate end-of-life care

In 2017, Mary Ann attended the Public Health Palliative Care International conference in Ottawa, Canada, where she met Dr. Julian Abel and Professor Allan Kellehear. It was the early days in the formation of compassionate cities. Over a meal, Allan sketched a simple formula for launching a public health social movement around loss, death, dying, and grief: engage three community sectors, incorporate academic research, and involve government to "give out the bobbles." These steps

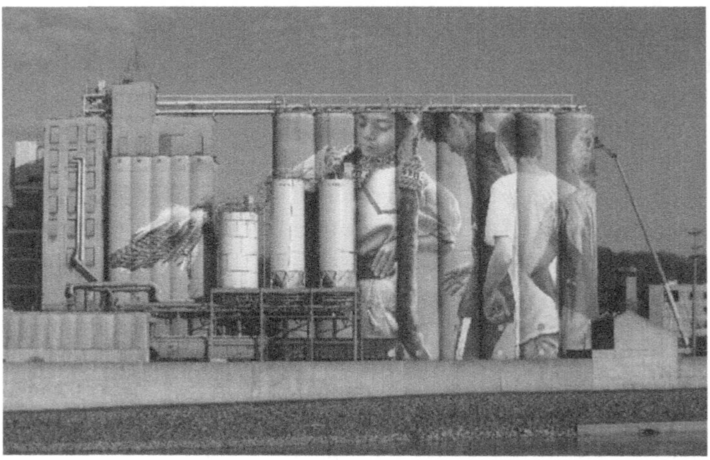

FIGURE 8.2 Silo Art

Source: Photo Courtesy of Twin Rivers Council for the Arts. Silo art by Guido van Helten

would form the foundation of a compassionate city charter, the cornerstone of a compassionate community. Later that year, Professor Kellehear presented at a town hall forum in Mankato, Minnesota (figure 8.2), where Déva had lived much of his life.

Mankato rests on the sacred and traditional lands of the Dakota people. During the Dakota-United States War of 1862, it was the site of the largest mass execution in US history, where 38 Dakota men were hanged. Today, a vibrant movement focused on remembrance and reconciliation is underway, providing even greater motivation to foster a compassionate city here. Dakota elder Glen Wasicuna met with Mary Ann several times. Among the teachings he shared, one stood out to her as especially significant: "Mary Ann, you don't have to bring compassion here, the land remembers." Then she shared her vision of community circles, spaces where people could offer their stories, be received without judgement, advice, or fixing, and together draw from the community's lived wisdom. Glen paused for a long, thoughtful moment and then looked up and said, "We've been waiting."

The town forum, led by Kellehear, launched a vital public dialogue and community-building process centred on collective responsibility. It marked a turning point, an invitation to mobilise a public health movement where everyone has a role. This gathering also sparked the creation of Deva Nation, with its mission: to foster belonging and compassionate communities.

8.3 Gathering the voice and wisdom of community: a call to connection

8.3.1 The invitation to speak: what emerges when we're asked

Funded by a community foundation, the project began with a needs assessment and interviews with individuals experienced in aging, loss, caregiving, dying, and bereavement. These conversations revealed a striking truth: while many suffer alone, others are ready to help but often feel they need permission. Some hesitate to ask, not wanting to be a burden; others are unsure how to help or feel uncomfortable. What we don't understand, we tend to fear.

This fear reflects a broader cultural disconnect from death and dying, leaving people unprepared, isolated in grief, and uncertain how to support one another. As death became medicalised and grief professionalised, what were once communal experiences shifted behind closed doors. Communities lost touch with their shared capacity to help and to hold sorrow together. In this landscape, many feel uncertain about their role, unsure whether they're allowed to show up, speak up, or lend a hand.

Yet, the interviews also revealed a way forward. The stories affirmed that healing comes not from avoiding death, but from acknowledging it as part of life. In response, the community began reclaiming its ability to face loss together, with compassion, open dialogue, and shared practices. When people are invited to speak openly, to grieve visibly, and support one another without hesitation, isolation gives way to belonging. Fear is voiced, honoured, and met with understanding. In this way, the social fabric is rewoven around death, not as an end, but as a moment that deepens connection, responsibility, and shared humanity.

8.4 The work of compassion

8.4.1 A community journey from sacred circle to citywide commitment

In 2018, a small group formed *Sacred Circle Wisdom around Death*, monthly peer support gatherings for end-of-life doulas, death educators, hospice volunteers, and community members. By 2025, the network had grown to over 70 members, meeting regularly to share insights, deepen learning, and foster compassionate connection.

In 2019, Deva Nation supported the training of 29 end-of-life doulas, including 11 from Mankato. These doulas began building grief and death literacy through Death Cafés and educational events. That same year, with support from nursing faculty at Minnesota State University, Mankato (MNSU), the organisation initiated the Compassionate Charter for Mankato and North Mankato (Kato Towns). Using an evidence-based process, initial focus groups brought together leaders from 15 sectors. Breakout sessions followed, with each organisation. Facilitated conversations began by exploring the meaning of belonging, then moved into discussions about loss, what was helpful, what could have helped, and concluded by inviting participants to identify practices their organisations could adopt to better prepare for loss, grief, and death. These best practices were to be woven into the Kato Towns Compassionate Charter, alongside a shared commitment to ongoing compassion-building and annual review.

8.5 A compassionate community model

8.5.1 Building belonging and collective care in the Kato Towns

In 2020, Deva Nation launched *NicBluCares*, a compassionate community model serving Nicollet and Blue Earth Counties. Its mission: to build a safety net of support and strengthen the community's capacity to care during times of crisis and loss. Mary Ann served as director, supported by a dedicated Advisory Team.

One of the model's first initiatives was *NicBluCaresNow.com*, a local directory now featuring over 2,300 programmes for connection, care, social services, and resources related to dying, death, and bereavement. Developed by the community and funded by the Cities of Mankato and North Mankato, the directory reflects a core value: belonging as a key determinant of health. Its first taxonomy column highlights nontraditional social determinants, spaces where people find meaning, connection, and mutual support. This BELONGING category includes the Arts, Nature, Recreation, Neighbourhood Programmes, Social Justice, and communities representing Disability, BIPOC, LGBTQ+, Refugee and Immigrant, and Spiritual Life. The goal is for NicBluCaresNow.com to become the go-to place for discovering and engaging with the treasures of local resources that foster social connection, health, and well-being.

In 2021, the nine sectors involved in the research study on conversations around belonging and loss formalised their unique best practices, initiating the Kato Towns

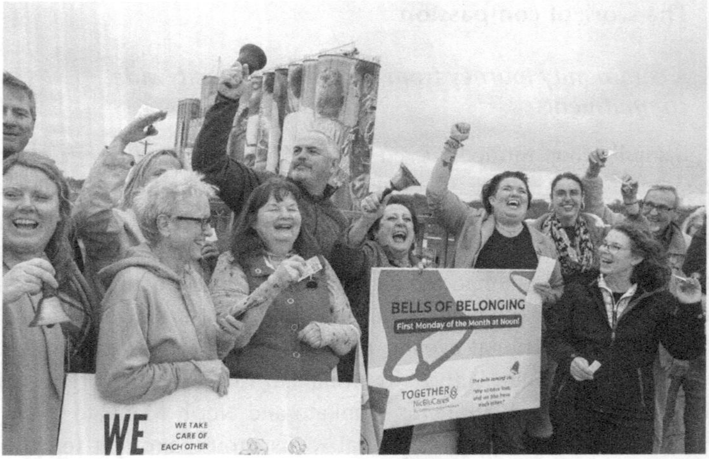
BELLS OF BELONGING
First Monday of the Month at Noon!
TOGETHER
WE
WE TAKE CARE OF EACH OTHER

FIGURE 8.3 Bells of Belonging

Source: Cities Mark Anniversary of Compassionate Charter. Photo by Casey Ek, The Mankato Free Press

Compassionate Charter. That November, on World Compassionate Communities Day, Public Health Palliative Care International recognised the Kato Towns as the first public health compassionate city in the United States.

One adopted practice crossing all sectors was the *Bells of Belonging*, a monthly ritual reminding residents they are not alone (figure 8.3). On the first Monday of each month at noon, bells ring citywide for one minute. During this shared pause, community members are invited to reflect on how they might offer a kind word, a listening heart, or a helping hand to someone in need. This ritual culminates annually on the first Monday of November, when the Mayors of Mankato and North Mankato meet at the centre of the bridge connecting their cities. Together with residents, they ring the bells to honour the Charter and the community's ongoing commitment to care.

That same year, the community launched *Elevate Compassion Kitchen Table Chats*, monthly global virtual gatherings for sharing stories, insights, and updates from compassion-centred work. These informal conversations offer space for reflection, inspiration, and solidarity. Also in 2021, the community created the Phone of the Wind, a contemplative installation at the Gustavus Arboretum. Developed with local artists, the Sacred Circle, and Gustavus Adolphus College, the quiet phone booth invites visitors to "call" a loved one who has died or is missing, a tender space for remembrance and healing.

With guidance from Compassionate Communities UK, additional initiatives deepened engagement and care: Talking Cafés, Community Connector Trainings, Connection Events, Conversation Circles, and Death and Grief Literacy presentations, all designed to strengthen relationships, build understanding, and foster a culture of compassion.

8.6 The Compassionate Community Centre

8.6.1 *Holding space for grief, growth, and the tensions of collective care*

For years, end-of-life doulas in the Kato Towns envisioned a welcoming drop-in centre where community members could gather, reflect, and connect. Designed for comfort and care, the space would include a resource library, informal seating, and grief and death literacy materials. Plans featured a quiet room for personal reflection, supportive practices like massage and reiki, private meeting space for doulas, and a multi-purpose hall for education, celebrations, trainings, and support groups such as Caring Circles and Sacred Circle Wisdom gatherings. A small kitchen would support retreats and workshops, while natural light and outdoor access would foster calm and connection. Administrative offices for the doula collaborative and NicBluCares would anchor the centre's mission to cultivate a compassionate ecosystem of care. Remarkably, on March 15th, the same day Mayo Health System closed its hospices, the vision became reality through the support of the Mankato Area Foundation and its Family Funds.

The Centre drew strong donor support with a clear mission: to provide nonmedical, community-driven holistic care for those navigating loss, grief, and the end-of-life. Beyond its services, it became a "Community Living Room," a space where gatherings and resources helped normalise conversations around death and bereavement. The timing felt right. The pandemic had softened cultural denial around death, and the doulas were ready to deepen their work. After eight years of steady growth, the movement reached a pivotal moment: not only was it time to move into the long-envisioned physical space but also to evolve structurally, from fiscal sponsorship with an Advisory Team to independent nonprofit status as a 501(c)(3) with a board of directors.

In its first month, donations continued as the centre transformed into the imagined setting. By the second month, doulas were hosting circles for widows and widowers, co-facilitating gatherings for women recovering from breast cancer, and parents of bereaved children. The large hall, formerly a church, was initiated with grief yoga and a workshop on herbs and oils, natural tools to support the grief journey.

Yet, beneath the celebration, tensions emerged. Some questioned the name "Compassionate Community Centre" and raised concerns about hosting gatherings not directly tied to death and dying. The doula team did not see the relevance of a circle for women in transition or a retreat for Spanish-speaking community members. A few leaders, new to the public health compassionate community movement, argued that expanding beyond grief and death would dilute the mission and confuse donors. They preferred to focus solely on the work of the newly formed *End-of-Life Doula Collaborative – Southern Minnesota.*

While the Centre moved forward as the movement's hub, the NicBluCares website was redesigned to reflect the new identity. Several members of the former Advisory Team remained engaged, recognizing that the compassionate community model extends far beyond service delivery. At its heart, it fosters belonging, builds trust, and nurtures shared responsibility across diverse sectors. These leaders understood that relationships, values, and community practices were the true infrastructure of the movement.

8.7 Decoupling purpose from infrastructure

8.7.1 A compassionate community movement at a crossroads

Now comes the pressing question: how do we continue cultivating a truly inclusive compassionate community initiative when a key branch, the end-of-life doulas, has stepped away, without fully embracing the relational and equity-rooted foundations of community development?

As momentum grew around the new Centre, with increased interest from funders and the formation of a formal board, the initiative entered a new chapter. For the first time, it had paid staff beyond the founder, who had often worked without compensation. The introduction of formal roles and financial support marked a significant shift in structure and visibility.

Before the pandemic, the Kato Towns Compassionate Community focused on fostering belonging, acknowledging loss, and building resiliency, an intentional approach to gently engage with the deep cultural fear of death. In the pandemic's wake, public openness to end-of-life conversations increased, and stigma softened. This cultural shift gave the movement new energy and urgency.

Seizing the moment, the community placed the end-of-life doula collaborative at the centre of its efforts, anchoring their work within the newly established Centre. Their presence brought professional legitimacy and offered a tangible expression of a public health-oriented compassionate movement. While the doulas became the visible hub, the broader work of cultivating belonging and trust, especially across diverse sectors, continued to expand outwards, forming the outer rim of the wheel that held the movement together.

As the vision of anchoring the movement in a physical Centre took shape, a quiet but significant shift unfolded: the doulas formally stepped away, choosing to pursue their work independently. The decoupling was real. It happened. After an outside consultant began supporting the doula collaborative's efforts towards independent sustainability, Mary Ann, still serving as director, was asked to return her keys and collect her belongings, which had already been boxed up.

8.8 When movements fracture

8.8.1 Lessons in leadership, clarity, and the limits of capacity

The decoupling of end-of-life doulas from the compassionate community movement reflects deeper structural tensions. Perhaps the vision was too expansive for those working in smaller, incremental ways. Or perhaps the movement lacked sufficient investment in community leadership, monthly Advisory Team meetings offered connection but not always enough voice or ownership.

Several factors contributed to this divergence:

- Limited organisational capacity. Without sustained funding, storytelling was intermittent, and consistent public engagement proved difficult. There was no communications staff, no outreach budget, and few pathways to elevate the work. As a result, transformative contributions remained largely unseen. Without visibility, signature efforts like the Bells of Belonging, Community Resource Directory, Circles of Care, and Talk Listen Connect Series risked being overlooked, not for lack of meaning, but for lack of amplification.
- Disrupted momentum during the pandemic. Sixty planned in-person focus groups in March 2020 became just 15 virtual ones. The Compassionate Charter remains a landmark achievement, evidence-based, presented at major conferences, and celebrated by civic leaders. Yet, individual sector follow-through proved inconsistent, and the initial energy gradually waned.
- Missed opportunities for shared leadership. Charter sector leaders were not invited into the Advisory Board. Greater ownership might have deepened practices, strengthened accountability, and fostered shared stewardship.
- Lack of policy integration. As Allan Kellehear reminds us, conversations are essential, but sustainability comes when dialogue moves to policy. The Charter needed ongoing care, renewal, and reflection to remain transformative.
- Strain on leadership presence. Without full-time staff or empowered volunteers, the founder carried much from afar. Living 200 miles away, she could only be present eight to ten days a month. Remote leadership has limits. Movements need proximity, presence, and shared stewardship to thrive.

Doulas' departure may feel like a rupture, but it also marks a clarifying moment. Rather than a loss, it's an inflection point: a chance to return to the movement's foundational purpose and recommit to the values that make community care transformative. Movements evolve. Sometimes, evolution requires divergence, not to fracture, but to allow new forms of care, leadership, and belonging to emerge. This decoupling may ultimately strengthen the ecosystem of care, making space for parallel paths rooted in shared values, even as they take on distinct roles.

8.9 Take the win

8.9.1 Lessons in compassion, loss, and the long arc of change

Bill Manahan, a pioneering physician and visionary elder, has spent a lifetime bridging holistic medicine, community healing, and compassionate end-of-life care. As a mentor to the compassionate community movement in his hometown of Mankato, he offered this grounding reminder: "You know, change takes about fifty years. Don't be concerned about success. Just enjoy the ride and the beautiful people you meet along the way."

In the wake of great loss, meaning can still emerge through what didn't work, through passion, energy, and commitment that may not yield the hoped-for outcome. Even when efforts fall short, there is always a win if you look for it. Take the win. And keep going.

8.10 The cliffhanger: where compassion meets possibility

8.10.1 From fracture to festival, renewing the compassionate community movement through Ubuntu's call to belonging

During the creation of the Compassionate Community Centre, and the subsequent fracture of the movement, several original members of NicBluCares continued working on community development. Over time, it became clear that engagement with the region's diverse communities remained limited. Through her work with the Charter for Compassion, Mary Ann discovered the Spirit of Ubuntu Movement, and an opportunity to centre a community festival around shared humanity and collective care.

Leaders from diverse sectors co-created a free, public festival to celebrate local compassion and strengthen collaboration. Sponsored by MNSU, Mankato and the Glen Taylor Nursing Institute for Family and Society, the festival aimed to foster belonging and trust. Planning involved a wide range of voices, including South Central College (SCC), the Living Earth Centre, MNSU's American Indian Affairs, MNSU's Centre for Global Engagement, Greater Mankato YWCA, Greater Mankato Diversity Council, Mankato Area Public Schools, the Cities of North Mankato and Mankato, and the Mankato Día de los Muertos Collaborative. Twenty Ubuntu Festival Planning Team members met regularly from November 2024 to the three-day festival held October 9–11, 2025.

Grammy-nominated musician Pato Banton and world-renowned reggae keyboardist Antoinette Rootsdawtah brought their uplifting messages to help launch the Ubuntu Movement in Greater Mankato (figure 8.4). Another featured performance was a drumming and traditional dance engagement led by Indigenous community leader Leo Gunner Baker, who performed alongside his son Leo as a powerful drumming and singing team, and his daughter Lakota, who brought intergenerational storytelling to life through Dakota acting, dance, and cultural expression.

At the heart of the festival was *The Spirit of Ubuntu*, a documentary by Pato and Antoinette that has received 26 international awards. The film highlights transformative leadership across ten African nations through love, service, and collective care. Their journey has taken them to Amsterdam, Mexico, Canada, and across Africa, and now, for the first time, they hosted their work in the United States. The October 2025 event at MNSU marked the inaugural Spirit of Ubuntu Festival in America.

The Ubuntu Collaborative, through the Greater Mankato Diversity Council at MankatoDiversity.org, will continue nurturing the spirit of belonging and growing the Ubuntu Movement in Kato Towns, welcoming more organisations and sectors through ongoing partnerships with MNSU, SCC, local schools, businesses, faith communities, and neighbours.

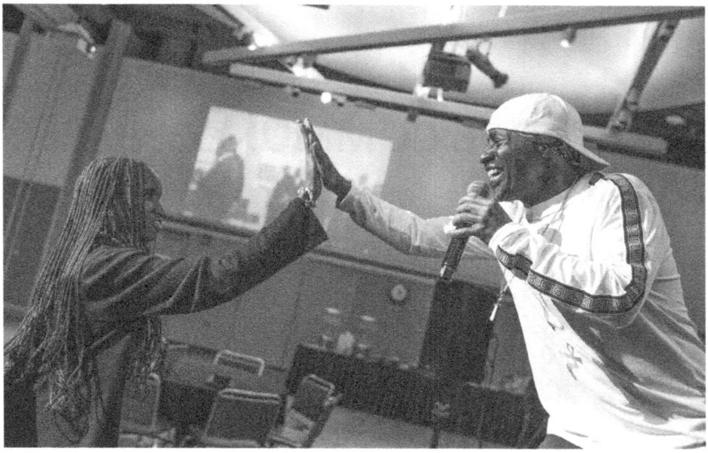

FIGURE 8.4 Ubuntu

Source: Ubuntu Brings Joy to Community. Photo by Casey Ek, The Mankato Free Press

Ubuntu is a deeply rooted African philosophy that celebrates our shared humanity. It means *I Am Because We Are; We Are Because I Am*, a recognition that our individual well-being is tied to the well-being of others. Ubuntu invites us to live with intention, knowing that through relationships and connection, we discover strength, happiness, and healing. Ubuntu reminds us of a profound truth: we are not alone. In a world that often pulls us apart, Ubuntu calls us back to community, to compassion, and to the deep understanding that *I Am Because We Are*.

Acknowledgements

With heartfelt appreciation to the Family Funds at the Mankato Area Foundation including the Lowell and Nadine Andreas Fund, Dotson Family Charitable Fund, Greg and Donnette Wheelock Fund, Tim Lidstrom Family Fund, and Kathy Van Tol. We are also deeply grateful to the Glen Taylor Nursing Institute for Family and Society, the City of Mankato, the City of North Mankato, and all those whose contributions continue to elevate compassion across the Kato Towns. A special thank you to Mary Ann's husband, Stephen, and Déva's sister, Bernadette Fox.

Reference

1. Deva Nation, "Deva's Story," [Online]. Available: https://www.devanation.com/devas-story. [Accessed 23 October 2025].

9

OASIS OF HOPE COMMUNITY-BASED ORGANISATION

Building compassionate communities in Kenya

Leonard Kiprono and Erin Das

Abstract

Kericho County is renowned throughout Kenya for its rolling tea plantations, vibrant culture, and thick church networks. But under the green landscape lies a less spoken reality: there are hundreds of families who struggle under the everyday burden of critical illness, cancer, renal disease, complex HIV, stroke, and non-communicable diseases such as diabetes and hypertension. For most, the very first hurdle is access. Specialist care is based in county referral hospitals or private facilities that are financially out of reach.

In such circumstances, the family, most often women, daughters, grandmothers, and now young girls, assume caregiving duties. Culture also makes caregiving more complex. Taboos in many communities in Kericho prevent men from providing intimate care to women, especially older kin. Religion and spirituality play a dual role, not only sustaining but also at times postponing candid discussion about severe and serious illnesses.

It is here that Oasis of Hope CBO started a community-level solution to a desperate need.

Oasis of Hope, Kericho County was endorsed as a compassionate community by Public Health Palliative Care International in October 2025.

9.1 Introduction – Our beginnings at Oasis of Hope

Shortly, this chapter will break down the areas of activity in our compassionate community; first, it is important to share a founding story.

DOI: 10.4324/9781003621348-10

9.1.1 *Rebecca*

On a quiet afternoon in Litein, Kericho County, the Oasis of Hope team walked up the narrow footpath leading to the home of 80-year-old Rebecca Cheruiyot. She had been living with advanced cancer and renal disease, conditions that drained her body and tested the resilience of her family. Inside the small homestead, the air was heavy with the smell of traditional herbs and the silence of uncertainty.

Rebecca's primary caregiver was her 14-year-old granddaughter, a form one student at the local day school. Each morning, the girl tried to balance school attendance with caring for her grandmother. She would wake up before sunrise to fetch water, prepare porridge, and clean Rebecca's wounds as best as she could. After school, instead of spending time with friends or doing homework, she hurried home to manage her grandmother's pain and provide company. The weight of responsibility far exceeded her years, yet she had little choice.

In many African communities, caregiving for the elderly, especially women, often falls on daughters and granddaughters. Cultural taboos limit the involvement of men in intimate care tasks such as bathing, wound care, or helping a woman change clothes. For Rebecca, this meant her adult sons and male relatives, though deeply concerned, remained physically distant, reluctant to cross cultural boundaries that discouraged men from "handling" their mothers' or grandmothers' bodies. What should have been a shared responsibility became the burden of a young girl, leaving both caregiver and patient vulnerable and isolated.

When the Oasis of Hope CBO team arrived for their home visit on 3rd November 2024, the atmosphere shifted. The visit included a nutritional evaluation, teaching on physical and wound care, and the provision of spiritual support for Rebecca and her caregivers. A trained nurse demonstrated safe wound cleaning techniques using simple, locally available materials. The chaplain listened as Rebecca shared her fears of being a burden to her family, offering prayers and words of encouragement that lifted her spirit. A social worker engaged the granddaughter, affirming her efforts and connecting her to a caregiver support group where she could learn from others in similar situations.

These interventions brought immediate relief. Rebecca's pain and wounds were better managed, her nutrition improved with locally adapted advice, and her granddaughter felt empowered rather than overwhelmed. Most importantly, the family rediscovered hope: dignity was restored to Rebecca, and the isolation that once defined their household began to dissolve as community volunteers and support groups stepped in.

Rebecca's story reflects a broader reality in Kericho County and across rural Kenya. Families often face serious illness with limited medical access, deep-rooted cultural taboos, and overwhelming caregiving demands. Yet, her case also demonstrates the transformative power of community-based palliative care, a model that respects culture, empowers families, and ensures that no one should face life's hardest moments alone.

9.1.2 The Kenyan context

Kenya has made significant progress in recognising palliative care as a vital part of health care. The Ministry of Health launched the Kenya National Palliative Care Policy (2011–2015, later integrated into broader health strategies) to guide services for people living with life-limiting illnesses. The policy emphasised equitable access, integration into the healthcare system, and capacity building for providers. In practice, however, implementation has been uneven. Large urban centres such as Nairobi, Eldoret, and Mombasa have specialist palliative care units, yet rural counties like Kericho remain underserved.

For many, the first challenge is access. Specialist care is concentrated in county referral hospitals or private facilities that are financially out of reach. Transport from remote villages to facilities is expensive, and patients often delay or abandon treatment altogether.

In such circumstances, caregiving becomes the responsibility of families, often women, grandmothers, daughters, and increasingly young girls. While family support is highly valued in Kenyan society, the demands of palliative care are complex: wound management, pain control, emotional reassurance, and sometimes navigating stigma from neighbours who associate illness with curses or sin. Caregivers are rarely trained to handle these responsibilities, leaving patients vulnerable and caregivers overwhelmed.

Cultural factors further complicate caregiving. In many communities within Kericho, taboos prevent men from offering intimate care to women, especially older relatives. Tasks like bathing, changing clothes, or cleaning wounds are seen as inappropriate for sons or grandsons. As a result, elderly women like Rebecca are often cared for almost exclusively by female relatives, even if those relatives are children. This creates an imbalance where care is gendered, isolating men from the process and placing disproportionate strain on women and girls.

Religion and spirituality play a dual role. Churches are central to community life in Kericho. They provide emotional and spiritual support, but at times, faith communities have been slow to openly discuss serious illness, death, and palliative care. Some families initially resist palliative care services, fearing that accepting them means "giving up hope." At the same time, once engaged, religious leaders can become powerful allies, helping congregations understand that palliative care is about compassion, dignity, and quality of life.

Despite these barriers, Kenya's palliative care landscape is slowly expanding. The Kenya Hospices and Palliative Care Association (KEHPCA) has been instrumental in advocating for training, integrating services into county hospitals, and building partnerships with organisations like Oasis of Hope. Yet, the gap remains wide. In Kericho, with a population of over 900,000, only a handful of trained professionals and volunteers are consistently available to deliver services, leaving large swathes of the county without structured support.

It is in this context that Oasis of Hope CBO emerged, a grassroots response to a pressing need. While policy frameworks exist nationally, local realities demand community-driven solutions. By training caregivers, equipping volunteers, and partnering with health facilities and churches, Oasis of Hope seeks to bridge the gap between policy and practice.

The Kenyan context is marked by promise and paradox: national recognition of palliative care as a right, but local communities still struggling with limited access; strong cultural and religious values that both inhibit and empower care; families carrying deep burdens, yet resilient when equipped with skills and support. It is within these tensions that compassionate community models like Oasis of Hope thrive, demonstrating how grassroots action can complement national policy and ensure that palliative care reaches those who need it most.

9.1.3 A community-based organisation, history, and needs assessment

Our community-based organisation (CBO) was formed as a response to the mounting health, social, and economic problems among households within our community. Founded in the year 2013, the organisation was a brainchild of a team of dedicated members of our society, who saw the need for a coordinated, caring response to problems such as poverty, healthcare disparities, education barriers, and inadequate social support systems.

Over the years, the CBO has emerged as a trusted community partner, by the community and for the community, with values of health empowerment, sustainability, and inclusivity. We are in close liaison with schools, churches, health centres, government offices, households, and local leadership in trying to respond to burning issues while constructing hope and resilience.

Before launching our flagship programmes, the organisation carried out a community needs assessment to find out more about the members of the community where we live and support one another, in particular, their problems and their priorities. Household surveys, focus group discussions, key informant interviews, and observation were used in conducting the needs assessment.

The needs assessment revealed several priority areas:

1. Healthcare gaps – Most of the households had no access to affordable health care, and chronic disease prevalence, maternal complications, and palliative or supportive care were limited.
2. Food and nutrition insecurity – They had frequent food shortages, malnourished children, and limited income streams.
3. Educational needs – Disadvantaged households had problems with school supplies, uniforms, and school tuition fees.

4 Psychosocial and spiritual support – Trauma, grief, and mourning were felt by most of the households, especially those who were sick, lost loved ones, or were impoverished.
5 Economic empowerment – The majority of the women and youth were vulnerable due to rampant unemployment and in need of skills training and livelihood activities.

It was from this robust understanding of the community and areas of need; we began to craft some responses. We prioritised several things as a group of community-based volunteers and leaders starting with home visiting and community health care. Community resilient initiatives like kitchen gardening support were starting, we engaged with primary school health and advocacy opportunities and focused on bereavement, grief, and psychosocial support groups. Other needs also came up which we were able to respond to through a support group for caregivers and families as well as community advocacy in media outlets and being the main community members to identify health needs of families and then make the required referrals and linkages.

9.1.4 The founding story

The Oasis of Hope CBO narrative is rooted in both this formal assessment and life experience. In 2013, the founding team members were engaged in active membership in local churches, hospitals, and community organisations in Kericho County. Again, they encountered families like those the assessment had identified, struggling in silence, with no access to specialty care, and with little more than prayer, herbs, and untrained family caregiving. These were not random incidents. They illustrated a chronic gap: serious illness was pushing families towards despair, poverty, and social isolation, and there were precious few local resources mobilised to respond with compassion.

The moment of truth came when one of the founders, Leonard Kiprono, a clinical nursing/palliative care trained chaplain and counselling psychologist, was called to the bedside of a neighbour in the terminal stages of cancer. The family had exhausted all their finances on hospital visits, transport, and traditional medicine. All that remained was a debilitated grandmother, a grieving home, and caregivers who felt abandoned by both the health system and society. After praying with the family and giving some general instructions on wound care and nutrition, Leonard left with a conviction: something more permanent had to be done.

From that realisation, the conversation began among friends, colleagues, and church leaders. The team understood that Kericho, like most rural counties, needed more than occasional hospital visits. It needed a community-based model of palliative care, one that combined clinical care, psychosocial support, and spiritual care, provided right at the household level. The seed of Oasis of Hope was planted.

Even though the vision was there as early as 2010, the organisation remained informal for the first few years, sustained almost solely by voluntary effort and goodwill. By 2013, Oasis of Hope was duly registered by the Government of Kenya as a CBO. Even then, much of its activity depended on community volunteers, church partners, and small community contributions. For nearly a decade, the activities were largely self-supporting until the breakthrough in 2023 when Hospice Care Kenya awarded Oasis of Hope its first small grant. This enabled the launch of the Palliative Care Empowerment programme, increasing caregivers' training and expanding household coverage. In 2024–2025, Das Consulting Ltd provided an additional small grant to operations, ensuring continuity of care and organisational sustainability.

By this time, Oasis of Hope had expanded from a volunteer group to a multicultural, professional staff:

1. Palliative care nurses – 4
2. Technical advisor – 1
3. Clinical oncologist – 1
4. Oncology nurse – 1
5. Chaplains – 2
6. Counsellors – 2
7. Nutritionist – 1
8. Medicine dispenser – 1
9. Caregivers – 36
10. IT support – 1
11. Accountant – 1
12. Youth mobiliser – 1

This internal team is supported by close working relations with community leaders, community chiefs, county assembly members, village managers, and local administrators, who enable mobilisation of families, break cultural taboos, and promote acceptance of palliative care as a community concern rather than an individual burden. The team's vision is to see more community team members who have passion and skills.

Early work was simple but profound. Home visits were made by volunteers, recruited mainly from local churches, health workers, and community youth, taking prayer, food aid, and basic health education. Most were untrained professionally in palliative care, but they offered what was most essential: empathy, the desire to listen, and the willingness to learn. Small-scale training workshops followed, equipping volunteers and family caregivers with practical skills such as safe lifting, wound dressing, nutrition basics, and counselling.

The community response was overwhelming. Families who had once felt abandoned discovered they were not alone. Widows who cared for bedridden husbands were encouraged by support groups. Elderly patients, who had resigned themselves to pain and loneliness as their fate, began to receive regular visits and emotional support. Even children, some as young as community caregiver's own granddaughter were trained in training sessions so that they would feel empowered rather than helpless in their role as caregivers.

From the very start, Oasis of Hope positioned itself as a bridge, knowledgeable community members and leaders linking families with formal health systems where referrals were needed. Partnerships with Kericho County Referral Hospital, dispensaries, and the KEHPCA began to form. What had started as a volunteer group grew over the years into a structured programme with clear areas of concentration: home-based palliative care, capacity building for caregivers, community health sensitisation, advocacy for the differently abled, and resilience-building activities.

Oasis of Hope began modestly, but it was defined by this one suffocating fact: when communities claim both their hurt and their capacity, transformation becomes possible. What first was a response to one neighbours' anguish has now grown into a movement, extending to hundreds of families across Kericho and beyond.

9.2 Building a compassionate community model

At Oasis of Hope, we realise that authentic care must be holistic. Illness is never just physical but impacts emotions, spirituality, family, and the broader community. For this reason, our interventions go beyond medication to encompass a holistic model that meets patients and families where they are, including five key areas of a community-based model of support:

9.2.1 Home-based care

At the heart of our work is home-based supportive care. Distance, cost, or immobility bars many patients in Kericho and surrounding counties from reaching specialist hospital care. Bringing the care to their doorsteps ensures no one is left behind. Our trained health workers and community volunteers conduct regular home visits, offering pain control, wound management, nutritional care, and emotional and spiritual support.

These visits are as relational as medical. To sit in a patient's home, to listen to their fears, to pray with them, or to simply hold their hand is to speak respect and dignity. Home-based care also removes the burden from families of daily hospital trips, allowing patients to remain within the comfort of their communities for their most vulnerable days.

9.2.2 Empowerment of community family caregivers

Caregiving is invisible and undervalued, yet palliative care's lifeline. In rural Kenya, it is typically left to women, children, or elderly spouses with no training. Oasis of Hope educates caregivers in practical care training workshops in safe lifting, hygiene, basic first aid, wound care, nutrition, palliative care training, and stress management. Some of the people being trained are family caregivers, religious leaders, and Community Health Promoters.

We also recognise the emotional cost of caregiving. In this regard, we have set up caregiver support groups, safe havens where individuals can vent their challenges, learn coping strategies, and be empowered by others who walk a similar journey. Empowered caregivers not only provide better quality care but also protect their own health and well-being.

9.2.3 Community health

We approach health as a community responsibility. Our community health initiatives include outreach programmes, medical camps, and partnerships with local clinics. These programmes provide health education on chronic illnesses, cancer screening, HIV awareness, mental health, and preventive practices such as nutrition and hygiene.

By demystifying disease and offering accurate information, we counter myths and misconceptions that often worsen suffering. For example, some communities interpret cancer as a curse or punishment, leading to stigma and neglect. Our education campaigns help break down these barriers, replacing fear with knowledge and compassion.

9.2.4 Constructing resilience

Serious illness can plunge families into poverty and desperation. It is for this reason that Oasis of Hope integrates resilience-building activities into its model. These vary from income-generating activities for vulnerable households, savings clubs, and community gardens that build nutrition as well as livelihood.

Resilience is also spiritual and emotional. We help families, through chaplaincy services, counselling, and community fellowships, to find meaning, hope, and strength during pain. In supporting resilience, we ensure that patients and caregivers are not just surviving but are also learning to live well despite their challenges.

9.2.5 Supporting the abled differently

Disability remains highly stigmatised in most rural areas. Oasis of Hope takes an inclusive approach, empowering the differently abled through advocacy, assistive devices, capacity building, and sensitisation of communities. We promote the reality that disability does not equate to inability.

This not only enables individuals with disabilities but also transforms communities as cultural taboos and negative stereotypes are shattered. Children born with disabilities, who were once hidden in shame, are now being enrolled in schools, and adults are gaining the confidence to participate in social and economic life.

9.2.6 Advocacy and sensitisation

The final thread of our work is advocacy and sensitisation. Some of the challenges patients and caregivers experience, cultural taboos, resource limitations, or policy lacunae, must be transformed at a systems level. Oasis of Hope engages with local leaders, religious institutions, schools, and policy-makers to raise awareness about palliative care and the rights of patients and caregivers.

With community forums, radio programmes, and partnerships with county departments of health, we ensure that palliative care is not a luxury but a basic human right. Advocacy also begins to shift cultural norms. For example, through open dialogue about the male role in caregiving, we slowly dismantle taboos that prevent sons and husbands from offering the care their loved ones need.

A new area for our team recently is to respond to a need that has come from our community members focusing on children with serious illness and their families. At Oasis of Hope, we recognise that children with life-limiting illnesses have unique needs requiring ongoing support, compassion, and sensitivity. Childhood serious illness not only affects the child patient but also places an overwhelming emotional, financial, and physical burden on the family. For this reason, focusing on children and their families with extensive needs takes high priority in our compassionate community development approach.

Through extending our home visitation to children and their families, they can be supported from the comfort of their own homes. Our community volunteers and staff provide safe places where siblings and other family members are free to express their emotions and learn how they can best care for one another.

Recognising that some children require more advanced interventions, Oasis of Hope is also a bridge to specialty care. We work with Kericho County Referral Hospital and paediatrics wards to facilitate timely referrals. Wherever possible, we connect families with organisations that provide medical equipment, nutritional supplements, and financial support.

In everything we do, we believe that children are not small adults. They deserve care that respects their stage of development, their rights to happiness and play, and their family's need for comprehensive care. Prioritising children's complex needs, Oasis of Hope ensures that no child suffers in silence and families are never alone in this difficult journey.

Finally, through our community-led bereavement and mourning support, we can offer an initial response to the grieving family soon after the loss to condole and assess immediate needs, providing condolence support such as care packages. We collaborate with community leaders to be present at services, providing practical and spiritual support. At a community level, we can also engage in one-on-one grief counselling, support groups, and children and youth special sessions are provided. We follow up through home visits on a regular basis, check-in calls, and annual memorial events so that no family is ever forgotten. In these moments, we as a community also provide immediate relief like food baskets, financial assistance for funeral costs, and referrals to other services are provided.

9.2.7 Healthcare providers capacity building

One of the core strategies of Oasis of Hope is strengthening the capacity of healthcare providers so that patients and families facing serious illness receive quality, compassionate, and holistic care. While the organisation began primarily with volunteers and community caregivers, it soon became clear that sustainable impact required training and equipping health professionals to address the unique needs of palliative care.

Through structured workshops and on-the-job mentorship, Oasis of Hope has trained a wide range of healthcare providers, including nurses, clinical officers, counsellors, chaplains, nutritionists, and community health volunteers, on both the clinical and psychosocial dimensions of palliative care. The key training modules include:

1. Pain and Symptom Management – equipping providers with knowledge on safe opioid use, non-pharmacological approaches, and managing distressing symptoms such as shortness of breath, nausea, and fatigue.
2. Spiritual and Psychological Care – drawing on Oasis of Hope's chaplaincy background, providers are trained to integrate emotional support, grief counselling, and faith-sensitive care in their practice.
3. Effective Communication – building capacity to break bad news compassionately, listen actively, and maintain dignity-centred dialogue with patients and families.
4. Holistic Care Planning – helping providers coordinate with families, community leaders, and hospitals for continuity of care.
5. Caregiver Support – training providers to recognise caregiver burden and equip them with strategies to build resilience in households.
6. Ethical and Cultural Sensitivity – exploring local beliefs around illness, death, and dying, while teaching respectful approaches that affirm dignity.

These training sessions are delivered in partnership with Kericho County Referral Hospital, KEHPCA, and other health institutions, ensuring that providers not only gain practical knowledge but also connect with a broader referral and support network.

By investing in provider capacity building, Oasis of Hope is creating a multiplier effect: every trained nurse, counsellor, or community health volunteer becomes a channel of hope for dozens of patients and families. This approach ensures that palliative care moves beyond the walls of hospitals and becomes a community-owned service, rooted in both professional expertise and compassionate human connection.

9.2.8 Emphasis of children palliative care needs

At Oasis of Hope, we recognise that children with life-limiting illnesses face unique challenges that require specialised attention, sensitivity, and support.

Serious illness in childhood not only affects the young patient but also places a profound emotional, financial, and physical burden on families. For this reason, children's palliative care is a core priority in our approach to compassionate community development.

Our work begins with parents and caregivers, who are often the primary providers of day-to-day care for their children. Oasis of Hope conducts targeted training sessions that equip them with practical skills in:

1. Pain and symptom management for children, tailored to their age and needs.
2. Nutrition support, especially for children with cancer or chronic conditions.
3. Psychosocial and spiritual care, helping families address the emotional strain of caring for a sick child while also nurturing the child's hope and dignity.
4. Communication strategies, enabling parents to better understand their child's needs and to advocate for appropriate care in hospital settings.

Beyond training, our teams, including palliative care nurses, chaplains, counsellors, and community caregivers, conduct home care visits. These visits allow families to access support in the comfort of their homes, reducing the burden of frequent hospital travel. During these visits, our team not only provides medical and psychosocial care but also creates safe spaces where siblings and extended family members can express their feelings and learn how to support one another.

Recognising that some children require advanced interventions, Oasis of Hope also serves as a bridge to specialised services. We work closely with Kericho County Referral Hospital, paediatric units, and KEHPCA to facilitate timely referrals. When possible, we connect families with organisations that provide medical supplies, nutritional support, and financial assistance.

In every encounter, we affirm that children are not simply small adults. They deserve care that respects their developmental stage, their right to play and joy, and their family's need for holistic support. By prioritising children's palliative care needs, Oasis of Hope ensures that no child suffers in silence and that families know they are not alone on this difficult journey.

9.3 An integrated community-based model of care and support

What is unique in this model is that each strand informs the other. A home visit generates caregiver empowerment. A caregiver training session identifies the need for disability support. A community health forum sparks advocacy on local health policy. The model is responsive and fluid, based on listening to communities and responding with compassion.

We believe at Oasis of Hope that holistic care restores dignity, strengthens families, and heals communities. This is what sets our work apart and drives our mission daily.

9.4 Stories from the field

Behind every programme statistic is a human story. At Oasis of Hope, these stories are the heartbeat of our mission. They remind us that palliative care is not just about services but about restoring dignity, strengthening families, and opening doors of hope.

9.4.1 Leonard Kiprono – a founder's conviction

Oasis of Hope was born out of the deep conviction of Leonard Kiprono, a clinical nurse, palliative care, ordained clergy, and counselling psychologist. Having walked with patients at the bedside, prayed with grieving families, and counselled caregivers overwhelmed by exhaustion, Leonard witnessed firsthand the gaps in palliative care in rural Kenya. He saw how cultural taboos, poverty, and lack of awareness compounded suffering, leaving patients isolated and families unsupported.

For Leonard, palliative care was not only a medical calling but also a spiritual and social mission. He founded Oasis of Hope to bridge the gap between clinical practice, pastoral care, and community empowerment. His vision was clear: that every patient, regardless of status or location, should experience dignity, comfort, and love in the most vulnerable seasons of life.

9.5 Mirriam's journey – from burden to confidence

For Mirriam, caregiving had begun as a heavy, isolating burden. As the only willing and available family member, she bore the responsibility of tending to her grandmother's wounds, bathing her, and ensuring she ate, all while struggling to keep up with schoolwork. The emotional weight was immense, and at times, she felt trapped between being a student and being a caregiver.

Through Oasis of Hope's caregiver training, Mirriam's story took a new turn. The training equipped her with practical skills in hygiene, nutrition, safe lifting, and emotional care. More importantly, it helped her understand the value of what she was doing and see caregiving not as a shameful or solitary task, but as a meaningful act of love.

Her confidence grew. No longer unsure or fearful of making mistakes, she began providing hygienic, professional-level care. The transformation was not hers alone; her confidence inspired other family members to step forward. With Leonard's encouragement, uncles and cousins who had once withdrawn due to cultural taboos began helping. Caregiving became a family effort, not Mirriam's private cross to bear.

Today, Mirriam balances school with caregiving without feeling torn apart. She studies comfortably, knowing her grandmother is well supported, and when she is home, she joins in with skill and pride. What once looked like a story of strain has become a story of empowerment. In her words during a feedback session:

> "I now know I am not alone, and what I do matters."

9.5.1 Reverend Koskei – a clergy's expanded ministry

Palliative care not only transforms families, but it also reshapes leaders. Reverend Koskei, a local clergy member, encountered Oasis of Hope through a community training. Initially, he joined with the expectation of learning how to provide spiritual comfort to the sick. What he discovered was far broader: palliative care was a ministry of presence, advocacy, and practical love.

The training opened his eyes to the power of integrating pastoral care with hands-on support. He learned how to help with feeding, mobility, and emotional counselling, alongside preaching hope. For Koskei, this was a paradigm shift. In his words: "Before, I would only pray and leave. Now, I roll up my sleeves and serve."

Since then, Reverend Koskei has become a strong advocate in his church and community. He preaches openly about the need to support the sick and their families, challenging cultural taboos and urging men to take an active role in caregiving. He also joins home visits, where his presence as both clergy and caregiver helps bridge the gap between faith and health. Through his ministry, others have caught the vision that palliative care is not charity but an expression of God's love and justice.

9.5.2 Threads of hope

Rebecca's renewed comfort, Mirriam's regained confidence, and Reverend Koskei's expanded ministry represent just three threads in the tapestry of Oasis of Hope. Each story shows how holistic care transforms not only patients but also caregivers, families, and entire communities.

At Oasis of Hope, we do not measure success only by the number of trainings held or visits conducted, but by these stories of change, where despair gives way to hope, where burdens become shared, and where dignity is restored.

9.6 Partnerships, collaborations, and learning

From the very beginning, Oasis of Hope recognised that palliative care cannot thrive in isolation. Illness touches entire families, and solutions require a web of support that extends beyond any one caregiver or organisation. Building partnerships has therefore been at the heart of our compassionate community model.

One of the most important collaborations has been with the Kericho County Health Department. While Oasis of Hope operates as a CBO, alignment with county health structures ensures that our services complement and strengthen existing health systems rather than duplicate them. Through regular meetings and joint trainings, Oasis of Hope has helped frontline health workers integrate basic palliative care into their daily practice. In return, the county has provided referrals, technical support, and opportunities to scale training to remote dispensaries.

Churches and faith leaders have also played a vital role. In Kenya, where most of the population identifies strongly with their faith, clergy are often the first people families turn to during illness or bereavement. Oasis of Hope has therefore intentionally trained pastors, catechists, and imams in both compassionate care and advocacy. Rev. Koskei's story is one among many where pastoral leaders, after receiving training, have been able to extend their ministry into both advocacy and practical care. This faith-based partnership has opened doors into homes and communities that might otherwise have been hesitant to engage with medical or psychosocial services.

Collaboration with schools and young people has been equally significant. Training adolescents like Mirriam to care for loved ones has proven that palliative care education can transform not only the immediate caregiving situation but also empower a new generation to break cultural taboos around illness and gendered caregiving. By engaging teachers and community youth groups, Oasis of Hope is planting seeds for a more resilient future.

Oasis of Hope maintains active national collaborations and partnerships, including registration with the National Non-Communicable Disease Programme, Kenya, the National Association of Christian Chaplains, and membership with the KEHPCA. In addition, team members are individually affiliated with their respective professional bodies such as the Nursing Council of Kenya, the Oncology Nurses Association, and other relevant associations. These collaborations not only enhance credibility but also provide opportunities for training, advocacy, and integration into national palliative care and health initiatives.

Finally, international connections have strengthened learning and credibility – through institutions such as KEHPCA, IAHPC (International Association of Hospices and Palliative Care), and Das Consulting Limited. Oasis of Hope has exchanged experiences with colleagues across the world. These networks remind us that while our context is uniquely Kenyan, our challenges are shared across borders, and our local innovations can inspire others globally.

9.7 Lessons learned and practical insights

Over the years, several lessons have emerged from Oasis of Hope's journey:

1 Start small but start where it matters most. Our work began in living rooms, with single families like Rebecca's. Change often starts with one caregiver empowered to act, and that ripple spreads wider than any programme design on paper.
2 Culture cannot be ignored; it must be engaged. Taboos around male caregiving, discussions of death, or stigma of illness do not disappear by confrontation alone. We have learned to approach these issues with respect, dialogue, and demonstration. When men see another man (like Leonard) offering professional yet dignified care, they realise it is possible for them too.
3 Training is empowerment. Whether for caregivers, clergy, or adolescents, knowledge transforms fear into action. Even basic skills in hygiene, wound care, or nutrition can restore dignity and confidence both to the patient and the family.

4 Partnership is sustainability. No single organisation can meet all the needs of families facing advanced illness. Building links with county health systems, schools, churches, and global networks ensures continuity and resilience.
5 Compassion is contagious. Once one family member steps forward, like Mirriam, others often follow. Compassionate care creates a culture where more people feel safe to help, breaking isolation and burden.

These lessons are not theoretical; they are lived experiences that any community, whether in rural Kenya or urban Europe, can adapt in their own way.

9.8 Conclusion and way forward

The story of Oasis of Hope is still being written. What began as one nurse-clergy-psychologist responding to visible suffering has grown into a community movement touching hundreds of lives. By blending professional care with cultural sensitivity, faith-based engagement, and grassroots empowerment, Oasis of Hope demonstrates that compassionate communities are possible even in resource-limited contexts.

Looking ahead, the vision is to deepen partnerships with government health structures, expand training programmes into more counties, and develop a stronger network of youth and faith leaders equipped for compassionate action. The long-term goal is not just to provide palliative care to those in need, but to cultivate a culture where no one suffers alone, and where dignity at the end-of-life is considered a shared responsibility.

As we reflect on Rebecca's story, on Mirriam's transformation, and on Rev. Koskei's expanded ministry, one truth stands out: compassion is practical. It is a skill that can be learned, a responsibility that can be shared, and a gift that renews hope in the darkest seasons of life.

Oasis of Hope's journey affirms that compassionate communities are not built overnight, but through steady acts of love, learning, and partnership. And in each act, however small, lies the seed of a more humane and hopeful world.

10

FROM BALLOONS TO BONDS

The journey of the students' initiative in palliative care

Saif Mohammed

Abstract

This chapter traces the evolution of the Students' Initiative in Palliative Care (SIPC), a youth-led movement that emerged in Kerala, India, from *scattered acts of symbolic commitment* into a sustained, community-based engagement with illness, dying, and caregiving. Drawing on lived experience rather than a prescriptive model, the chapter illustrates how young people can meaningfully contribute to palliative care through presence, companionship, creativity, and collective action. Situated within Kerala's long-standing public health and community-oriented palliative care ecosystem, the story of SIPC explores how trust, decentralised care, and cultural openness created fertile ground for young people to step into roles traditionally seen as outside their domain.

Through stories of patient–student relationships, community events, and reflective learning, the chapter examines the reciprocal impact of this engagement: how patients and families experience dignity, connection, and renewed meaning, and how students themselves are transformed in their understanding of suffering, care, and responsibility. Introducing the concept of a "loop of compassion," the chapter argues that care is not a one-way act but a mutually sustaining exchange that shapes individuals and communities alike. Rather than offering SIPC as a blueprint to be replicated, the chapter invites readers to consider broader lessons for public health palliative care, including the power of small, consistent acts; the role of youth in shaping cultures of care; and the possibility of organising compassion as a collective, enduring social practice.

DOI: 10.4324/9781003621348-11

10.1 Introduction

In a quiet corner of Calicut, a northern city in Kerala, under the sprawling trees at the Institute of Palliative Medicine (IPM), something beautiful and quietly profound unfolded one October morning in 2010. It was just past 10:10 AM on the tenth day of the tenth month when 100 college students from ten local institutions gathered in quiet anticipation. There were no banners or microphones, no formal speeches or media crews, just a moment of shared purpose.

Each group carried a bundle of ten balloons. On cue, they let them go into the sky, ten bundles of ten, gently rising into the morning light. That was it. No performance, no slogans. Just balloons, and a question held in the air: *What if young people made space in their lives for those who are ill, suffering, or dying?*

That simple act, symbolic as it was, marked the birth of what would grow into the Students' Initiative in Palliative Care (SIPC), a youth-led movement rooted in presence, compassion, and quiet courage.

We called the launch Ten-Ten. The idea was modest: Each student would commit to giving ten hours a month to palliative care and raising ten rupees a week to support patient services at IPM. It wasn't about grand ambition. It was about planting a seed. The hope was that even small, regular acts, of time, attention, and kindness, could amount to something meaningful.

Back then, we had no blueprint, no fixed model, and honestly, no clear plan for what SIPC would become. But what we did have was a shared feeling. We had seen patients who felt forgotten. We had met families stretched thin, emotionally and financially, while caring for a loved one at home. And we had met students, bright, curious, idealistic, who were looking for something real to pour their energy into.

SIPC emerged from that meeting point. It wasn't imposed from above. It grew from the ground, quietly, like many good things do.

I still remember the energy of that first morning. Most of the students didn't know exactly what they were signing up for. But there was something about the simplicity of the gesture, and the clarity of the invitation, that spoke to them. The balloons carried no slogans, but each one symbolised a possibility: That care isn't just a professional task; it's something young people can offer too.

In the years since, SIPC has grown beyond what we imagined. Today, it brings together hundreds of students each year from more than 20 colleges. They offer their time, creativity, companionship, and most of all, their willingness to walk with people through some of the hardest moments of life.

10.2 Where it takes root

To understand how SIPC took root and grew, it's important to understand the soil it was planted in. Kerala's palliative care movement has long been recognised for its unique, community-based approach. From the very beginning, it was never framed as something solely for hospices or clinics. Instead, it was seen as something that belonged to the people, a social response to human suffering, with a medical component, not the other way around. This approach made a significant impact.

When care is seen as the responsibility of society, not just of professionals, it opens the door to participation from every corner. In Kerala, that meant not only nurses and doctors, but also retired teachers, autorickshaw drivers, shopkeepers, and students could find a place in the work of palliative care. Everyone had something to offer. And everyone was needed.

At the IPM, this way of thinking deeply shaped how we envisioned SIPC. We never saw young people as too inexperienced or too young to contribute. In fact, we saw their youth as a strength. They brought with them energy, adaptability, and a kind of emotional honesty that made them deeply effective in connecting with patients.

This is how we reach out to youngsters: We would reach out to local colleges and ask if we could hold a short awareness session, usually about an hour and a half. These weren't lectures. They were conversations. We would talk about palliative care, what it means, and why it matters. There was no pressure to sign up. At the end of each session, we'd simply offer a choice: *If this speaks to you, you're welcome to join us.*

And students did. Some hesitantly, others with quiet conviction. But they came. Once they registered, they would attend a short orientation at IPM. This was called *Samvedanam*, which loosely translates to "shared feeling." It wasn't a technical training. It was an introduction to what it means to be present with someone in distress. We spoke about communication, active listening, the emotional landscape of illness, and the basics of caregiving. For many students, this was their first time encountering these ideas.

Those who wanted to take it further could opt into a 20-hour caregiver training course, developed by IPM, based on WHO guidelines. Others joined a six-month psychosocial support programme, making weekly home visits and attending regular reflection circles. Some gravitated towards community outreach, organising events, writing newsletters, raising awareness through art or social media. There was no one path. SIPC welcomed many kinds of engagement.

What surprised us most was how naturally the students took to the work, not just the logistics, but the emotional weight of it. They weren't afraid of silence. They didn't look away from pain.

One student, after her first few home visits, said to me,

> "I used to think being helpful meant fixing things. But here, I've learned that sometimes, the most helpful thing you can do is sit quietly next to someone who's scared. Just so they know they're not alone."

That's the kind of insight we hope stays with them long after their volunteering days are over.

We don't expect students to become experts. What we hope is that they start to see caregiving as something deeply human, not the exclusive domain of professionals, but something that lives inside all of us, waiting for the right moment to be called forward. And when that happens, when a young person discovers they can bring comfort not just with knowledge, but with presence, it becomes more than training. It becomes transformation.

10.3 A story I carry with me

Over the years, I've seen many students grow through SIPC. I've watched them stumble through their first visits, return with red eyes and full hearts, and gradually find a steady, grounded rhythm in the work. But there are a few stories that stay with me, not just as a teacher or mentor, but as a fellow human being. One of those is the story of Ravi.

That wasn't his real name, of course, but I remember him vividly. Ravi had once lived what many would call a successful life. He worked in the corporate sector, travelled across countries, and spoke several languages fluently, including French. But when he arrived at IPM, he was in a wheelchair, living with multiple sclerosis. The illness had limited his body, but more than that, it had shrunk his world.

He was reserved, just closed. Like a door that had been quietly shut for a long time. The medical team tended to his symptoms, but we could all sense that something deeper was missing, a connection, a reason to wake up in the morning.

One day, a few student volunteers, mostly young girls, were spending time with Ravi, as suggested by the clinical team. During their conversations, they discovered something remarkable: Ravi was multilingual. He could speak seven languages, including French.

Within minutes, the conversation turned into an invitation: "Would you help us as a translator for our international visitors at IPM, to speak with patients and their family members?"

Ravi agreed – maybe out of politeness, maybe out of curiosity. But something shifted in him after that.

Over the next two weeks, we saw him rolling through the corridors in his electric wheelchair, a gift from IPM, offering to translate, helping visitors find their way around the institute, and even giving language lessons to the young volunteers. The change was quiet, but unmistakable. His eyes were brighter. He laughed more. He asked questions.

The illness was still there. The pain hadn't vanished. But something inside him, something that had been tightly coiled, began to loosen.

That's what companionship can do. That's what it often does.

It wasn't medicine that softened Ravi's loneliness. It wasn't therapy. It was the fact that a few students took the time to see him, not just as a patient, but as a person with gifts, with knowledge, and with a life still worth sharing.

To this day, when someone asks me, what students can really do in a palliative care setting, I think of Ravi. I think of how he wheeled himself through the ward, not just receiving care but offering it.

10.4 Creating joy in the middle of it all

One of the most surprising things about SIPC, at least for people who encounter it from the outside, is how much joy lives at its centre.

When people think of palliative care, especially in the context of youth involvement, they often imagine quiet, heavy rooms and emotionally draining encounters. And yes, there are moments like that. But what we've seen over the years is that joy and grief are not opposites. In fact, they often live side by side. SIPC has taught us that it's entirely possible, and even necessary, to make space for both.

We've seen this especially through the creative ways students choose to engage with their communities. There's something deeply refreshing about how young people approach caregiving. They don't carry the baggage of how it's "supposed" to look. They come with ideas, with playfulness, and with a desire to make things meaningful and memorable.

Let me give you an example: the Biryani Fest. On the surface, it's a fundraising initiative. But, in reality, it's much more than that. In a single day, student volunteers across colleges came together to cook and sell 14,000 packets of biryani, all in support of palliative care. Each packet carried a handwritten note: "You've helped someone through pain today."

I remember one woman who bought a biryani packet at a traffic signal, read the note inside, and came to IPM the very next day asking, "How can I be part of this?"

Another powerful example is *Curios*, a three-day festival that has become something of an annual landmark in Calicut. On those evenings, the courtyard of IPM transforms. There are music, food stalls, storytelling corners, art installations, and quiet spaces for reflection.

Patients and families attend, as do neighbours, students, and complete strangers. Conversations happen, some light, some tender, some unspoken.

It's not about putting a positive spin on suffering. It's about making compassion something you can see, taste, and walk through. It's about saying that care isn't just a response to pain, it's a celebration of connection.

Many of these events are completely student-led, from the planning to the execution. And what's remarkable is how much love goes into the details. Whether it's decorating a food stall or crafting a playlist, the intent is always to create an experience where people feel welcomed, uplifted, and part of something larger than themselves.

There's a kind of healing that happens in those moments. A kind of softening. People who might never have spoken about death before find themselves at a stall writing postcards to someone they've lost. Children laugh beside patients in wheelchairs. Strangers share meals at long communal tables. The boundaries between caregiver and cared-for begin to blur.

That, to me, is the quiet genius of SIPC: It reminds us that care doesn't always have to look solemn. It can look like a shared plate of biryani – a handwritten note, a song echoing through a courtyard, a student dancing with a patient.

10.5 What students take with them

One of the most profound aspects of SIPC is that it doesn't just change the lives of the patients and families it touches. It transforms the students themselves. Over the years, I've watched young people arrive uncertain, quiet, and hesitant, unsure of what palliative care even means. And I've seen them leave, months or years later, not just with more knowledge, but with more humanity.

What do students take with them from this experience? It's rarely just the facts or skills. It's something deeper.

Many speak of how their perspective on suffering has changed. Some come in afraid, afraid of illness, of ageing, of being in the presence of someone who is dying. But as they spend time with patients, that fear gradually gives way to something else: empathy, steadiness, and a willingness to stay present even when things feel uncertain.

One former volunteer, now a doctor, told me recently,

> "When I sit with a patient now, I don't rush to write a prescription. I try to see the whole person in front of me. I learned that first in SIPC."

Another student, who went on to work as a social worker, said something that struck me: "This is where I learned how to hold silence. How to listen without needing to respond. And that's something I use every day now."

Not every student becomes a healthcare professional. And that's never the expectation. What matters is how SIPC shapes their sense of self in the world. It nurtures qualities that are increasingly rare: slowness, attention, and a commitment to walk alongside others, even when there's nothing to solve.

There's also the matter of friendship, deep bonds that form in unexpected places. Many students speak of how the relationships they built within SIPC felt different from any they had before. When you work together in a setting where vulnerability is present, where people are speaking openly about pain, loss, and love, something shifts. You start to show up as your full self. And you begin to see others more fully too.

That's a kind of education you don't get in classrooms.

Some students, after years of volunteering, return to IPM not as interns or trainees, but as mentors to the next generation. They come back to guide, to share stories, and to sit in the same courtyard where they once hesitated to speak. That continuity is one of SIPC's quiet strengths: It doesn't just grow volunteers, it grows a community.

When we ask students what they remember most, it's rarely a big event or achievement. More often, it's a moment, a patient's smile, a family's thank you, a song sung softly at a bedside.

And almost always, they say the same thing in different ways: "This changed me."

10.6 The loop of compassion

Over time, while observing the relationship between our student volunteers and the patients they serve, we noticed something powerful, a pattern. It was quiet, almost invisible at first, but unmistakable once you saw it. I now call it the Loop of Compassion.

It begins simply. A student signs up to volunteer. They're not professionals. They don't have any special training in medicine or counselling. What they bring is something more basic and more profound. They show up.

They show up at the bedside of a woman in pain. They sit with a grandfather who can no longer walk. They hold the hand of someone facing the end of life. And they do this not for reward or recognition, but because they believe it matters.

And then something begins to happen.

In return for their time and presence, these students receive something unexpected. They're met with gratitude. With trust. With stories, smiles, and sometimes even silences that feel sacred. They realise that their presence has weight, that it brings comfort. That they, even as students, have the power to make someone feel seen.

That emotional exchange, the offering of care and the receiving of trust, creates something deeper: a sense of meaning. A sense of purpose.

One of the most touching reflections on this dynamic came from Mr. Kumar, a paraplegic patient registered at IPM who was regularly visited and supported by SIPC volunteers. When asked what the students meant to him, he paused and said,

> "We are like banana plants which keep falling as they grow. These students support us to keep us straight and firm."

The image is simple, yet deeply resonant. In Kerala, where banana plants are a familiar sight, it is well known that as they grow taller, their soft trunks can't always bear their own weight. So, farmers place slender bamboo sticks beside them and gently tie the plants for support, not tightly, but just enough to keep them upright through sun and wind. That's what SIPC students become in the lives of those they accompany: not fixers or rescuers, but quiet supports who walk alongside, offering just enough steadiness for someone to hold their shape a little longer.

And as Mr. Kumar's words remind us, support in SIPC flows both ways. The students offer care, but they receive something just as sustaining in return: trust, perspective, and the humbling knowledge that even simple presence can matter. This reciprocity is not incidental; it is the very soul of the Loop of Compassion.

10.7 Lessons for the world

As we look at the world around us, a world where healthcare systems are stretched, loneliness is on the rise, and young people often feel disconnected, it's worth asking: What can we learn from SIPC?

10.7.1 Care can be decentralised and still be deeply personal

SIPC is not built on specialists alone. Its strength lies in ordinary people, especially students, being invited into the circle of care. What this tells us is that compassion doesn't need a professional title. It needs an invitation, a little support, and the space to act.

Across cultures and countries, we could be asking: *How might we involve students, neighbours, retirees, and schoolchildren in the work of caring, in daily life?*

10.7.2 *Young people don't need to be protected from suffering, they need to be trusted with meaning*

There is often a tendency to shield the younger generation from illness, ageing, and death. But what SIPC has shown is that when young people are given the chance to be present in these moments, they don't collapse. They rise.

They respond with creativity, energy, and a fierce, quiet kind of love. They bring joy where we expect silence. They build connections where we expect detachment. The key is to offer them a role, not just in service, but in shaping the culture of care itself.

10.7.3 *Small, consistent acts, more than grand gestures*

What sustains SIPC is not a one-time campaign or viral moment. It's the rhythm of students showing up week after week, writing notes, making visits, cooking meals, organising events, or simply sitting with someone who needs company. This kind of everyday care, when done collectively, has power.

In a world that celebrates speed and spectacle, SIPC reminds us of the quiet dignity of showing up.

10.8 Care is contagious

When one student chooses to care, others follow. When a campus begins to talk about palliative care, the conversation spills into families, streets, and social media. A single act can ripple outward into a cultural shift. That's not a theory, it's what has happened, again and again, in the SIPC journey.

What if we designed our systems, healthcare, education, and even urban planning, with that kind of ripple in mind?

10.8.1 *Compassion can be organised*

This is perhaps the most hopeful lesson of all. We often think of compassion as spontaneous, something that happens in rare, beautiful moments. But SIPC shows that compassion can be cultivated, structured, and scaled. It can be trained, supported, and passed from one generation to the next.

In other words, compassion isn't just a feeling. It's a culture. And cultures can be built.

SIPC may be local, but its lessons are universal. In a world looking for new ways to reconnect, to rebuild, to recover, perhaps it's time we stop asking how much one person can do and start asking what happens when many people choose to care, together.

Because when care becomes collective, it becomes powerful. And that's a lesson the world can carry forward.

10.9 Sustaining the spirit: how we keep it going

People often ask us: How have you kept SIPC alive all these years? What makes it work, not just once, but repeatedly, across batches, across colleges, across time?

We don't have a secret formula. But when we look back, what has helped us sustain this work comes down to three things: the message, the people, and the opportunities. Simple words. But in our experience, they've made all the difference.

From the beginning, we knew that for SIPC to take root, we needed a message that mattered, not just to us, but to the students we were inviting in.

And so, we began with a truth that's easy to forget:

Most people don't die suddenly. For the vast majority, there's a period of illness, of increasing dependence, of emotional and social strain. And in that in-between space, between diagnosis and death, there is immense need.

Need for presence. For companionship. For dignity. For connection.

We shared this message everywhere we went in classrooms, in campus auditoriums, in quiet corners of conversations. We spoke not with urgency, but with honesty. We said: *This is real. This could be your parent. Your friend. You.*

And if that's true, then caring isn't something extraordinary. It's something essential.

Not a charity, but a life skill. Not a professional domain, but a shared human responsibility.

And like any skill, the earlier you learn it, the better you become at offering it, not just in volunteering, but in life.

The heart of SIPC has always been its people. But we didn't just wait for them to find us; we went to find them.

We reached out to local colleges, not with recruitment drives, but with conversations. We walked into classrooms, not with PowerPoint slides, but with stories. And at the end of every awareness session, we extended a simple invitation: *If this speaks to you, come see us.*

Some students signed up on the spot. Others returned after days, or years. Some came curious, others cautious. But when they showed up, we welcomed them not for what they already knew, but for what they were willing to learn and feel.

We've seen repeatedly that participation grows when there is real, meaningful work to do, and when students feel trusted to try, to create, to lead.

And in that way, SIPC has never been a programme students pass through. It's been a space they help build. A place where care isn't performed, but practised, week after week, in many forms, with many hands.

10.10 Care that echoes beyond

As the journey of SIPC continues to unfold, what remains most striking is not just its scale but its soul. It was never about building an organisation; it was about shaping a culture, a way of being in the world where presence is power, where quiet commitment outweighs performance, and where young people are not just participants in care, but co-creators of its meaning.

SIPC reminds us that systems can change when values are deeply lived, and that even the most complex challenges, like suffering, isolation, and grief, can be met with simple, sustained acts of humanity.

As this chapter closes, we are left not with a model to replicate, but with a question to carry: *What would it look like if every community trusted its young people to be part of the work of care?*

SIPC offers us a glimpse, tender, resilient, and radiant, of what becomes possible when compassion is decentralised, when joy is invited to sit beside grief, and when care becomes a shared, living practice.

The students may graduate. The seasons may change. But the echo of their care lingers, like the memory of balloons rising into the sky, carrying more than just air…carrying hope.

11

CARING COMMUNITY KÖLN, GERMANY

Raymond Voltz, Georg Bollig, Karin Ohler, Sabine Eichberg, Anne Kreische, Birgit Weihrauch, Julia Strupp and Kerstin Kremeike

Abstract

The Caring Community Köln (CCK) is part of a systematic approach in a city of more than 1 million inhabitants to improve death and grief literacy, both on the side of professionals as well as the citizens. This chapter outlines the overall Plan-Do-Study-Act cycle of the systematic approach and summarises the various ongoing interventions of which CCK is one. In detail, we will describe how CCK was set up, how its structure works, how we have gathered support and what topics the current working groups and projects are addressing. These include bereavement and last aid at the work, the innovative buddy intervention, projects in schools, death café and the care city map.

CCK also was a major factor why in the process of implementation of the National *Charter for the Care of the critically Ill and the Dying in Germany*, where this topic of caring communities was prioritised for 2024/2025, and Cologne was chosen as the place for the first separate congress of the German-speaking countries in November 2025 on this subject. This chapter will include the lessons learnt so far and conclusions we draw for future development of CCK.

11.1 Introduction – "If I had just known this before...": improving death and grief literacy is necessary

How often do we hear this quote, certainly around the globe, from patients and relatives when they finally encounter palliative and hospice care and then feel so supported. One could ask back: Why did *you not* know about this support structure before? Certainly, on the one hand, there is the issue of a healthcare service, which does not

DOI: 10.4324/9781003621348-12

communicate severe illness and prognosis openly enough. On the other hand, however, this corroborates with a population still lacking basic death and grief literacy.

In our city of Cologne, with more than 1 million inhabitants, we, facilitated by the local Department of Palliative Medicine, started with several health service research projects that were embedded in the establishment of Cologne as a model region for health and social services research [1]. In these projects we have, for example, asked patients, relatives and bereaved family caregiver about their experiences in the last year of life, or what was needed to enable dying at home [2].

Based on this data, we could then go one step further on this regional Plan-Do-Study-Act cycle by designing various interventions on the part of the healthcare system. For example, we looked at improving the initial conversation about serious prognosis through a MINI intervention (surprise question plus patient prompt sheets) [3] or sought improvement of care of the dying in our hospitals [4]. We also, based on the health services research data, established an innovative additional support service, we call it the buddy system, a combination of volunteer and professional buddies who will support patients and relatives earlier than palliative and hospice care would do [5].

However, we were very aware from the beginning that interventions only targeting the healthcare system would not be enough. It also needed interventions targeting the healthy population to increase their death and grief literacy, it needed a public health movement in Cologne, which we decided to call "Caring Community Köln" signalizing connection to the international movement. As to the decision of the term: this English term "caring" would be more appealing to Germans than "compassionate".

11.2 Insight No 1: it´s a marathon, no sprint

Back in 2018, after listening to a lecture by Allan Kellehear, we wrote a research proposal on a "Caring Community Köln". We came up with the first basic structures that would give this idea a sustainable future for a large city, i.e., setting up a round table, led by a steering group and supported by the city. We also established working groups on topics which were already very active in the city (see Figure 11.1). For this, we drew on ideas from external "critical friends", especially Prof. Werner Schneider, a German sociologist and Prof. Andreas Heller, an Austrian palliative care specialist with experience in similar Austrian projects. In addition, we collected "letters of intent" for the research proposal from several relevant interest holders in the city. When the proposal was rejected, we were very sad, but all the partners decided together to go ahead anyway; we had the ideas and the people and just started. So, even a rejected proposal may help a good idea move forward! Since then, seven years later, people have changed, and everything takes longer than initially thought, but the concept is still evolving up to this date, the right idea at the right time in the right city. So be prepared for a year-long process with ups and downs, many successes and repeated setbacks, which will probably never be completely finalised.

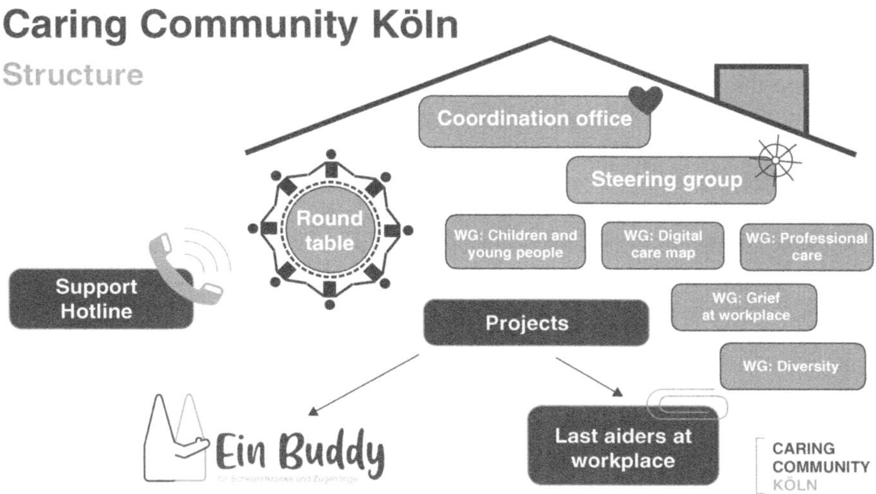

FIGURE 11.1 The Structure of Caring Community Köln

11.3 Insight No 2: political support by community is essential

When we approached the City of Cologne in 2018, we did so as the local professional palliative and hospice care network Köln (PHNK) that had been established more than ten years earlier. As municipal finances were (and still are) very tight, we "only" asked for political support of the idea, which was immediately taken up by our mayor and especially by the Head of Social Affairs, Dr Harald Rau, and all the three directors of the local health authority since 2018, Drs Bunte, Niessen and Denfeld. In 2018, the City Council, Health Committee, dealt with the subject of a CCK and expressed consent to the further development. The CCK was then officially launched by the mayor with an official kick-off in the ancient town hall in January 2020 (Corona then hit and slowed things down a bit). We have set up an annual workshop, hosted by the City of Cologne, on Care for the Severely Ill, for all relevant health and social care services in the city, and we are receiving massive hands-on help from two members of the health authority, e.g., in the steering group. So, a Caring Community initiative may start by the palliative and hospice movement, but as we want to reach all citizens, the political support of the city, responsible at the same time for many public services, is essential. This was also one of the main findings when we studied barriers and facilitators of setting up our CCK [6].

To emphasise its roots in the local palliative and hospice network (PHNK) and the support of the City of Cologne, we always mention both of them and refer to them as the initiators of the CCK.

As CCK is one of the longest-lasting in Germany, we receive many requests from other cities and regions in Germany on how to approach this topic.

Because of this growing national interest, our national consensus process on the "Charter for the Care of the critically Ill and the Dying in Germany" has taken up this issue for 2024/2025, and nationally consented recommendations on how to set up a Caring Community were published in 2025. The city of Cologne had already signed the Charter in 2013, and representatives of the CCK-Process were now engaged in preparing these recommendations. Furthermore, in November 2025, we hosted the first separate Caring Community congress of the German-speaking (Germany, Austria and German-speaking Switzerland) section of Public Health Palliative Care International in Cologne, with a follow-up planned in Austria in 2027.

11.4 Insight No 3: caring community goes beyond but also includes healthcare structures

As CCK, we set ourselves the following aims, to increase in the city of Cologne

1. Death and grief literacy for everybody
2. Knowledge about support structures in severe illness and the last year of life
3. Knowledge about grief and support structures
4. Death and grief literacy in health and social care structures

When in the compassionate cities′ movement the 95–5% time rule is cited, the focus, understandably, lies on the 95%; however, the 5% health and social care structures should not be forgotten in our initiatives. They often initiate and build a safety net for any compassionate/caring city/community. We therefore established as one of the initial working groups also one on health and social care structures (see Figure 11.1). Of course, there is overlap with the PHNK: while the PHNK coordinates the exchange among professional care structures in the city, the CCK activities aim at the citizens: e.g., How do they get more information about what is available? How can a rebalancing of care be supported by the patients and relatives themselves?

The question was, how to go beyond traditional healthcare structures: by working together on specific issues. We have done this by setting up various working groups with local experts. Particularly noteworthy are

1. The working group on grief in the workplace with various well-known Cologne companies such as banks and insurance companies, as well as the local Chamber of Crafts and the Chamber of Industry and Commerce,
2. The group on children and young people,
3. The Care City Plan working group,
4. The already mentioned group on health and social care structures,
5. The newly founded group on diversity.

Each working group has two spokespersons and proceeds according to the following steps:

1 What is the initial situation?
2 Where do we want to go? What goals are we pursuing?
3 What specific actions can we take to achieve our goals?
4 How can we implement our actions?

The working groups offer, for example, events, a film project, recommendations for action, questionnaires or literature lists that are open to the public.

The structure of our CCK-process is now as follows: a coordinating office, a steering group, a round table and various working groups in which people come together on a voluntary basis, except for the coordinating office. But we are also involved in large projects, such as

- The research project "Last Aid at the Workplace" as a sensitive approach to death and grief, which is anchored at the Department of Palliative Medicine at the Cologne University Hospital,
- The buddy project mentioned above or
- The counselling hotline on hospice and palliative care, offering information and advice to the citizens of Cologne.

The common goal is to strengthen society in dealing with serious illness, dying, death and grief.

11.5 Insight No 4: so many interest holders need coordination

Very quickly, the idea of a CCK attracted many institutions in the city; besides institutions representing health and social care, others represented public and school education, large companies, smaller businesses like undertakers. Mostly, it is individuals who are motivated to work together in CCK; however, for the working groups or as official representatives in the different CCK committees we ask them to get the mandate from their overarching organisation or institution, so that CCK gets a growing and sustainable representation within the society.

To handle all the correspondence, to organise the meetings and symposia as well as to keep the highly motivated people together and connected, of course this need coordination power [6]. Fortunately, right from the official beginning in 2020, two main Cologne foundations have given us financial support for such a position, namely the Imhoff and Familie Ernst Wendt foundations. We are most grateful to them for their visionary support!

Of course, support by foundations is mainly focused on finite projects, so we are currently in the process of developing CCK from an informal project into a sustainable, formal structure. In the German system, the first step was to establish a non-governmental organisation ("eingetragener Verein") so that every single citizen of Cologne and Cologne institutions may become an official member of CCK and by this become part of the process within the urban society. To handle larger projects in a more flexible way, however, we have also set up a non-profit limited liability association ("gemeinnützige Gesellschaft mit beschränkter Haftung, gGmbH"). This will allow us to manage larger projects that previously had to be organised in indirect ways.

11.6 Insight No 5: take advantage of regional specifics

Especially as we had chosen an English term for our CCK, we felt it was very important to make a connection with Cologne´s particularities. So, we chose the colloquial "Förenander do" as a subheading to CCK, which means "to be there for each other" in Kölsch, the local dialect. In addition to football, and this may be an advantage over other cities in Germany, Cologne has a very deep-routed carnival tradition. In addition to spring, summer, autumn and winter, Cologne has a fifth season, carnival, including specific well-known music groups and traditional and modern carnival songs that everyone in Cologne knows and sings along to. What many people do not recognise is that many songs remind us of our finiteness, with a hidden Cologne "memento mori". For example, when the very popular music group Kasalla sings "Alle Jläser hu" ("lift up all glasses"), it is NOT a traditional drinking song but the singer's way of honouring his father who had died suddenly. In this way, we try to build bridges to the carnival to address and reach people in a way they understand and by this increase people's skills in dealing with serious illness, dying, death and grief. The current head of the Cologne carnival is a well-known undertaker. So, enjoying life in the face of one´s own mortality seems to be deeply rooted in Cologne culture, and CCK can build on this tradition.

11.7 Insight No 6: use a (visual) language which does not scare people away

Probably also building on this specific death-accepting spirit, Cologne has a long-standing palliative and hospice tradition. In 1984, Germany´s first palliative care unit was established at Cologne University Hospital (at that time within surgery!), and in 1986/1987 the first three in-patient hospices for Germany were founded in Aachen, Recklinghausen and Cologne (all three close together in the Rhineland/Westfalen area). CCK therefore can build on that tradition of well-established hospice and palliative care. Having said that, in the meantime also across Germany, hospice and palliative care are well-established structures in the healthcare system and well known to basically everybody. However, the terms hospice and palliative are, obviously, associated primarily with death and dying,

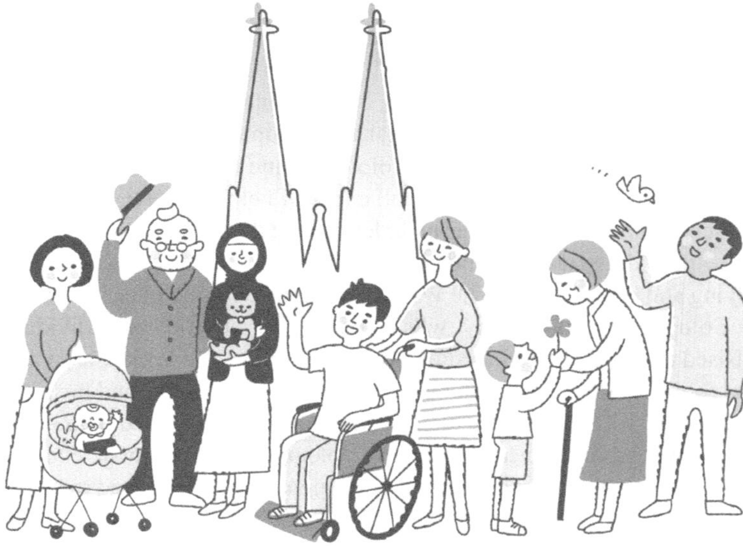

FIGURE 11.2 Visual Language of Caring Community Köln

and so many, especially healthy people shy away. It is a healthy reaction not to talk about death, dying and bereavement, until needed, but that makes improving death and grief literacy across the population a challenge. Basically, we must work against human psychology!

We therefore feel that we need to use innovative terminology to reach those in society who have not yet been reached by hospice activities so far. This includes novel terms such as CCK, or buddy, or last aid, and also a visual language that differs from the usual palliative and hospice colours and designs (see Figure 11.2).

11.8 Insight No 7: combine top-down with bottom-up – participation through action

CCK was initiated as a "top-down" project with a round table established under the leadership of the City of Cologne and the PHNK, supported by a steering group (see Figure 11.1) [7]. This steering group approached local organisations representing various aspects of society, calling in further participants if this was considered helpful. At the round table, currently 35 organisations from very different parts of the urban society are represented, including health insurance companies or the Cologne Chamber of Crafts. It is intended as a permanent institution to exchange experiences and discuss new approaches and stand for the participation of urban society. The two initiators, the City of Cologne Health Department and the PHNK, play a special role in the round table. We believe that this "top-down" structure, which also involves the City of Cologne, is necessary to establish a sustainable change, especially for such a large city.

However, when it came to deciding on the contents of the working groups, we opted for a "bottom-up" approach, taking up topics (and experts) where there had already been projects ongoing in Cologne, some of them for a long time. For example, the WG "Children and Youth" expands help for bereaved children and existing school projects. The latter includes project days at primary and secondary schools to provide space for guided discussions on the topics of serious illness, death/dying and bereavement. The WG "Grief at the working place" started around a large Cologne-based company, which, on the initiative of an individual, took action based on the results of a company-wide survey. The WG "Care City Map" based its further actions on an established database of palliative and hospice facilities. Finally, the WG "Care Structures" coordinates actions based on the results of a large research project, "last year of life, Cologne" [8]. Of course, challenges of cooperation, transparency and citizen involvement remain and need to be reflected on constantly [6].

Despite this combination of a top-down and bottom-up approach, we feel that there is still a long way to go to really see changes at the level of every citizen. However, we have noticed that things start to change concretely when action is initiated jointly, the understanding of dying as a relational process is strengthened and all relevant parties are involved in a resource-oriented way [9].

For example, we have attracted three years' finances by the German TV lottery for an innovative "buddy" support for patients with severe illness who at this stage would however refrain from palliative or hospice support. This "buddy", the idea of which is again based on research [5], will offer both low-level psychosocial support through a volunteer "buddy" and institutional support through a professional "buddy", the "buddy" as Caring Community in person coming to you when you are in need. In setting up this project, we can already see that a participatory approach to this action project resonates very well both in the participating institutions as well as on social media level, where we are planning a crowdfunding and participatory concept change campaign. Therefore, participation through action is probably the best way to achieve our common goal.

In conclusion, increasing death literacy in your community is indeed possible. However, it takes time.

In Cologne, we were fortunate to be able to build on a research network and a care network. In addition, there were already many initiatives in the community, and the City of Cologne Health Department was very open to the topic. So, it's always worth looking at what's already out there and then connecting the dots.

Working on concrete projects in a combined top-down-bottom-up setting is a realistic way to achieve this goal [7]. It is an endeavour that is worthwhile and of great importance and fun, as it brings the community together on topics that are so human and close to everyone. It is worth the energy!

References

1. Karbach U, Ansmann L, Scholten N, Pfaff H, Albus C, Jessen F, Kuntz L, Rietz C, Schubert I, Schulz-Nieswandt F, Stock S, Strupp J, Voltz R. (2017). Bericht aus einem laufenden Forschungsprojekt: CoRe-Net, das Kölner Kompetenznetzwerk aus Versorgungspraxis und Versorgungsforschung und der Value-based Healthcare-Ansatz. *Zeitschrift für Evidenz, Fortbildung und Qualität im Gesundheitswesen, 130*, 21–26. https://doi.org/10.1016/j.zefq.2017.11.005
2. Kasdorf A, Voltz R, Strupp J. (2024). Dying at home: What is needed? Findings from a nationwide retrospective cross-sectional online survey of bereaved people in Germany. *Palliative Support Care.* 1–9. Advance online publication. https://doi.org/10.1017/S1478951524000440
3. Strupp J, Kasdorf A, Dust G, Hower KI, Seibert M, Werner B, Kuntz L, Schulz-Nieswandt F, Meyer I, Pfaff H, Hellmich M, Voltz R. (2021). CoRe-Net. Last Year of Life Study-Cologne (LYOL-C) (Part II): Study protocol of a prospective interventional mixed-methods study in acute hospitals to analyse the implementation of a trigger question and patient question prompt sheets to optimise patient-centred care. *BMJ Open, 11*(7), e048681. https://doi.org/10.1136/bmjopen-2021-048681
4. Kremeike K, Ullrich A, Schulz H, Rosendahl C, Boström K, Kaur S, Oubaid N, Plathe-Ignatz C, Leminski C, Hower K, Pfaff H, Hellmich M, Oechsle K, Voltz R. (2022). Dying in hospital in Germany - optimising care in the dying phase: Study protocol for a multi-centre bottom-up intervention on ward level. *BMC Palliative Care, 21*(1), 67. https://doi.org/10.1186/s12904-022-00960-1
5. Kasdorf A, Voltz R, Strupp J. (2024). The Buddy intervention: Designing an additional support system for the last year of life. Qualitative insights from triangulated interviews and focus group discussions. *Journal of Public Health, 32*(10), 2001–2013. https://doi.org/10.1007/s10389-023-01950-0
6. Meesters S, Ohler K, Voltz R, Schulz-Nieswandt F, Eichberg S, Strupp J, Kremeike K. (2024). How can a community be successfully empowered to deal with death, dying, and bereavement? *Annals of Palliative Medicine, 13*(4), 778–779. https://doi.org/10.21037/apm-23-598
7. Voltz R, Meesters S, Ohler K, Weihrauch B, Kreische A, Niessen J, Heller A, Strupp J, Kremeike K. (2024). Top-down and bottom-up or participation through action? How to build a compassionate community - the experience of Caring Community Cologne. *Palliative Care and Sociale Practice, 18*, 26323524241238230. https://doi.org/10.1177/26323524241238230
8. Voltz R, Strupp J, Ditscheid B, Schippel N, Dust G, Rietz C, Stock S. (2020). Improving regional care in the last year of life by setting up a pragmatic evidence-based Plan–Do–Study–Act cycle: Results from a cross-sectional survey. *BMJ Open, 10*(11), e035988. https://doi.org/10.1136/bmjopen-2019-035988
9. Sallnow L, Smith R, Ahmedzai S.H., et al. (2022). Report of the Lancet Commission on the Value of Death: Bringing death back into life. *The Lancet, 399*(10327), 837–884. https://doi.org/10.1016/S0140-6736(21)02314-X

12

TALKING ABOUT THE INEVITABLE

Community-led change in end-of-life conversations from Northern Ireland

Jenny Marshall

Abstract

This chapter shares the story of Mid & East Antrim Agewell Partnership (Agewell) a small charity based in Ballymena, Northern Ireland. It provides support to older people living in the wider Mid and East Antrim area using an assets-based community development approach to improve health outcomes through a variety of health interventions, which help older people feel better physically, better emotionally and be better connected.

The key to Agewell's success is its focus on partnership working, which brings together key stakeholders including the community and voluntary sector, statutory bodies, the private sector and, most importantly, older people themselves, harnessing lived experience for a true co-production model. This collaborative working model doesn't just help with everyday health and well-being; it also uses the power of local communities, to facilitate a safe and welcoming space for discussion around challenging subjects such as death and dying.

12.1 Mars Bar & Apple Sandwiches and other stories

12.1.1 Building compassion through culture, connection and conversation in Northern Ireland

Mars Bar & Apple Sandwiches is a storytelling project delivered by Agewell, which uses food and storytelling alongside end-of-life and funeral traditions to spark conversation about death and difference. Against a fractured backdrop of sectarian division in Northern Ireland, this book has brought together voices from

DOI: 10.4324/9781003621348-13

a wide range of cultural and religious backgrounds to explore how we mourn and grieve, and how we connect with each other at the end of life. With recurring themes of honesty, humour and heritage, the initiative has shown how death can bring together communities from different backgrounds and inspire compassion, regardless of what background or religion someone comes from.

12.2 Northern Ireland: a fractured backdrop

Mid and East Antrim is a predominantly rural area in Northern Ireland shaped by the legacy of the Troubles, where social divides, often alongside religious and cultural lines, still influence community dynamics at a local level. For many, especially, older adults, death has been a part of daily life, yet also a subject wrapped in silence, taboo or tradition particularly in the picture of the divided Protestant and Catholic communities of Northern Ireland.

Amid these tensions, Agewell, as a local charity, which supports older people, sought a new way to bring communities together: through storytelling, shared experience and one unforgettable sandwich.

12.3 Origins: a Sandwich sparks a story

It all started with a laugh. During a light-hearted community discussion about funerals at a local older people's community group in Larne, someone quipped,

> You know you're at a Presbyterian funeral when you get Mars Bar and apple sandwiches!

That offhand remark, half-joke and half-truth, sparked a wave of laughter and recognition. Suddenly, from around the room, memories were shared: stories of wakes, traditions, quiet rituals and superstitions. From that moment, a unique idea took root, a community-authored book exploring death and traditions, supported by the Mid & East Antrim Borough Council's Community Relations Fund and working in partnership with Mid & East Antrim Inter Ethnic Forum.

The goal was simple: to use storytelling as a gentle way to explore differences in grief, end-of-life, death and everything beyond for those who believe in an existence after death.

The Mars Bar & Apple Sandwich itself may not be traditional, but for many in the Presbyterian community, it holds a fond place at funeral teas. Quietly beloved, especially by children, it was rarely seen outside solemn or special occasions, making its appearance feel both meaningful and special.

The recipe is as strange as it is memorable: slices of sickly-sweet Mars Bar – a chocolate bar with nougat and caramel coating, the ultimate childhood indulgence, paired with sharp green Granny Smith apple, layered between soft wholemeal bread thickly spread with real Irish butter. An unlikely combination, yet somehow it worked: sweet and sharp and just a little bit naughty!

Always made with care, the sandwiches were cut into neat fingers or dainty triangles, their presentation reflecting the reverence of the occasion. And for those who remember them, the taste brings back more than just flavour; it evokes hushed conversations, warm kitchens and the quiet closeness that follows a final goodbye.

12.4 Activities: writing, remembering and reconnecting

12.4.1 Community story collection

Facilitated by Agewell and working in partnership with the local ethnic minority charity – Mid & East Antrim Inter Ethnic Forum, older people were invited to share memories of funerals and end-of-life traditions. Contributions ranged from childhood memories of attending Irish wakes in rural County Tyrone to Hindu cremation ceremonies and Polish Catholic customs.

As part of the initiative, one woman recalled her childhood memories of attending a traditional Irish wake:

> My Granny died at home, and Granny Mulryan from the community came to wash her body. She had a suitcase with everything needed. Rosary beads were threaded through her hands, and a veil was placed over her face. You'd lift the veil to kiss her goodbye, on the face or hands, not something we'd have the wains do now!

12.4.2 Cultural exchange

Stories were collected from Older People from a variety of backgrounds stretching across the globe, including from the Hindu Culture.

> "In Hindu Culture, a Hindu priest and senior family members conduct the cremation ceremony ('mukhagni'). Various death rituals are carried out with family & friends prior to the cremation. These include:
>
> - Washing the body with ghee, honey, milk, and yoghurt
> - Placing essential oils on the head of the deceased (turmeric for females, sandalwood for males)
> - Placing the palms in a position of prayer and tying the big toes together
> - Dressing the deceased's body in smart clothes (contemporary) or wrapping it in a white sheet (traditional)
> - Placing a garland of flowers and 'pinda' (rice balls) around their loved ones
> - Putting a lamp near the head or sprinkling water on the body"

12.4.3 Humour, humanity and the unexpected

Amid solemn traditions were tales of comic chaos. One woman remembered a humorous experience:

> At one of my aunt's wakes, Granny Mulyryan washed her body and gave the dish of water to someone to throw out. For some reason they thought it was a good idea to empty it into the sink that the good cups and saucers were being washed in! What an uproar that caused!

Another shared:

> I can remember my Daddy saying that as a boy him and his friends always sneaked into wakes to get the free cigarettes that were sitting out in all the rooms and that corpses when he was young had old pennies covering their eyes (possibly as a means of holding the eyes closed)

Stories like these helped humanise the grieving process, offering space for both reverence and release.

12.4.4 Outcomes: what changed?

Although not formally evaluated, the project had strong anecdotal impact in several key areas:

For many participants, this was the first time they had openly shared funeral memories or talked about death.

> Being able to record my experiences of losing my parents before and during the Covid pandemic in Mars Bar and Apple Sandwiches meant that somehow my mother's death was recognised, especially when we hadn't been able to have a proper funeral for her, when we had been able to pay that tribute for Dad, just six months beforehand. It meant a lot to me and my brothers and sisters.

The book illuminated surprising overlaps between cultures, like covering mirrors or stopping clocks. As one participant put it:

> Turns out, Polish and Jewish people cover mirrors too. We're not as different as we thought.

This built empathy across divides, especially in a region still navigating sectarian separation.

For isolated older adults, the project was more than a book, it was a chance to connect. They were listened to, laughed with and lifted up as keepers of cultural knowledge. One participant commented

> Reading the stories of others experiences of end-of-life, helped me to feel less alone in the world.

12.4.5 Conclusion

In a country shaped by difference and division, *Mars Bar and Apple Sandwiches and Other Stories* reminded people that regardless of our religion, background, race or class, we will share the same fate in that someday we will die.

Through stories both sacred and silly, the project showed how compassion can start with something as small as a sandwich and grow into something that helps entire communities face death, and life, with more honesty and humanity. As one participant summed up:

> My wish to be cremated is my last hope for a smoking hot body!

A strong reminder that even in death, humour can light the way.

12.5 Northern Ireland's First Funeral Festival

12.5.1 Building courage through conversation

In the autumn of 2022, something quietly significant happened in Ballymena. Agewell, opened the doors to Northern Ireland's first-ever Funeral Festival, a forward-thinking and brave event, that invited local communities to come together and talk openly and safely about death and dying. It was an event which answered several questions that many people for a long time felt they could not ask.

The event encompassed a warm buzzing atmosphere of chatter, laughter and the sound of questions being asked and long sought-after answers provided. It was a turning point in which suddenly those in attendance felt safe to explore their own views, thoughts and expectations around death and dying.

12.5.2 Activities

The idea was simple in its creation; it was about bringing professionals from the end-of-life industry together to create a safe and welcoming space for people to be curious, to ask questions and to encourage the normalisation of talking about death and dying.

Inside the Ballymena venue, the atmosphere felt more like a wedding fair than anything death-related. Rows of stalls offered information and examples of everything from traditional oak coffins to biodegradable willow caskets and ashes turned into glass jewellery. Local Funeral Directors chatted over tea with visitors and answered questions. Florists demonstrated farewell arrangements bursting with colour and meaningful symbolism. Local solicitors quietly guided people through wills and power of attorney. Palliative Care Nurses spoke gently but practically about comfort, dignity and choice at the end-of-life.

A recent addition to the local landscape was a new Crematorium built by the neighbouring Antrim and Newtownabbey Borough Council. As only one of two crematoriums across the region of Northern Ireland, the staff team were inundated with questions and curiosity about the cremation process and how residents of the Mid and East Antrim area could access the facilities when needed.

Northern Ireland Humanists, part of the wider Humanists UK organisation, highlighted the option of non-religious ceremonies and the increasing interest and appetite in Northern Ireland for this type of ceremony to celebrate lives lived and their legacies left behind. Their presence demonstrated just how many people and organisations are dedicated to supporting individuals and families through the end-of-life journey.

What was most poignant about the event was that there were no whispers. No hushed conversations under the dark cloak of taboo and no over-the-shoulder looks of shame at the prospect of talking about death. There were open conversations, warmth and sprinklings of laughter. One participant commented:

> I had no idea what to expect but it was so relaxed and comfortable, everyone was chatting and laughing, not at all scary or negative. It was great to have the opportunity to actually see and touch the coffins, and now I have a clear idea of what I would like and what I wouldn't like for my own funeral. Once I have my plans in place, I will have peace of mind knowing that my family's burden will be lightened as I will have made the majority of difficult decisions for them. It has also given me the confidence to make an appointment with my local solicitor to organise my will and power of attorney.

Within the room, there was an air of warmth and tranquillity. The professionals around the room facilitated a sense of understanding, which allowed people to ask the questions that they wouldn't normally feel they could ask.

Whilst keen to challenge the taboo, Agewell also recognised that the subject of death can often be upsetting and at times a trigger for grief. Therefore, it was important to the team that a safe space was provided with professional support on hand for anyone who felt overwhelmed. This was facilitated by Agewells' counselling partner, Selina Allen at Lead Counselling, Carrickfergus. Selina was on hand throughout the day with tea, compassion and emotional support where required.

12.5.3 Outcome: what changed?

The public response revealed just how important a safe space such as this was needed. For many attendees, it was the first time they had ever spoken openly about their own funeral wishes or touched a coffin in real life! One woman admitted she had expected something sombre, even morbid, but instead found empowerment. The relaxed, wedding fair-like atmosphere, with laughter, conversation and hands-on exploration of coffins and music choices, allowed her to touch a willow coffin and realise what felt right for her.

Individuals returned home and began conversations with families and friends that had been long postponed. Some wrote down their funeral music choices, others made legal plans and many expressed relief, an unexpected emotion to come from a festival about death.

The festival changed the narrative around death and became a topic for community discussion rather than hushed whispers; planning ahead became an act of care and empowerment rather than a morbid obsession and funeral choices became expressions of identity rather than hastily made decisions by a grief-stricken family. In Northern Ireland, the timeline between death and a funeral is a short one, with funerals normally taking place only two or three days after death. This means that in an incredibly short period of time, a family must make several important decisions about their loved ones wishes including burial or cremation, a religious or non-religious service, music, flowers, readings, type of coffin, and casket or urn. All these decisions are also entangled with overwhelming feelings of grief and often stress due to the organisation of family and friends travelling home from abroad to attend the funeral. Events such as Agewells Funeral Festival provided the much-needed prompt and opportunity to encourage individuals to write their wishes down and take some of the pressure off their families for when that inevitable time comes.

12.5.4 Conclusion

The Funeral Festival didn't glorify death or showcase morbidity; it gave people a voice in what their life might look like at the end, how they will be remembered and what legacy they might leave. It proved that with openness, honesty and compassion, we can facilitate end-of-life conversations that can feel natural, soft and part of our every day.

With a safe, warm and comforting environment, Agewell provided a spark which has been the catalyst for future conversations and projects which continue to challenge the narrative about the subject of death being taboo.

12.6 The dying art of conversations

12.6.1 Using creativity to speak the unspeakable

The Dying Art of Conversations began with a simple but bold idea: to carve out space for the conversations we avoid the most. Funded by the Arts Council of

Northern Ireland in partnership with The National Lottery Community Fund and The Baring Foundation, and delivered by Agewell, the project invited older people in local communities to explore life, death and legacy, not through formal methods, but through creativity and social connection.

In a society where death often remains unspoken, the project offered an alternative. Using art as vessel, the use of creativity opened up conversations that previously had been locked away for fear of stigma or superstition that talking about death would somehow speed up its inevitability.

12.6.2 Activities

The journey began with curiosity. When Agewell called for local community groups and care homes to take part, six groups stepped forward each unsure of what was to come, yet willing to try. To guide them through such sensitive territory, Agewell partnered with Arts Care NI to recruit three pairs of professional artists. Each artist worked with one community group and one care home, weaving creativity and conversation together across the lifespan of the project. Each group experienced a different art form, and each found its own path into difficult but meaningful conversations.

12.6.3 Music: memory in *melody*

For two groups, it began with song. Participants brought in favourite tunes, hymns from childhood, school assembly chants, rebel ballads whispered at céilís and love songs danced to in earlier years of youth. Each song was a story that helped unfold memories. Together, groups wrote their own songs, pieces that held not only their words but their lives, bringing them together in shared experience where it felt safe to open this challenging but significant conversation.

12.6.4 Movement: the dance of life

Another two groups explored life through movement. Drawing inspiration from the quiet wisdom of a tree, from seed to root to full bloom, they began to explore the idea that life, like nature, moves in seasons. There was no need for words as participants used gesture and movement to express their feelings. Their journey culminated in a collective performance set to 'What a Wonderful World', a tribute not to life coming to an end, but to the memory of a life that had been lived to the fullest and everything that entailed.

12.6.5 Visual art: stories in *colour*

The final two groups picked up brushes, scissors and ink. In one group, participants created a series of framed artworks inspired by the four seasons, each piece a vision of life's story. In another, a local bridge became a metaphor for the journey of life, its three arches symbolising childhood, adulthood and the final crossing. One step at a time, memories were collaged into place, ticket stubs, pressed petals, old photographs, fragments of conversations and the unspoken weight of goodbye. Just as important as the art forms themselves were the conversation over tea breaks that opened feelings, memories and plans for what end-of-life might look like for each of them.

12.6.6 Outcome: what changed?

At first, there was hesitation. Death had long been a topic participants were taught not to discuss. "Keep it to yourself", some recalled being told. "No sense in upsetting people", said others. But as the sessions took place, the participants relaxed into an easy relationship with each other and an unspoken agreement that this was a safe space to express how they felt about the journey we call life.

One woman shared that she had previously tried to talk to her children about her wishes, only to be met with resistance. By the end of the programme, she had not only held the conversation but also written a will. *Now they won't have to guess,* she reflected. Others discovered strength and identity in unexpected ways. At the final celebration, participants saw their creativity come to life, painting, poetry, storytelling and performance revealed talents they hadn't acknowledged in years. A quiet resident from one of the local care homes, previously non-verbal and withdrawn, expressed herself through art, surprising staff who learned she had once been a secondary school art teacher. This project didn't just allow expression; it helped participants be seen, recognised and valued.

By the final session, death was no longer a subject for discussion behind closed doors. It became part of normal, everyday conversation. Participants returned to families and loved ones having started long-avoided conversations, wrote down their wishes, chose music and flowers. Using art as a vessel for discussion around life's journey left them feeling empowered to make these decisions and be prepared by communicating them with those who needed to know.

12.6.7 Conclusion

The Dying Art of Conversations proved that when approached with compassion, creativity and courage, conversations about death don't diminish life, they deepen it. Through art, the participants stepped into important conversations. They left the project not afraid but empowered and connected to make decisions about how they would like the end of their life to look.

There is no doubt that death is a challenging and difficult subject, but this project demonstrated that with compassion and creativity, it is amazing how we can support people to dip their toes into the conversations that really matter.

12.7 Reflections

The role that community organisations such as Agewell play in conversations about death and dying is paramount to creating a world where death is not a forbidden subject. Within local communities, there is an opportunity to create a safe space, which offers warmth, compassion and understanding about a subject that undeniably and unapologetically affects everyone, no matter what age, gender, race or religion. Whilst there is still some way to go in making death an everyday subject, communities have an opportunity to use creativity, curiosity and compassion to open these discussions and pave the way for a future where conversations about death and dying are as normal as talking about the weather.

13

THE COMPASSIONATE OTTAWA STORY

Monica Patten and Jim Nininger

Abstract

Compassionate Ottawa (CO) is a community model of caring established in November 2016 at a gathering of community leaders who enthusiastically agreed that caring for one another at times of life-threatening illness is everyone's responsibility.

Word spread of the new initiative quickly, and before long, over 80 individuals volunteered to become involved in building the new organisation. Workshops were held to create a vision, mission, and infrastructure to support the volunteer-led organisation. Initial teams were created to develop programming to offer workshops in Advance Care Planning and Grief and Bereavement in both French and English.

An advisory council consisting of healthcare providers, social service agencies, and academics was created to offer guidance and support. This proved to be invaluable. To be eligible for government grants, a not-for-profit legal entity was created along with a board of directors.

Over time, new programmes were added to our offerings, along with enhanced infrastructure, including an evaluation framework and relationships with faith communities, schools, and public health agencies. A major research project called HELP (Healthy End-of-life Project) and funded by a local foundation was launched in association with Carleton University.

The pandemic forced us to change course. We offered our workshops virtually and introduced a new online webinar called Conversations with Leaders. As soon as we could return to in-person events, we hosted a city-wide celebration to honour those who had died and to mark the return to more normal community life.

DOI: 10.4324/9781003621348-14

Today, we work both online and virtually. Almost all our activity is undertaken with a partner, including some within healthcare providers. Our focus on diverse communities is an asset in a city made up of residents from around the world who have chosen Canada as a place to live.

CO has earned respect and recognition throughout the community. While we are ever conscious of the challenge of financial and organisational sustainability, we remain confident that our work is contributing to the capacity of citizens to be more compassionate.

13.1 Introduction – our story

The capital city of Canada, Ottawa's population is just over 1,000,000. A city of great diversity, Ottawa is a bilingually French and English city and welcomes many newcomers from around the world each year. While the government is its main employer, education, health care, and high tech are also prominent. And like many other places, Ottawa, with its rivers and hills nearby, attracts many older adults.

Our story covers the period from November 2016 to the fall of 2025 and describes how our initiative evolved over this period.

13.1.1 Part 1: 2016–2019

13.1.1.1 Initial exploration

A small number of community leaders developed an interest in end-of-life care from a community perspective and met several times to explore the topic of compassionate communities and community development. These discussions were informed by the writing of Dr. Allan Kellehear, and his focus on the role of the community in end-of-life care. Discussions were held with health providers to get their perspective on the role of the community, which was very supportive.

This initial exploration led to the decision to hold a community round table in November 2016 to discuss the idea of Ottawa becoming a compassionate community for end-of-life care. In total, 45 community leaders attended this meeting, which resulted in very positive support for launching a community development initiative.

Following this very positive outcome, the small leadership group spent the next few months meeting with a wide range of community organisations and health providers to further test interest and support. The result of this work was the sense that there was a real gap around community support for those facing life-threatening illness.

A second community workshop was held in May 2017, which drew 85 participants. The aim of this meeting was to develop a vision, mission, and initial programme priorities for a new organisation. It was clear that the support for a community-led initiative was growing.

13.1.1.2 Creating structure for the new organisation

A small steering committee was created to provide guidance for the next stage of development. This included working with volunteers to create the following.

13.1.1.2.1 Our vision for Ottawa

A CO supports and empowers individuals at any age, their families, and their communities to live well and to die and grieve well. Note that this was our vision for Ottawa and not our organisation.

13.1.1.2.2 The mission of Compassionate Ottawa

CO is a movement that builds the capacity of the citizens of Ottawa to be more capable and confident of helping themselves, their families, and their communities to live well and to die and grieve well.

Our goals are to

1. Change attitudes and behaviour. Change the way we think about dying and death so that we can be better prepared and thus improve our quality of life. Encourage individuals to prepare their end-of-life wishes and communicate these to their families and others.
2. Educate, support, and empower. Engage Ottawa's many and diverse communities and provide support as they develop their own approaches to becoming compassionate communities. Develop a shared understanding in the broad community of the need to work together to help Ottawa become a compassionate community.
3. Engage community partners. Work with partner organisations with common interests to increase the impact of our collective work. Engage with health providers, social organisations, and other community partners to enhance connections and reduce isolation.

Our values

1. We believe in supporting each other in times of serious illness and loss and are generous in both giving and receiving.
2. Living well and dying well. We accept death as part of the continuum of life and human experience and believe that it is possible for each person to live fully in their situation and die comfortably.
3. Leadership in an engaged community. We embrace volunteerism and service to individuals, groups, and communities.
4. Building on evidence. We take guidance from research and empirical knowledge, learning from wisdom and experience in the community.

5 Collaboration. We are relationship-based, working in partnership to build communities and networks.
6 Inclusion. We are dedicated to equity, diversity, and inclusion, and through all our work will contribute to dismantling the systemic oppression, racism and exclusion of all groups that experience discrimination.

13.1.1.3 Compassionate Ottawa programme activities

We have several programme activities we offer to the Ottawa community. They include our workshops in ACP and Grief and Bereavement. These are our largest offerings and are conducted in English and French. We were very fortunate in attracting several volunteers who wished to become facilitators. One, a registered nurse, had led the development of a national ACP programme for a government-funded agency and she became our lead in overseeing the growth of our community offerings. Another retired nurse had extensive experience in grief and bereavement facilitation, and she played a key role in overseeing our workshops in this area.

13.1.1.3.1 Healthy End-of-life Project

This CO-sponsored three-year initiative was designed to create a collaborative end-of-life culture. Based on the successful approach at La Trobe University (Melbourne, Australia), the project was located in Carleton University and engaged two faith sites and two community health centre sites. Its goal was to strengthen links between people who are frail, living with serious illness, experiencing grief, or acting as caregivers and to mobilise and prepare community members to be capable and confident in offering and providing help. Numerous resources were created through HELP.

13.1.1.3.2 Let's Talk about Later Life

Another project, Let's Talk about Later Life, was funded by the Canadian Frailty Network and consisted of four components. These are described on our website under the heading Resources and include a short video, a handbook describing our journey, a discussion guide, a book chat guide, and a series of digital stories describing the experiences of seven storytellers giving and receiving help.

13.1.1.4 CO infrastructure activities

We created several initiatives to help us build a strong organisation. One such initiative was our evaluation model. A team of volunteers with an interest in research created an evaluation model to help us focus on the results of our work. This logic model requires us to focus on outcome measures, both short and long term. Other infrastructure work initiatives involved volunteer engagement, financial sustainability, marketing and communications, governance and leadership, and building partnerships. It was a challenge keeping an eye on these important internal projects given the demands on a small staff of two excellent professionals.

13.1.1.5 Some initial lessons

After three years of activity, we decided to spend some time reflecting on our experiences and what we had learned to that point in time. We sought the advice of some of our volunteers with extensive experience in community change management. We thought it would be helpful to share these lessons at this point in our story.

Keep in mind that there are several ways of structuring a compassionate community initiative. A lot will depend on those involved in establishing the initiative. Some initiatives are created in association with residential hospices, and there are a variety of such initiatives in Canada. Others are affiliated with hospitals. As well in Canada, several provinces have sponsored the establishment of compassionate communities. There is no one right way of doing this. CO, however, was developed as a community-wide, volunteer initiative without affiliation with another organisation. This was not based on a preconceived plan but evolved as we progressed with our development. From our experience, there are fewer of these types of compassionate communities in Canada.

13.1.1.5.1 Lesson 1

Why create a compassionate community? The focus that initially brought several of our volunteers together was the unfortunate state of palliative care in Canada, and the heartbreaking impact this has had on the experiences of many dying Canadians and their families. The need to improve people's experience at the end-of-life was supported by published studies, the work of several associations, conversations with palliative care physicians, and researchers. It was clear that palliative care was inadequate in three areas: access to services, the equity of access to these services, and the quality of care.

We learned from healthcare providers that they could not deal with these issues alone. As we look back, we can see how real the need was when we came together in 2016. This need has been exacerbated by the ageing of the population on the one hand and by the pandemic on the other. The impact of the pandemic on long-term care homes and other vulnerable populations has been devastating.

Our work has also led us to better understand the importance of living well as we age. One of our volunteers described it this way:

> How do we live as long as we can as well as we can with the supports in the community that can make this happen?

Our work in understanding the role of the community has been greatly enhanced by Professor Allan Kellehear who has written extensively on the subject.

13.1.1.5.2 Lesson 2

We found that there are several important factors that had an impact on engaging the community and developing support for the initiative. One is developing an inspiring vision and mission. We spent a lot of time on this, as volunteers had quite different ideas on our role and work. We held a large community forum where 85 volunteers discussed this critical matter. The effort was worth the labour as we reached a strong commitment to our vision and mission.

Another factor is the readiness of the community to embark on such an initiative. Some of us desire to move quickly, but the pace of movement needs to be tempered when working with the schedules and priorities of volunteers and desired partner organisations.

13.1.1.5.3 Lesson 3

Developing a compassionate community needs to be viewed as a long-term journey. Compassionate communities need to be rooted in community development principles and practices, the understanding of end-of-life as a public health issue, and a social model of caring. Raising awareness, let alone changing attitudes in a city of 1 million citizens, is no small task. Some experts talk about such an undertaking as taking at least a decade or more.

13.1.2 Part 2: 2020–2025

13.1.2.1 The pandemic hiccup

Perhaps more than a hiccup, the pandemic forced us to pivot dramatically in both our thinking and our action. We knew that the cry for compassion would build as people, including those experiencing serious illness or living with grief or as caregivers, faced isolation and anxiety. We also knew that we could not continue to hold workshops in person, and that the availability of volunteers would decline as they too were faced with illness or deep worry. A quickly created Rapid Response Team developed ideas to help us continue offering support and encouraging others to as well. A newspaper story stressing the importance of caring for each other in this time of stress was helpful. So too was the redesign of our workshops for virtual delivery and to include references to the distress created by the pandemic.

And, perhaps most importantly, we introduced Conversations with Leaders, which involves our volunteers virtually interviewing local, national, and international experts on a field related to compassion. These forums, which are broadcast internationally, bring leading-edge experiences to our community.

The impacts of the pandemic were several. Our workshop offerings thrived and indeed we learned how valuable they were to many during this stressful time. Conversations with Leaders was an immediate success as people could listen and learn from their homes. It continues today to attract significant audiences who provide positive and helpful feedback. In fact, each forum attracts about 500 viewers, combining those who attend live and those who watch later, on YouTube.

Towards the end of the pandemic, we began to plan for a city-wide event to bring people together after the long period of isolation, to honour those who had died, reflect on our shared experience, and anticipate a more hopeful future. In spring and summer of 2022, we hosted Together Ottawa Ensemble (TOE).

Over 30 groups participated in TOE, welcoming people of all ages to activities as diverse as picnics, a stroll through a cemetery, a musical evening in a park, or a specific cultural community centre event. While there were many learnings for CO from hosting this event, one stood out: our inclination to do our work in partnership was proven to be right on. Our current partnerships are described in the following sections.

But it would be incomplete to leave the effects of the pandemic without describing the more concerning ones. Some volunteers who had been with us since the start of CO moved on to other interests. Some volunteers stayed with us but did not want to do in-person workshops. New volunteers were harder to find, a challenge shared by many in the community sector. Our attempts to host in-person events for volunteers were largely unsuccessful. Funding was more difficult to secure in a more competitive environment. And some settings we had begun to explore as sites for workshops, such as workplaces and schools, were no longer readily available to us. But we carried on, successfully, in large part because of the relationships and partnerships we had developed over the few years of our existence.

13.1.2.2 Stories of relationships and partnerships

13.1.2.2.1 Advance care planning and grief workshops

Forging relationships with local organisations has always meant a steady flow of workshop locations. Our focus has been on groups serving older adults, faith communities, retirement homes, ageing-in-place initiatives, libraries, and cultural groups. The latter have been made possible through our relationship with Ottawa Public Health, a high-profile organisation throughout the pandemic with significant relationships in all parts of Ottawa. With them we have reached communities otherwise unlikely to be easily accessible to us. With a community college training retirement home managers, we partnered to reach into retirement homes to offer workshops.

Most recently, through our partnership with Academic Family Health Teams, we have reached nearly 700 individuals for ACP workshops. Working in partnerships with healthcare professionals has long been a goal, one that seemed to be difficult to achieve given well-known pressures on health care for time to engage with others and what we occasionally sensed was ambivalence about community work. Today, we feel confident that we are on the way to forging continuing partnerships with this sector, a collaboration that stands out as an example of close professional relationships from the past and the present, and of the high respect CO has earned in the community.

Our grief workshops have taken place in various settings, including in faith communities where we have worked closely with faith leaders to understand the interests of their communities. This work was assisted by an invitation to present to a well-known Ottawa theology programme for lay people, as well as a cross-faith training programme for pastoral care.

13.1.2.2.2 Care for life

This innovative project is in partnership with the Social Planning Council of Ottawa. They host a network called the Ottawa Ethno-Cultural Seniors Network, which consists of older adults from 30 culturally diverse groups. Following an introduction to the group, we collaboratively developed a programme to encourage compassion in their respective communities. A survey identified areas of high interest, materials to most appropriately respond to their interests were introduced, and recently over 20 volunteers from six communities began training to become facilitators. More will follow. This community development approach, led by a CO volunteer, will, we hope, be replicated elsewhere.

13.1.2.2.3 The Death Literacy Index

With encouragement from colleagues in Australia, we have completed a first phase of the Death Literacy Index with a small sample of people completing the survey and participating in focus groups. The interest was keen enough to lead to a partnership with the University of Ottawa and go deeper into this work. More research and efforts to Canadianise the instrument, including within Francophone communities, are underway. An article on our work has been accepted for publication. Our partnership with the university builds on several years of strong relationships where we have been a placement for students to, as one example, develop evaluation approaches for our programmes.

Other partnerships, such as TOE and HELP, which started before the pandemic, informed our approach to developing partnerships. We know that all the work we do in the future will benefit from doing it with others.

13.1.2.2.4 Convening groups serving older adults to explore new possibilities

During our workshops and conversations, we often heard about loneliness, isolation, and anxiety. We asked ourselves what we, as an organisation encouraging compassion, can do to tackle these almost universal concerns. To help us think about that, we have recently convened a few partner groups to explore what we can do collaboratively. Inspired by the 2024 Bern Declaration [1], we are exploring ways to share stories, host learning opportunities to build compassion and connectedness, and make more visible the need for compassion.

Our communications activity is not only about our own programmes but almost as much about the work of our partners. Often, the most viewed social media post in any given month is about someone else's work!

13.1.2.3 Building our own capacity

Over time, our approach to organising our work has changed, largely because of the pandemic impact. Rather than work in teams, we have taken a more holistic approach, with board members and volunteers stepping up to lead particular work, along with other volunteers, some from the community who share a particular interest. The convening initiative described above is an example of this, as is Care for Life.

Attending workshops and conferences, staying on top of current literature in our field, and understanding the realities in our city have also built our capacity. So too has the growing skill of our small but dedicated staff.

In 2025, we find ourselves facing significant board turnover. The founding board is making way for a new group of leaders, working in transition to make sure the mission and vision of CO remain, while the programming might grow and change over time.

Not only are there new board members, but there are also new volunteers in our programmes. And we are beginning to rebuild excitement and energy around events to bring volunteers together in person.

13.1.2.4 Measuring our success

In an earlier section of this chapter, we described our evaluation approach. As well, feedback is invited from participants in all our workshops and Conversations with Leaders forums, helping us continually adapt and adjust.

We have been successful in bringing hundreds of people into our key programmes, offering information, resources, and follow-up. We have made connections with others in Ottawa serving those who are seriously ill or living with grief, helping to enrich the overall environment in our city.

As evidenced by our growing social media presence and website traffic, we have raised awareness about the importance of compassion, the need for caring for each other, and the ways in which care is offered.

But we have not yet evaluated the impact of our organisation as a whole. We know from the many relationships and partnerships that we enjoy that we are highly respected and have considerable credibility. Feedback on our programmes is universally positive. But if we didn't exist, what would happen?

13.1.2.5 Lessons learned in the post-pandemic world

Measuring capacity is difficult. A challenge we have faced is describing our work in an environment where the emphasis is on measurable outcomes. We don't offer concrete services, but rather work towards raising awareness, levels of knowledge, and understanding, all hard to measure.

Sustaining organisational capacity is challenging. Funding for new not-for-profit organisations is always a challenge. We have been fortunate to have significant support from a private donor, from foundations and government grants, as well as from our annual request to the public for contributions. We do not charge for any of our services, so keeping our eye on the bottom line is always important. This focus takes a lot of our time.

In a milieu where formal health care is positioned to be where and how people are cared for, conveying the role of community in caring for others can be challenging, especially to the healthcare community (and its funders) itself. But the example of our partnership with a Family Health Team gives us confidence that time in forging partnerships with health care or indeed any potential partner is never a waste of time.

Reference

1 Public Health Palliative Care International, "The Bern Declaration." Available online: https://www.phpci.org/berndeclaration. [Accessed 27 Jan 2026].

14

COMPASSIONATE COMMUNITIES AND PUBLIC HEALTH PALLIATIVE CARE FOR CHILDREN'S HOSPICES, AN EXAMPLE FROM QUEENSLAND, AUSTRALIA

Elham Day, Cara Doherty and Leigh Donovan

Abstract

This chapter offers reflections on how Hummingbird House, Queensland's only children's hospice, has sought to integrate Compassionate Communities and Public Health approaches into paediatric palliative care through key partnerships and community development. Set against the backdrop of a vast and decentralised state, this chapter situates this work within a decade of advocacy, collaboration, and system-level change, describing the evolution of community-centred approaches to care across great geographic areas.

It outlines the development of a Community Development Framework grounded in participatory practice and reflective praxis, presents practical examples, and illustrates how interdisciplinary collaboration has shaped key initiatives. These include building social connection, amplifying family voices, fostering grief and death literacy, and embedding community capacity-building within both hospice and healthcare settings.

This chapter reflects critically on lessons learned, challenges encountered, and the importance of sustaining meaningful relationships with families, communities, and professionals over time. It presents a radically relational, grassroots model of paediatric palliative care, one that supports families to maintain connection with their communities before, during, and after a child's death.

Ultimately, it argues that community development should not be seen as an adjunct to clinical care, but as a vital, integrated practice essential to high-quality, compassionate paediatric palliative care.

DOI: 10.4324/9781003621348-15

14.1 Introduction – Paediatric palliative care: background and context

The death of a child remains largely incomprehensible in high-income countries. This reality leaves families of children with life-limiting conditions increasingly isolated, both during the child's life and after their death. In Queensland, Australia, this isolation is magnified by geography: a vast state of approximately 1.7 million km^2 where only one tertiary children's hospital and one children's hospice (both in Brisbane) serve the entire population. Despite significant numbers of children with life-limiting conditions across the state, only a fraction receive palliative care services, and even fewer access hospice care [1].

For families, the burden of long-term care is profound, with impacts spanning emotional, psychological, financial and existential domains [2,3]. Parental relationships are strained, siblings become disenfranchised, and social networks either gradually withdraw or are eroded by the demands of care. Commonly, the loss of relational networks and community support also extends to family experiences of death (and after-death care), which are typically highly medicalised. The Lancet Commission report The Value of Death [4] highlights how dying has become primarily dominated by professionalisation. Subsequently, families and communities (in many highly industrialised countries at least) have become increasingly deskilled in responding to death and grief within their own communities. Their report proposes five principles to 'radically reimagine' support systems, the most relevant to this chapter being:

1 establishing networks of care to support people who are dying, caring, and grieving and
2 normalising conversations about death, dying, and grief.

Despite these important recommendations, the specific experience of children dying remains largely neglected, as do the voices of their parents, caregivers, and families.

Following a child's death, parents, particularly mothers who typically serve as primary caregivers, experience a severe disruption in relation to their grief, yet secondary losses in relation to their identity after years in a caregiving role [5]. Re-entering the natural rhythm of life becomes challenging whilst processing grief and adapting to life without their caregiving responsibilities, often compounded by the context of the professional and social support during the child's illness having also withdrawn.

Society remains ill-equipped to witness and respond to this chronic sorrow, anticipatory grief, and mourning that extends throughout parents' lifetimes, and grief responses are too often pathologised and medicalised as a means of assimilating bereaved parents back to 'normal'.

Significant numbers of caring, grieving, and bereaved family members could have many of their needs supported by well-equipped grief- and death-literate communities; yet, a lack of public understanding or service-reorientation (towards communities) leaves families isolated, faced with the additional labour of trying to educate their own support networks, while navigating the pain of their own grief [6]. To change this, there is an urgent clinical and ethical need to invest in community capacity before a child dies – ensuring bereavement care is not an afterthought but part of a continuum that extends beyond the institution and into the hands of a prepared, grief-literate community [7].

14.2 The progression of paediatric palliative care in Queensland

In keeping with the establishment of children's hospices globally, effective collaboration and supportive relationships were critical in the foundation of Hummingbird House Children's Hospice in Brisbane, Australia. From the hospice co-founders to families (both bereaved and those living with a child with paediatric palliative care needs), community organisations, grassroots advocacy, philanthropy, and support from multiple levels of government, Queensland's only children's hospice is a success story built on relational partnerships. Of specific relevance to capacity-building approaches to care has been the relationship between Hummingbird House and the state-wide Paediatric Palliative Care Service (PPCS).

From its inception in 2009 at the Royal Children's Hospital in Brisbane, paediatric palliative care identified equity of access as the most significant barrier to care for Queensland children with life-limiting conditions [8]. From the time the Hummingbird House vision was first shared with paediatric palliative care in 2013, to the hospital services' extensive support of the hospice through clinical and holistic education as the hospice build was completed in preparation for opening to guests in 2016, increasing access and enhancing community capacity has been and remains a shared priority.

Ongoing collaboration between hospital and various community services has proven vital in cultivating the groundwork for future Public Health Palliative Care (PHPC) development. While PHPC and Community Development Frameworks were integrated into Hummingbird House over time, a commitment to collaboratively resourced, community-centric care was present from the outset. A key example of this was Hummingbird House being invited to partner (with Qld Children's Hospital) in a state-wide telehealth project, which included collaborative resourcing for a community development and telehealth project worker (see activities section 14.4.3.1).

Concurrent to nurturing multiple hospital and health partnerships, Hummingbird House was also intentional in initiating active relationships outside institutional contexts. Though typically small in scale and organic in nature, such efforts were significant in the early years of the service. Some highlights included partnerships with local arts organisations (to honour and celebrate family experiences of paediatric palliative care through visual, installation, and performance art projects), engaging progressive funeral directors and death doula educators (to support training and resourcing for a then-emerging model of Participatory After Death Care). These examples of practical cross-sectoral initiatives in service delivery are snapshots in the broader 'radical reimagining' of the role of a children's hospice in enhancing community-centred approaches to dying, death, and grief care for Queensland families.

While the detailed internal development of Hummingbird House as a service is specific to our context and therefore less applicable to share, Section 14.4 outlines key milestones in the strategic and operational development of community development approaches. These milestones illustrate how research analysis, targeted consultation, expert insight, and context-specific knowledge informed the evolution of the Family Support team into the Family and Community Support team. This shift was much more than tokenistic change in language – involving specific framework development and solidifying our commitment to embedding community development approaches across the entire service, in order to support shaping sustainable future service models into the future.

While the broader context of Australian Palliative Care benefitted significantly from founders and innovations in the PHPC movement for adults (Prof. Allan Kellehear, The Groundswell Project, La Trobe University's HELP Project, etc.), there were significant gaps in guidelines for applying PHPC work directly to children's hospice care when we began to explore these approaches in the 2010s. We sought to synthesise existing family-centred models of children's hospice care, with broader (adult) PHPC examples and policy recommendations by combining the existing interdisciplinary hospice and healthcare expertise between our teams, with that of highly regarded and experienced community development practitioners, Professor Peter Westoby [9] and Paul Toon [10]. The next section demonstrates how this work progressed and may be relevant in principle to many other Compassionate Community contexts. We are immensely grateful for all the groundbreaking work that has emerged from Australia across the disciplines of Community Development, PHPC, and Compassionate Communities, which continues to support the evolution of network-centred care partnerships across communities.

14.3 Key milestones in developing community development and PHPC approaches at Hummingbird House

14.3.1 2017

A study was commissioned by the leadership team at HH, to inform developing key service components of a Queensland-specific hospice family support programme [11]. An integrated project approach combined a review of relevant literature with international service benchmarking, and an analysis of family lived experience. This integrated Hummingbird House's first 30 holistic family assessments.

For families receiving paediatric palliative care, social networks often contracted over the course of a child's illness and are often replaced by clinical (transactional) relationships. With limited opportunity for sustained social connection, the loss of ongoing social networks can also increase family bereavement risk. This awareness guided decisions regarding the application of limited staff resources to focus not only on individual family well-being but also towards addressing inter-family isolation and connection. In addition, recommendations included developing a hub-and-spoke model for sustainable service delivery and to recruit community development workers to provide service guidance on strengthening local capacity around families.

Impact and outcomes

1 Resulted in a business case to pilot a trial of a community development worker at Hummingbird House (2019).
2 Challenged organisational assumptions relating to professional resourcing for bereavement care (i.e. psychology and expert led) in contrast to models of a peer-support bereavement mentoring programme, later established at Hummingbird House (2022/2023).
3 Guided staff to specifically explore opportunities for inter-family connection.
4 Led to decisions further supporting resourcing care for families state-wide.

14.3.2 2020

A CD Issues and Options Paper was commissioned, to provide strategic guidance for the initial investment in a community development worker. Despite recurrent literature recommendations on the integration of CD in adult palliative care, and although some innovative projects already existed in adult services in Australia, there were no guidelines, examples, or roadmaps found supporting the application in paediatric palliative care or children's hospices.

Three key recommendations from this report led to: (i) increased leadership understanding and support to embed CD practice across Hummingbird House, (ii) a move from iterative practice of CD in individual teams to a more strategic effort to embed CD into the core practice of Hummingbird House (inter-team), and (iii) engaging pilot project-oriented explorations at 2–3 'test sites' outside of the urban and metro areas of Brisbane.

Impact and outcomes

1 Subsequently, this took shape as a collaborative partnership with paediatric palliative care to jointly resource the CD role (and a complementary, state-wide telehealth project officer).

2 Establishing regional partnership sites, two of which were sustained over two years.
3 Expansion of existing child-centred HNA process to a family- and network-centred holistic assessment.
4 Development of a Community Development Framework specific to Hummingbird House context.

14.3.3 2022

We identified the need for systematic strategic planning to consolidate cross-team approaches to state-wide care through Hummingbird House, based on a PHPC framework. This *Regional Development Strategy* project utilised a three-phase methodology involving rapid literature review; service mapping of complimentary models or frameworks guided by a PHPC/CC approach and scoping conversations with national and international colleagues [12].

This resulted in guiding principles intended to directly inform the development of state-wide approaches to care; key questions for the leadership team to support clarifying the value proposition of the hospice *beyond the house* to frame the mission forward, including relationally and financially sustainable approaches to network-centred care for families with PPC need.

When published internally in 2022, a confluence of internal and external factors led to the indefinite delays with progressing the HH Regional Development Strategy. These included major changes in senior management; leadership fatigue from two years of supporting EoL and ADC during the COVID-19 pandemic; coupled with ongoing pressure and uncertainty regarding service funding sustainability. Despite challenges with implementation internally, this work has however proved to be a useful reference for other hospice and palliative care organisations (both interstate and beyond Australia) as one evidence-informed example for implementing inter-disciplinary approaches to sustainable PHPC in the context of work with children and families.

Impact and outcomes

1 A Regional Development Strategy served to roadmap strategic opportunities and increase understanding of innovative CD approaches beyond only the FCS team.
2 Supported the continuity of specific intentional partnerships with regional stakeholders
3 Presented innovative better practice aligned with a PHPC approach, with specific relevance to Hummingbird House and Qld context.
4 Delivered detailed and nuanced recommendations regarding culturally safe engagement with Aboriginal and Torres Strait Islander families and communities across Queensland.

14.4 Community development from a children's hospice: participatory practice

There are five pillars in the Community Development Program Framework at Hummingbird House (See Figure 14.1). Each pillar reflects a distinct focus, encompassing a range of engagements – working alongside families, collaborating with community stakeholders, and embedding a community-centred approach within the organisation. This framework was designed to be intentionally dynamic, continuously reviewed, and adapted to remain responsive to changing needs and opportunities. It allows space for experimentation, for planting seeds and seeing what takes root, and for moving at the pace of the people, rather than to a service-driven timeline.

Below, we outline each programme area with a practice example to illustrate the approach.

14.4.1 Working with community in places

This first pillar is one of the most familiar in CD and involves building relationships and connecting with Hummingbird House families, local groups, and organisations in their communities across regions in Queensland. Hummingbird House staff periodically travel to different regions, facilitating connections between interested families who have shared experiences of care. These peer connections foster

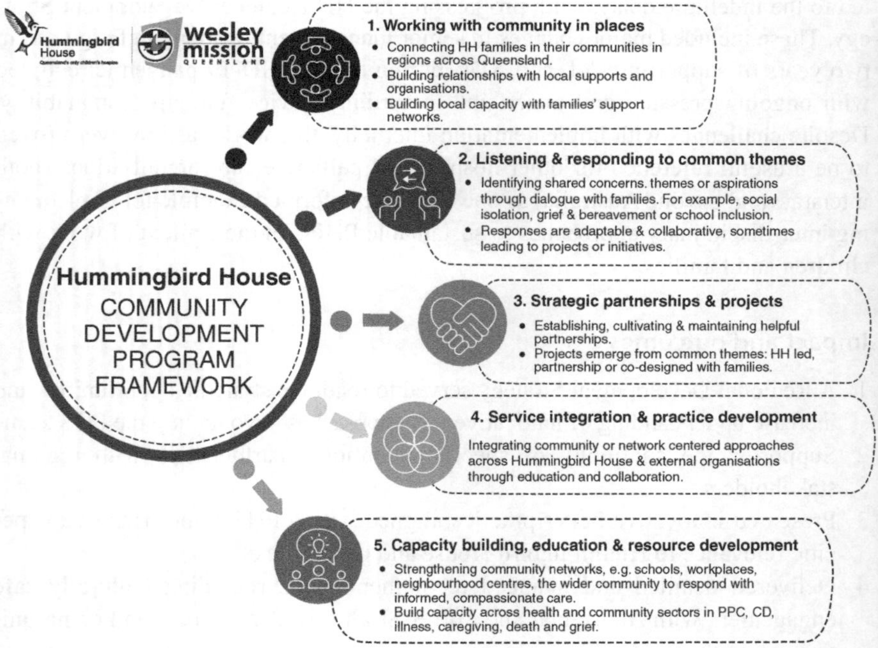

FIGURE 14.1 Hummingbird House, Community Development Program Framework

support, exchange of valuable local information, and new friendships. It has not been uncommon in some regional towns, for families living only a few streets apart, both caring for children with life-limiting conditions, to have not known each other prior to making a Hummingbird House connection. Additionally, by establishing and nurturing relationships with local community networks, health, and community services, we ensure that families are more effectively linked to the local support and resources that are supportive in their day-to-day lives.

14.4.1.1 Hummingbird House connecting group of Bundaberg

Since 2021, a Hummingbird House CD worker has been visiting Bundaberg in the Wide Bay-Burnett Region (360 km north of Brisbane) to build relationships with families and key stakeholders. This initiative began with Hummingbird House staff listening to the experiences and perspectives of families in regional Queensland. A common theme emerged as a shared sense of social isolation, and a desire for greater connection with other families walking a similar path. The Hummingbird House CD worker invited families in the region to come together at the local neighbourhood centre. This grassroots approach led to the creation of the *Hummingbird House Connecting Group of Bundaberg*, a family-led initiative, of which Hummingbird House is a partner. The group meets several times a year, where families find a sense of mutual support, connection, and the sharing of valuable information.

Beyond the family gatherings, a broader initiative also emerged. A working group of families, professionals, and community members came together to organise a Compassionate Communities forum focusing on enhancing community grief and death literacy, centring the voices of families through a discussion panel.

This work has fostered strong relationships with local hospitals, schools, and community services, leading to improved collaboration and greater local capacity to support families of children with life-limiting illness. Grounded in a participatory, strengths-based approach, it empowers families and builds community connections by working alongside, not on behalf of, the community. It shows that communities hold innate capacities to support one another, beyond traditional service models.

14.4.2 Listening and responding to common themes

A key part of our community development approach is listening deeply to families' shared experiences. Through ongoing dialogue, we identify common themes and reflect on these before collaborating on responses which are adaptive and always developed in partnership with families. These may include advocacy, creating spaces for connection, or layered support tailored to the concern. *Collective Narrative Approaches* have been significant in this area, with two examples shared below:

We often draw on narrative therapy in community work, an approach that centres people as the experts in their own lives. Narrative therapy is based on the belief that individuals possess the skills, values, and knowledge to navigate life's challenges, and that shared storytelling can be a powerful tool for connection and empowerment [13]. The first example is the NDIS *Collective Narrative Report (2021)* that captures the experiences of families navigating the National Disability Insurance Scheme (NDIS) while caring for children with life-limiting and complex conditions. Emerging from a series of dialogues with a group of Hummingbird House parents and caregivers, key themes included profound social isolation, the system's failure to understand complexity, the double burden of caregiving, and the administrative toll of accessing support. Managing NDIS plans and paperwork was described as equivalent to a full-time job, with calls for better systems such as team-based care models, resulting from the feeling that their children are viewed as costs rather than valued as individuals.

The document also highlights collective wisdom, including strategies for effective advocacy: telling the full story, using Family and Carer Impact Statements, knowing your rights in meetings, understanding NDIS jargon, and seeking peer and formal support. Families emphasised the need for systemic change and stronger advocacy to ensure that all children and families are respected, supported, and included. This report was helpful to share with other families experiencing similar challenges and has helped reduce the systems-isolation which can often also be present for families.

The second example is a Bereaved Grandparents Group, which emerged from ongoing conversations with grandparents who felt their grief was often unseen though multifaceted. This group was co-created as a partnership, rather than a traditional support group facilitated by professionals. While it commenced quite organically, after three years of quarterly gatherings, the group wished to articulate what they felt made their community so meaningful. A narrative therapy-based workshop was developed between a family support worker and a community development worker, using the metaphor of a Tree of Life, allowing grandparents to define their values, share their wisdom, and shape their collective story.

This summary will be used in future to share invitations to more recently referred and/or bereaved grandparents, giving greater visibility to a previously unseen aspect of family grief. This approach illustrates an example of how we engage in deep listening with families and respond in ways that are collaborative and empowering, relating to families as partners rather than *patients*.

14.4.3 Strategic partnerships and projects

We cultivate partnerships with organisations and peak bodies to foster collaboration, knowledge exchange, and coordinated support for families. Projects emerge organically in response to identified community themes or as opportunities for capacity-building. Some are Hummingbird House-led, while others are co-developed with key stakeholders. Two brief examples follow:

14.4.3.1 E-PPCS: expanding access to paediatric palliative care in Queensland (strengthening inter-service partnerships and regional capacity)

Originally titled the Paediatric Palliative Care Outreach Collaborative, the E-PPCS project was established in 2020, with the aim to improve access to paediatric palliative care for children with life-limiting conditions outside south-east Queensland. By delivering telehealth and outreach services, key outcomes include enhanced patient experiences, upskilling of local health professionals, and reduced preventable hospital admissions. An interprofessional team offers weekly telehealth clinics, ad hoc reviews, and 24/7 clinical phone support. Hummingbird House plays a smaller role in the larger project – through its community development practitioner and telehealth project officer who work alongside the telehealth project by supplementing place-based regional initiatives and capacity-building engagements with families. Collaborations with local services and other NGOs ensure holistic support, while a partnership with Queensland University of Technology supports the academic evaluation of the programme. Through E-PPCS, children and families in rural and regional areas receive more equitable, compassionate care, embedded in their own communities.

14.4.3.2 Grief-informed schools initiative (linking sector stakeholders, hospice, and community)

This initiative commenced in 2024 as a partnership with peak body Palliative Care Queensland and was born from two distinct areas of awareness. First, the recognition of the important role schools plays in the lives of families and in a Compassionate Community, and second, as a hospice team, we repeatedly encounter a vast inequity in grief and death in the schools which Hummingbird House families attend during illness and/or return to as bereaved students and staff. We initiated a listening and scoping project to seek to better understand the experiences of students, families, and staff experiencing grief and loss. The first phase of this project has been all about listening and learning, rather than coming in with predetermined 'solutions' for death and grief literacy, and subsequently what role a hospice may hold in this. Through focus groups and shared expertise, we hope to progress this work to co-design practical, evidence-informed resources that equip schools with the knowledge and confidence to support grieving students and families. By taking a partnership-driven approach, we ensure that any outcomes are rooted in real-world experience. This strengthens our collective capacity to cultivate compassionate, grief-aware school communities – where families feel supported by the networks they already belong to, across the full trajectory of serious illness.

14.4.4 Service integration and practice development

We have sought to integrate community development and principles of Compassionate Communities across all areas of our work at Hummingbird House. This has included fostering inter-team collaboration and promoting internal education on how to apply community support in palliative care. By embedding a community-centred approach to service delivery across teams, we enhance the organisation's capacity to provide holistic, network-centred care.

14.4.4.1 Mapping resources while assessing needs: from family to community-centred care

The routine use of network mapping for all clinical staff is a key recommendation for PC services incorporating a PHPC approach. Hummingbird House CD workers led a process of quality improvement in 2020, to integrate family network mapping into an existing Holistic Needs Assessment (HNA) tool. The HNA tool was designed by East Anglia Children's Hospice in England, adapting principles from existing holistic assessments in adult palliative care to better suit the needs, voices, and dynamics of children and families [14]. As an ethically aligned framework which sought to enhance holistic family well-being, the HNA process was well suited to naturally incorporate elements of network-centred care with the introduction of network mapping.

The impacts of introducing network mapping to the HA process resulted in expanded understandings from staff of the complexity and individual differences in family experiences. It also broadened possibilities for staff to imagine directing resources to enhancing family well-being beyond *service delivery* interventions directly with family members. Practically, this has ranged from grief education sessions for home carer teams who were struggling with anticipatory grief, to collaboration between hospice and school staff to improve grief literacy in response to a primary school's punitive approach to managing a student's behavioural changes in their first term back at school as a bereaved sibling.

This example of evolving an existing tool from child- or family-centred care to network-centred care seeks to challenge the dominance held by transactional relationships in family life and to invite conversations about networks of mutual support and aid between families and their community. While this process has not been without its challenges, we continue to see its importance as many families report how their lives remain dominated by the needs of transactional supports, placing further strain on the maintenance of networks of mutual care.

14.4.5 Capacity-building, education, and resource development

We actively contribute to capacity-building within the broader community by enhancing understanding of death, grief, and compassionate care through a range of actions. These include workshops and presentations on community development principles within the health and palliative care sectors, as well as through community engagement activities (e.g. webinars and resource development). By fostering community-wide grief and death literacy, we are keeping our hospice vision in clear view: *that every family in Queensland may be connected to a community that knows how to care for them in life, death, and bereavement.*

14.4.5.1 Collaboration and capacity-building with neighbourhood centres

Since our community development programme was implemented, we have collaborated and engaged with neighbourhood and community centres across Queensland in a variety of ways. In 2025, we hosted two state-wide webinars for neighbourhood centres. One session featured an initiative focused on building death and grief literacy in a community within the Sunshine Coast region. This work began as an effort to engage Sunshine Coast families connected to Hummingbird House but evolved, due to COVID-19, geographic spread, and family capacity challenges, into a broader community education initiative.

Supported by the local neighbourhood centre, a community working group hosted 'Compassionate Community Conversations' exploring topics around illness, death, bereavement, and grief. The webinar highlighted these experiences and encouraged other centres to pursue similar initiatives, sharing resources and learnings along the way.

There was strong interest across Queensland, particularly from regional centres where many Hummingbird House families live. Building these connections allows us to strengthen local support networks that can better serve families. In response to this momentum, Hummingbird House also delivered a grief-informed care workshop for centre staff and volunteers. Neighbourhood centres, natural hubs for connection when informed and resourced, can offer meaningful support during illness, caregiving, grief, and bereavement. The more resourced and confident our communities are, the stronger the networks of care become for everyone, including families caring for children with life-limiting conditions.

14.4.5.2 Community development workshops for health professionals

Hummingbird House also piloted a community development workshop with staff from the Queensland Children's Hospital (QCH) PPCS. Recognising that community development remains a relatively new concept in paediatric palliative care, this project, which was funded by QCH, explored practical ways to integrate these principles into various roles within the health sector.

Health professionals from diverse disciplines attended, building their understanding of the field of community development as well as learning strategies to build community support networks, reduce family isolation, and enhance holistic care beyond the clinical setting. Further, staff provided valuable feedback on workshop content ensuring it's relevant and useful in the paediatric health context.

Through these initiatives, Hummingbird House continues to advocate for education, connection, and community-led support around families navigating serious illness, death, and bereavement.

14.5 Conclusion

In this chapter, we've reflected across years of dialogue, service delivery, and evidence-informed explorations which have been central to our praxis in applying community development principles to paediatric palliative care at an Australian Children's Hospice. We've highlighted themes of partnership, innovation, adaptation, and the importance of sustained relationality at all levels. As we conclude, while much of our content has been presented through frameworks and historical summary, we wanted to share some key learnings in a reflective format framed through analogies from the natural world. It is our hope that these insights will not just document some of our learnings, but that they may hold relevant considerations across different contexts for readers. So let us begin, not with another framework but with a framing metaphor:

> When a gardener plants a fruit tree sapling, she may know what species the tree is and therefore what kind of fruit the tree will bear. Given we're writing from Queensland and there are three in the back garden of the hospice – let's imagine the gardener is planting a mango tree! From the first act of planting much remains unseen: who will one day eat the fruit of future harvests, how abundant those harvests will become, and how their fruits will be savoured and shared by others. The gardener can only wonder and imagine as she tends the soil and supports the young sapling to develop – will the ripe golden fruits be preserved and stored in the family pantry? Will many fruits fall untouched, to compost into the soils below? Will seeds be shared with neighbours, enabling them to cultivate food sovereignty within their own community?

As Hummingbird House approaches a decade of care (which coincides with the fruiting time for a seed-grown mango tree), the service is well established in the Queensland landscape of paediatric palliative care. We have much to celebrate in what we have delivered for Queensland families, and we continue to face many of the common ongoing challenges that many children's hospices do, from funding sustainability to workforce shortages – despite this, we have found the process of applying PHPC and CD to the hospice Family and Community Support work has taught us several valuable lessons.

14.5.1 What's beneath determines what blooms

Hummingbird House was able to invest in innovation during the hospice's early years because the soil it was planted in had been intentionally nourished over time with vital relationships and environmental supports. We have maintained a commitment to cultivating and sustaining interconnected networks of care which extend beyond traditional health service partners (e.g. WMQ, local hospitals, national children's hospices) to include those outside our locality (internationally with other hospices and org's aligned to PHPC) as well those beyond the infrastructure of the health system (natural funeral directors, neighbourhood centres, and community arts organisations). Just as trees are sustained not by their own roots alone, but by vast mycelial networks of connection beneath the forest floor, our commitment to fostering cross-sectoral, interdisciplinary relationships continues to strengthen both our own service and the wider paediatric palliative care ecosystem through both mild and harsh weather conditions (and Queensland has both, in abundance!).

14.5.2 Observe and interact, before you act

This principle of permaculture design [15] encourages pausing to understand the environment you are engaging with, recognising patterns and relationships before acting. Through the influence of CD in the early years of the service, the Hummingbird House leadership team embraced this mindset when considering family support and state-wide care models focusing less on dissecting parts in isolation and more on understanding the living whole. In practice, this included resourcing analysis from experienced paediatric palliative care and CD practitioners to synthesise practice wisdom, evidence, and context-specific knowledge at key points in service development (see Section14.4). As a result, Hummingbird House avoided (some!) common missteps such as applying one-size-fits-all models in communities where they may not align with local realities. Instead, we sought to identify antecedent conditions [16] learning from what already existed and seeking *to resource capacity* rather than rushing *to service*. Our work with families' attempts to continue reflecting this principle: we approach care not as intervention but as relationship, incorporating the lived experience of family voices into our ongoing learning and reflection cycles.

14.5.3 Staying Responsive Through Changing Seasons

In Queensland, we often gratefully remind ourselves in late January that there is no such thing as an endless summer! Growth, flowering, and fruition (and harvests) come in seasons. No matter how much we try to stretch or resist the turning of seasons, anyone tending a garden, or a community development programme, knows that as night follows day, seasons shift bringing change and loss and working with or against these cycles is a choice. The pace of CD work is often slow. Frustrating, yes, but necessary. Working at the pace of families, meeting them where they are, takes time. It demands we continually reassess not just what we do but how we think especially about what it means to partner with families, rather than simply deliver services. Families who are caring for a child with a life-limiting condition often face complexity and great uncertainty in lives which are shaped by shifting demands. This context resists quick fixes or linear solutions, just as you can't fast-forward through winter to bring spring back quicker. This approach asks us to sit with open questions, to stay responsive, and to work in ways that may not neatly fit with health-centric preferences for pre-designed outcomes prior to partnering with children and families in the reality of their lives.

As poet David Whyte writes: ‘Our human essence lies not in arrival, but in being almost there: we are creatures who are on their way, our journey is a series of impending arrivals’. Moving toward a truly community-centred approach has no fixed destination. We may never feel a full sense of arrival. There will always be more to hear, more to learn, and more reshaping, of ourselves and of the systems and cycles we are part of.

14.5.4 Roots and leaves grow at different speeds

Like all living systems, organisations grow in layers and at different speeds. At Hummingbird House, our Family and Community Support team embedded CD and grew a model rooted in participation and outward-facing work. This occurred while we were still establishing our hospice care; alongside other teams still finding their footing amid swirling demands of staffing, intensive clinical care and challenges with organisational resourcing and funding sustainability. The rhythms didn’t always align. Understandings of CD and PHPC principles across the hospice service encountered both cultural and structural tensions, particularly amid pressures of the newly rolled out NDIS system, navigating a global pandemic and latterly a national cost-of-living crisis. The nurse-led model at Hummingbird House has helped to shape some innovative and participatory aspects of care (such as a Perinatal Hospice Program) which may have been adopted more readily with the benefit of being more familiar to clinical staff. PHPC work however has called for ongoing reframing and re-education to help clinical staff recognise CD not as an optional extra but as core to holistic, sustainable care. Transforming a culture isn’t a one-time act, or a transplant of external models but rather long term, often inter-generational work. It involves sharing seeds, listening to local knowledge, and tending to what takes root. Outcomes may not be immediate; yet by learning to work adaptively during cycles of fast and slow movemnent, we affirm that change is most enduring when it grows from the ground up – with deep roots and open branches.

14.5.5 Nurturing ecosystems

A garden’s relationship to its wider environment depends greatly on its design and intention. While an ornamental and a permaculture garden may grow from seemingly similar ground, their impact diverges. The former often relies on artificial inputs, may disrupt surrounding species, and exists in relative ecological isolation. In contrast, the permaculture garden, though still requiring care, serves the broader web of life: supporting biodiversity, regenerating soil, and reducing dependence on external resources. To translate this into our practice context, by sustaining a founding commitment of the hospice to supporting families state-wide, we have kept ecological questions present (such as *How might Hummingbird House be of service, beyond the service?*). With a network-centred approach, we are expressing a commitment of care not only for families who can access our hospice building or connect virtually with our team but also for the wider environments in which those families live, grieve, and seek to thrive. As we build relationships with schools, funeral providers, neighbourhood centres, disability advocates and community fundraisers – these are all part of a nurturing living web – and our contribution to family well-being not made as a health service in isolation but as part of an interconnected, community-sustaining ecology of care.

References

1. A. Bowers, A. R. Herbert, R. Chan and P. Yates, "Estimating the prevalence of life-limiting conditions in Queensland for children and young people aged 0-21 years using health administration data," *Australian Health Review*, vol. 44, no. 4, pp. 630–636, 2020.
2. S. Ekberg, A. Bowers, N. Bradford, K. Ekberg, M. Rolfe, N. Elvidge and A. Vickery, "Enhancing paediatric palliative care: A rapid review to inform continued development of care for children with life-limiting conditionsournal of paediatrics and child health," *Journal of Paediatrics and Child Health*, vol. 58, no. 2, pp. 232–237, 2022.
3. L. Barrett, L. Fraser, J. Noyes, J. Taylor and J. Hackett, "Understanding parent experiences of end-of-life care for children: A systematic review and qualitative evidence synthesis," *Palliative Medicine*, vol. 37, no. 2, pp. 178–202, 2023.
4. L. Sallnow, R. Smith, S. H. Ahmedzai, A. Bhadelia, C. Chamberlain, Y. Cong and K. Wyatt, "Report of the Lancet Commission on the Value of Death: Bringing death back into life," *The Lancet*, vol. 399, no. 10327, pp. 837–884, 2022.
5. A. Karakul, D. Kıratlı, E. A. Akgul and T. Celik, "The experiences of parents of children in pediatric palliative care: A qualitative study," *Journal of Pediatric Nursing*, vol. 67, pp. 107–115, 2022.
6. J. Cacciatore, *Bearing the unbearable: Love, loss, and the heartbreaking path of grief*, Wisdom Publications, 2017.
7. W. G. Lichtenthal, K. E. Roberts, L. A. Donovan, L. J. Breen, S. M. Aoun, S. R. Connor and W. E. Rosa, "Investing in bereavement care as a public health priority," *The Lancet Public Health*, vol. 9, no. 4, pp. e270–e274, 2024.
8. N. Bradford, M. Bensink, H. Irving, J. Murray, L. Pedersen, J. Roylance and A. Herbert, "Paediatric palliative care services in Queensland: An exploration of the barriers, gaps and plans for service development," *Neonatal, Paediatric & Child Health Nursing*, vol. 15, no. 1, pp. 2–7, 2012.
9. A. Kelly and P. Westoby, *Participatory development practice: Using traditional and contemporary frameworks*, Practical Action Publishing, 2018.
10. P. Westoby, E. Day, F. Hawthorne, M. F. P. Toon and K. Oldham, "A community development story and portrayal of a phenomenological reflective practice in the field of paediatric palliativecare," *Community Development Journal*, vol. 58, no. 3, pp. 402–418, 2023.
11. L. Donovan, "Hummingbird House HNA Analysis Report," 2017.
12. L. Donovan, "Hummingbird House Regional Development Strategy: Issues and options to guide a sustainable state-wide approach for community, family and clinical support service," Collaboraide, Prepared for Hummingbird House, 2022.

13. Dulwich Centre, "What is narrative therapy?" [Internet]. Adelaide: Dulwich Centre; [date unknown] [cited 2026 Jan 27]. Available from: https://dulwichcentre.com.au/what-is-narrative-therapy/.
14. G. Hartley, Z. Berger and L. Maynard, "The development and evaluation of a holistic needs assessment within children's palliative care," *International Journal of Palliative Nursing*, vol. 22, no. 5, pp. 236–242, 2016.
15. D. Holmgren, *Permaculture: Principles and pathways beyond sustainability*, Permanent Publications, 2002.
16. M. L. Kelley, A. Williams and L. De Miglio, "Developing rural palliative care: Validating a conceptual model," *Rural and Remote Health*, vol. 11, pp. 178–189, 2011.

15

NATIONAL WORK TO SUPPORT COMPASSIONATE COMMUNITIES – LEARNING AND REFLECTIONS FROM 17 YEARS OF WORK IN SCOTLAND

Mark A. Hazelwood and Rebecca M. Patterson

Abstract

This chapter explores how the Good Life, Good Death, Good Grief (GLGDGG) initiative has worked in various ways to nurture communities in Scotland that support each other with death, dying, loss and care. It summarises key initiatives introduced by GLGDGG including the To Absent Friends Festival; EASE course; Demystifying Death Week; and Bereavement Charter Marks for workplaces and schools. It explores the philosophy and principles underpinning this work, the practicalities and challenges involved and some of the key learning gained from 17 years of work in this area.

15.1 Introduction

This chapter looks at the role a national organisation can play in nurturing communities that support each other with death, dying, loss and care.

We explore how the Good Life, Good Death, Good Grief (GLGDGG) initiative has worked across Scotland to:

1. Grow an infrastructure and networks that nurture local activity
2. Devise resources and projects that inspire and support community action
3. Value diversity and local knowledge while providing a scaffolding for cohesive activity
4. Take action across a wide range of relevant domains

Scotland is one of four nations making up the larger United Kingdom (UK) and has a population of around 5.5 million. Scotland has its own legal and education

DOI: 10.4324/9781003621348-16

systems, and the devolved Scottish Government is responsible for areas such as health, social care, housing and justice.

In global terms Scotland is a relatively wealthy country, with well-developed health and social care services including good specialist palliative care. However, cultures in Scotland often lead to reticence on the part of professionals and community members in thinking and talking about care giving, dying and grieving. Structures and conventions create barriers to members of the public providing care or support in their community. Many people lack knowledge, time, experience or confidence to support others, or to plan ahead for ill health or old age.

15.2 Background

15.2.1 Origins of Good Life, Good Death, Good Grief

In 2008, the Scottish Government's strategy for palliative care identified a need to explore how to address palliative care from a 'public health and health promotion perspective' [1]. This led to the Scottish Partnership for Palliative Care (SPPC) establishing Good Life, Good Death, Good Grief in 2011 [2].

15.2.1.1 Aims

GLGDGG is an alliance of individuals and organisations open to all and committed to making Scotland a place where:

1 People have the knowledge, skills and information they need to deal with the practical, legal, medical, financial, emotional and spiritual issues associated with death, dying and bereavement.
2 People have opportunities to talk about and plan ahead for ill health and death.
3 People have opportunities to offer and receive support relating to ill health, death, dying and bereavement as part of supportive communities.
4 Policymakers and service providers address the range of factors outwith formal health and social care services that affect people's experiences of death, dying, loss and care.
5 Public policies acknowledge and make provision for the needs of people who are caring, dying or grieving.
6 Health and social care service providers understand that they can help individuals and families by supporting future care planning, listening to people's needs and empowering people with realistic, practical information [3].

15.2.1.2 Practicalities

A small central team (currently 2 ½ people) at SPPC enables GLGDGG to provide support and ideas for people in Scotland who want to improve experiences of caring, dying and grieving within their community. We provide a network, resources, events, opportunities for learning/sharing, website, media comment, newsletter and practical tools. GLGDGG also advocates for better public policies. In addition, GLGDGG undertakes projects to enable communities and individuals to support each other through the difficult times that can come with death, dying and bereavement. GLGDGG's work is funded on a year-by-year basis by the Scottish Government and by the members of SPPC. More details about the work of GLGDGG can be found at www.goodlifedeathgrief.org.uk.

15.2.1.3 Philosophy

GLGDGG takes a 'community development approach'. By this, we mean that we aim to encourage and support individuals, communities and organisations to undertake the change they think needs to happen within their own communities.

The work of GLGDGG has been informed and inspired by leading academic thinkers such as Allan Kellhear, Libby Sallnow and Kerrie Noonan. We have also learned from and contributed to the sharing of practice between different countries. Our primary concern is how best to translate ideas into effective practical action which makes a difference in Scotland.

15.2.2 Good Life, Good Death, Good Grief: some key initiatives

15.2.2.1 To Absent Friends, a people's festival of storytelling and remembrance

Launched in 2013, To Absent Friends [4] is an annual festival which takes place across Scotland during the first week of November [5]. The festival creates opportunities for storytelling and remembrance. People who take part benefit from the solace which can come with remembering and telling stories. They also benefit from the strengthening of connections which can come with acknowledging the shared human experience of loss.

The festival gently models greater openness about the 'ordinary' losses we all carry. Beyond immediate solace, the aim is that it becomes easier throughout the year to acknowledge loss, thus reducing the isolation often experienced by bereaved people.

The festival is non-prescriptive, flexible and inclusive because everyone's losses are individual. The focus is not on grief. Instead, the festival emphasises celebration and remembrance of lives lived, but it acknowledges grief. We also acknowledge that remembrance can include memories of difficult relationships and regret. The events in the festival are created and organised by a wide range of different groups and organisations, able to understand what will work best in their context. GLGDGG staff publicise and promote the festival.

For some participants, the very fact of a 'proper festival' provides 'permission' to engage with a topic that is often shrouded in silence. GLGDGG staff provide easy-to-use resources; ideas and advice; an events guide and planning drop-in sessions; a website; events listings (which also act to share ideas); promotional materials and very small grants (when budgets permit).

15.2.2.2 End-of-life Aid Skills for Everyone

EASE is a free course for members of the public in Scotland. It aims to build people's comfort and confidence when dealing with death, dying and bereavement [6]. The course enables people to become better equipped to provide informal support to friends, family and community members. It also aims to make it easier for people to deal with these issues when they have to face them themselves, including learning about options for planning ahead.

EASE was initially developed and piloted by SPPC in 2019. The scope of the course is based on an understanding of what people need or want to know when faced with these issues. In addition to an informal review of published research we did some polling. We asked people who had experience of providing care and support what they wish they had known beforehand. We also asked people who had yet to provide care and support what they wanted to know [7].

For two reasons, EASE is designed so that it can be delivered by community members, within their communities. First, a course that can only be delivered by clinical expert's risks reinforcing the message that these issues are the sole preserve of professionals and institutions. Second, this community-led model enables the scale of delivery to snowball which wouldn't have been possible if dependent on the scarce and expensive time of professionals.

Once trained, the volunteer Course Facilitators deliver the course in pairs working from a structured manual. They are supported by SPPC's Community Development Lead. Regular feedback, evaluation and review provide a framework for quality assurance.

People have different learning styles, so EASE features multiple approaches. Group discussions are central to the ethos of the course; people bring their experiences and perspectives and learn together and from each other. EASE also features short films, group tasks, quizzes, presentations and handouts. EASE is available face-to-face or via an online learning platform combined with group discussion on Zoom. The course takes approximately 8–12 hours to complete over a period of four weeks. A shortened 'taster' version has been used to achieve initial engagement with more marginalised or disadvantaged groups.

15.2.2.3 Demystifying Death Week

Just like To Absent Friends, the annual Demystifying Death Week is a collaborative effort. The week aims to promote practical information about death, dying and bereavement in ways which builds public comfort and confidence around these issues [8]. Each year, the week provides a hook for all kinds of organisations and individuals to organise events for people to discuss and learn about death, dying and bereavement. For example, people have organised death cafes, discussion groups, lectures, photo exhibitions, film screenings, craft workshops, theatre performances, seminars and information stands.

GLGDGG staff support participation by providing organisations with a huge range of freely available resources; advice and support on event planning; a communications pack including press release templates and small grants. The week is non-prescriptive (it is not a 'campaign' which demands that people replicate-specific messages), so participants can focus on what is most important for them locally. Each year, GLGDGG tries to design and introduce a new resource which people can use. In 2025, this was an escape room.

15.2.2.4 The Truacanta Project

With funding from Macmillan Cancer Support, the Truacanta Project was set up to support local communities in Scotland who were interested in taking action to improve people's experiences of death, dying, loss and care.

The project took a community development approach. It ran from 2019 to 2023. Following an open call for expressions of interest, five very different communities were selected as participants. The project had some high-level intended outcomes, increasing knowledge and confidence to deal with and provide support to others around death, dying and bereavement; better access to information; more opportunities to plan ahead; more opportunities to provide (or receive) support; new and strengthened relationships between local organisations; new learning about how compassionate community initiatives work and can best be nurtured. Importantly, within this broad framework, each community had complete freedom to develop their own approaches to addressing the specific issues they felt were most important locally.

Each community received support and advice from SPPC's Community Development Lead, opportunities to share with and learn from the other sites and small grants. Activities undertaken by the participants included conversation cafes, social media campaigns, online discussions, creative arts workshops, public art installation, delivering the EASE course and participating in Demystifying Death Week and To Absent Friends.

An independent evaluation was conducted [9]. Despite the need to pause or reconfigure because of the COVID-19 pandemic, significant progress was made towards all the high-level outcomes. At local level, positive legacies were created and some elements of work were sustained beyond the end of the project period.

15.2.2.5 Bereavement Charter Marks

The Bereavement Charter for Adults and Children in Scotland describes a vision for how organisations and people can all work together to ensure adults, young people and children who are experiencing bereavement are supported [10].

To encourage and support organisations to put the principles of the Charter into practice, SPPC, in collaboration with others, is developing a series of Charter Marks. The first of these was the Charter Mark for workplaces [11]. This can be earned by any organisation which takes a few simple but meaningful steps to create a more bereavement-friendly workplace. SPPC has developed a Bereavement Friendly Workplaces Toolkit [12] to support employers. At the time of writing, 48 workplaces had been awarded the Charter Mark to date, and a similar Bereavement Charter Mark for Primary Schools was being piloted in partnership with St Columba's Hospice Care, the University of Strathclyde and ten interested schools [13].

15.2.3 Understanding the impact of Good Life, Good Death, Good Grief

The aims of GLGDGG are broad and varied, involving fundamental changes in attitudes and behaviours across Scotland. It is very difficult to evidence change at the population level, and even more difficult to show the contribution which GLGDGG initiatives specifically may have made to national change. All this work has been undertaken on a tight budget. There is often a stark choice between spending time taking action or spending time evaluating/measuring. Without the resources to conduct a series of population-level surveys, we've taken a pragmatic approach to understanding the value of our work using various methods.

15.2.3.1 Routine metrics

We use easily gathered data to inform reflection on our impact. This includes web downloads or views of resources; social media metrics; numbers of events taking place in Demystifying Death Week and To Absent Friends; number of organisational and individual members of GLGDGG; number of EASE courses, participants and facilitators; amount of media coverage and the type of organisations engaging with GLGDGG work.

15.2.3.2 Qualitative feedback

Wherever possible, we provide opportunities for participants and stakeholders to provide feedback. For example, this might be via a survey or as part of a short report on how a small grant has been used. We also use rapid informal methods such as '2 stars and a wish' around meetings and events. People often contribute helpful unsolicited feedback.

15.2.3.3 More formal evaluation

We commissioned an independent evaluation of the Truacanta Project. EASE participants complete 'before and after' surveys of their knowledge, skills and confidence relating to the course's learning outcomes. We are currently working with a post-graduate student of public health to explore the longer term impacts of EASE.

15.2.4 What have been the impacts?

15.2.4.1 Increasing scale of engagement

At its outset in 2011, GLGDGG consisted of a handful of like-minded individuals and organisations. By the end of 2023, 499 organisations and 1268 individuals had signed up as members committed to bringing about change. At the time of writing, 700 people have completed the EASE course, and 74 community members have trained as course facilitators.

15.2.4.2 Growing variety of engagement and participation

Our approach of supporting communities to develop activities which reflect their own circumstances and values has enabled a whole variety of people and their groups to engage with or participate in GLGDGG activities. The initial core of palliative care organisations has broadened out to a wide cross-section of civil society: schools, arts organisations, musical groups, sports clubs, craft groups, pubs, faith groups etc. Groups and people who are sometimes excluded have chosen to engage including people in prison, people bereaved by suicide, people with profound and multiple learning disabilities, people in the African-BME communities, LGBTQI+ groups, groups for people with drug and alcohol issues, people who are homeless, people living in some of the most socio-economically disadvantaged parts of Scotland, families bereaved through a death in prison and people with mental health issues.

15.2.4.3 Strengthened capacity

Our provision of networks, free resources and regular opportunities to act has encouraged and made it easier for other organisations to get involved in work around death, dying and bereavement. As a result, the collective capacity working for change in Scotland has grown.

15.2.4.4 Effective resources

Data shows that EASE is highly effective at building comfort and confidence (and waiting lists demonstrate that it is needed). Many of our resources are widely used and reused, suggesting efficacy.

15.2.4.5 Impactful moments and ripple effects

The most important things can be hard to measure. Beyond what it is possible to identify and record, we know that the impact of new connections, awareness, skills, comfort and confidence ripples onwards and outwards in unknown ways. Through qualitative feedback, we catch glimpses of moments which seem impactful and are sometimes perhaps transformative:

> Saturday was amazing, and it helped us so much, we really felt supported for the first time in this process.
>
> *To Absent Friends event participant bereaved by a death in custody.*

> I will take away a new strength in being able to help, plan and offer support
>
> *EASE participant*

> I was terrified of death and talking about it before the course. During the course I lost someone and through what I learned in the first 3 sessions, I had the confidence and peace to go and see the person who has passed. I never would have been able to have this experience; had I not attended this course.
>
> *EASE participant*

15.2.5 Key reflections

15.2.5.1 Doing a lot with a little – creativity and innovation

For most of its lifetime, GLGDGG has been run from the existing resources of the SPPC, a small Scottish charity reliant on membership subscriptions and the Scottish Government for its funding. Though occasional additional short-term funding has been hard-won, the absence of recurrent and predictable funding is an ongoing challenge.

The lack of financial resources has necessitated SPPC finding creative, opportunistic and innovative ways to support this work. Working within strict financial limitations ourselves means that we have an intrinsic understanding of some of the issues that community groups are facing financially. We've looked to harness people's enthusiasm and creativity while recognising that time and money are likely to be in limited supply. We have created resources and projects that require relatively small financial expenditure, but which engage, support and enhance the assets of alliance members.

Though there are several downsides to being under-resourced, one positive has been that, lacking the option of implementing a well-resourced top-down approach, we've had strong motivation to ensure our work is informed and led by an understanding of local context. GLGDGG's portfolio of activities and resources has been developed bearing in mind the challenge of translating theory into practical, scalable local action. Efforts have been made to offer ideas and practical resources which can be adapted for local use depending on context and time available. Where funding has been obtained, this has been spent on creating a sustainable infrastructure that is of practical use to those working on these issues locally.

15.2.5.2 Breadth of remit and lack of understanding

When GLGDGG began its work in 2011, the term 'compassionate community' was not in common usage, the term 'death literacy' had not yet been coined, and there was limited understanding of the aims or methods of 'health promoting' or 'public health' approaches to death, dying and bereavement. Though awareness has grown over the years, so have competing understandings of what is meant by these terms.

Though many people and organisations are passionate about improving experiences of death, dying, loss and care through community involvement, empowerment and development, there are many perspectives and priorities on what is most important and how to best take action to achieve positive change.

GLGDGG has successfully become a 'broad umbrella' for everyone interested in these issues in Scotland. People and organisations join GLGDGG for all kinds of reasons and bring with them a diverse range of agendas. For example, GLGDGG encompasses those who are interested in bringing death education into schools, reducing funeral poverty, improving informal community support for people who've been bereaved, enabling family to undertake care of loved ones at home after death, encouraging greater uptake of Power of Attorney, improving communication skills of health and social care staff, building compassionate communities and much more.

We consider this a success, GLGDGG is a hub of activity for a diverse range of people concerned about improving experiences of death, dying loss and care. However, GLGDGG's many-faceted nature, combined with the general lack of conceptual clarity within the wider field, can make it difficult to promote a wide understanding of our aims and approach.

Over the years, we have developed more clarity about our aims and methods and worked to communicate these in appropriate ways to different audiences.

15.2.5.3 Cultural/institutional/professional reticence

Within our work, we often encounter organisations and individuals who are very cautious about engaging with issues relating to death, dying and bereavement. This might be expressed as generalised concerns about 'sensitivities', more specific concerns about 'doing harm' or sometimes simply as a lack of engagement without explanation as to 'why'.

While there is no expectation or pressure for members of the public to engage with these issues, a lack of engagement from professionals, people in positions of authority, politicians, policymakers and 'gatekeepers' in general can be a real barrier to making progress on important issues. This risk aversion is well-intentioned but can be a barrier to action and lead to the harms which flow from these issues remaining hidden from the public domain.

Over the years, GLGDGG has modelled an openness about these issues and created 'tried and tested' resources and activities that others can use in public spaces, helping to build confidence and overcome risk aversion within the wider communities we work with. However, we still have a long way to go; perhaps, when we no longer encounter reluctance to engage, we will know our work is done!

15.2.5.4 Power and money

A community development approach would advocate for control/agency to reside within communities, yet money/influence tends to reside back to outwith communities. Funders usually have requirements in terms of outcomes, approach, evaluation and reporting which impose certain well-meaning restrictions on how money can be spent and projects set up. Funding requirements inevitably mould projects to some extent; funding can affect existing power dynamics between community members and the withdrawal of funding at the end of a project can have a negative impact on project sustainability.

Power dynamics are difficult to quantify but invariably play an important role in community projects, meaning that those who 'hold power' in these projects (often through access to money, role/status or decision-making) need to actively and consistently find ways of sharing power and control.

This was a complexity we did our best to address within the Truacanta Project by working to create a collegiate dynamic between funders and communities, and by providing accessible grants for communities to spend as they saw fit. However, though one can endeavour to change power dynamics, it isn't possible to remove them completely, and a key piece of learning has been the importance of using what small power we have in helpful ways.

15.2.5.5 How does 'a community' work?

Our work has highlighted questions about how researchers, funders, governments and formal service providers perceive what a 'community' looks like and how a 'community' behaves. In this context, phrases such as 'a whole community response' or 'active communities' paint a vague picture of a large, varied group of active citizens collaborating cheerfully to support each other. However, it is important that those operating in a theoretical or policy space allow for the dynamics of real people in communities. In the words of our Community Development Lead, Caroline Gibb:

> While I think that a 'whole community response' is a nice idea, in my experience, it is never a whole community or even most of a community that is involved. It is more often, a small group of people who take on a huge amount of work, and with it the weight of expectation. It is often people who are already

busy with other things, whether that's work or other volunteering or caring responsibilities, and therefore can't be sustainable.

The Truacanta Project also raised questions about where institutions and organisations fit within compassionate communities. Local projects were led variously by individuals who were volunteers, or employees of third sector, university, council or NHS organisations. Are these organisations part of communities, or separate from them? The boundaries between being a community member and being a paid employee of an organisation operating 'within' a community are blurred.

15.3 Moving from theory to practice – the evolution of a national approach that nurtures local action

The idea of nurturing communities where people support each other through the hard times that can come with death, dying, loss and care is intrinsically attractive and objectively worthwhile. However, achieving this in practice is 'easier said than done', and when we began this work, there were few practical examples to learn from.

In the 17 years we've been doing this work, we have grappled with many questions about how to turn this vision into a reality. How do we move from theory to practice? How can a national organisation take a community development approach? How can communities lead action without an unsustainable burden falling on one or two conscientious citizens? In the financial climate of rising costs of living and decreasing funding for the third sector, what is actually achievable?

Our approach and portfolio of work have gradually grown as we've experimented and learned more about what works and what communities find helpful. The work of GLGDGG illustrates that a national organisation can add value to local work by:

1. Making resources available that can be used locally and flexibly, for example, event templates, conversation menus, an escape room and photographic exhibitions.
2. Providing networking and learning opportunities, for example, a monthly e-bulletin, conferences and online get-togethers.
3. Creating motivation and a sense of community, for example, through meet-ups and conferences, and through a shared sense of purpose such as Demystifying Death Week.
4. Creating opportunities for local involvement in national initiatives, for example, To Absent Friends festival and the EASE course.
5. Providing financial aid, GLGDGG has only ever provided small amounts of money (up to £300) and sometimes it is less about the financial aid and more about the support, encouragement and validation of being part of a bigger project.

Communities will only use what is useful to them, so resources and opportunities provided by a national organisation must be developed in a sympathetic, collaborative and adaptable way, as exemplified by *Demystifying Death Week*, the *To Absent Friends Festival* and *EASE*.

Ideally, communities need both a national infrastructure *and* local support in order for community-led action to thrive.

15.4 Compassionate communities as part of a wider public health approach to death, dying and bereavement

Public Health Palliative Care (PHPC) aims to understand and influence the social and structural factors that affect people's experiences of death, dying, loss and care. PHPC is based on a belief that death, dying, loss and care are experiences shaped by all aspects of society including culture, economics, politics, schools, workplaces, communities and the media. PHPC is a broad field that encompasses work to effect change in a range of areas.

Over the years, GLGDGG has built up a portfolio of community-oriented projects and resources which aim to nurture more supportive environments, more opportunities to give and receive support and more knowledge and skills around death, dying, loss and care in Scottish communities. It has drawn on various approaches in its work, including public education, information provision, community engagement, health promotion, community development and policy influencing.

Our work illustrates that different approaches each have their place in work to improve experiences of caring, dying and grieving within communities. Built on the principles of self-determination, empowerment, collective action and learning together, a community development approach can help create a supportive and collegiate environment for work to take place, in which values such as social justice, equality and respect for diversity are prioritised. While 'community development' is an important grounding principle, other, more directed approaches, can also have an important and complementary role to play in working to nurture more compassionate communities.

15.5 Next steps

Membership of and engagement with GLGDGG continue to grow. Long-term annual initiatives such as To Absent Friends and Demystifying Death Week attract more participants each year, and from an increasingly diverse range of organisations and communities. The EASE course has proven itself to have huge resonance and utility, and course numbers are increasing. Recent years have seen GLGDGG's work branch out to support workplace and school communities through the development and promotion of Bereavement Charter Mark schemes. These are all areas that we will continue to develop in the future.

The portfolio of resources available for members to use free of charge also continues to grow. What began with 11 information leaflets now includes a conversation menu, origami game, event templates, loanable photographic exhibitions, guidance on holding events, two online toolkits and a DIY escape room.

Looking ahead to the future, GLGDGG's funding continues to be precarious. Searching for and applying for funding takes time and energy away from the work itself and raises uncertainties about long-term sustainability. We continue to adapt, finding ways of explaining our goals and projects in ways that appeal to potential funders while maintaining true to the core principles of the work.

Our model relies on organisations, community groups and enthusiastic individuals taking relevant action within their community. However, different communities have different levels of social capital and various inequalities and inequities exist in Scotland. Without dedicated resource, it is a challenge for GLGDGG to undertake the sensitive groundwork needed to bring our work to communities that are currently underserved and marginalised. We continue to work on this as a priority and remain committed to ensuring that our work benefits the people who need it most.

References

1. Scottish Government, "Living and dying well," *Scottish Government*, 2008.
2. M. Hazelwood and R. M. Patterson, "Scotland's Public Health Palliative Care Alliance," *Annals of Palliative Medicine*, vol. 7, Suppl 2, pp. 99–108, 2018.
3. Scottish Partnership for Palliative Care, "Good Life, Good Death, Good Grief," [Online]. Available: https://www.goodlifedeathgrief.org.uk/. [Accessed 22 October 2025].
4. Scottish Partnership for Palliative Care, "To Absent Friends," [Online]. Available: https://www.toabsentfriends.org.uk/. [Accessed 22 October 2025].
5. R. M. Patterson, R. J. Peacock and M. A. Hazelwood, "To Absent Friends, a people's festival of storytelling and remembrance," *Bereavement Care*, vol. 36, no. 3, pp. 119–126, 2017.
6. Scottish Partnership for Palliative Care, "End of Life Skills for Everyone (EASE)," Scottish Partnership for Palliative Care, [Online]. Available: https://www.goodlifedeathgrief.org.uk/plan-illness-ease/. [Accessed 22 October 2025].
7. R. M. Patterson, C. Gibb and M. A. Hazelwood, "End of Life aid Skills for Everyone in Scotland," *Palliative Care and Social Practice*, vol. 16, 2022. doi:10.1177/26323524221076511.
8. Scottish Partnership for Palliative Care, "Demystifying Death Week," *Good Life, Good Death, Good Grief*, [Online]. Available: https://www.goodlifedeathgrief.org.uk/members-dmd/. [Accessed 22 October 2025].
9. J. Biggar, R. McFarlane, C. Gibb and R. Patterson, "The Truacanta Project: Evaluation Report," 2023.
10. Bereavement Charter for Scotland Group, "The Bereavement Charter for Adults and Children in Scotland," *Good Life, Good Death, Good Grief*, [Online]. Available: https://www.goodlifedeathgrief.org.uk/about-charter/. [Accessed 22 October 2025].

11. Bereavement Charter for Scotland Group, "Bereavement Charter Mark for Workplaces," *Good Life*, *Good Death*, *Good Grief*, [Online]. Available: https://www.goodlifedeathgrief.org.uk/about-charter-mark-employers/. [Accessed 22 October 2025].
12. Scottish Partnership for Palliative Care, "Scottish Bereavement Friendly Workplaces Toolkit," *Good Life*, *Good Death*, *Good Grief*, [Online]. Available: https://www.goodlifedeathgrief.org.uk/members-resources-workplaces/. [Accessed 22 October 2025].
13. Bereavement Charter for Scotland Group, "Bereavement Charter Mark for Primary Schools," *Good Life*, *Good Death*, *Good Grief*, [Online]. Available: https://www.goodlifedeathgrief.org.uk/about-charter-mark-schools/. [Accessed 22 October 2025].

16

TRANSLATING COMPASSION INTO ACTION

Building an ecosystem for Compassionate Communities Singapore

Bee Hia Sim

Abstract

This chapter shares Singapore's unique approach to localising the Compassionate Communities movement within a highly urbanised, multi-ethnic city-state. As Singapore faces the realities of a rapidly ageing population, the need to mobilise communities in end-of-life care has become increasingly urgent. Every town in Singapore has its own network of grassroots, healthcare, and social service partners—an asset that makes it more ready to embrace Compassionate Communities Singapore to provide support for caregivers, dying, grieved, and bereaved, as part of everyday life. Led by the Singapore Hospice Council (SHC), the initiative began with understanding needs from the ground, engaging diverse stakeholders, and co-developing the vision, mission, and user guides. The official launch of Compassionate Communities Singapore on 12 October 2025 marks a key milestone in building a shared responsibility for care in the community. This chapter outlines Singapore's journey, key strategies, lessons learned, and a call to action: to grow and sustain a compassionate ecosystem, one community at a time.

16.1 Introduction

The demand for palliative care, caregiving support, and end-of-life services is expected to increase drastically in the coming years, and it is widely expected that the Singapore healthcare system alone cannot meet these needs.

DOI: 10.4324/9781003621348-17

TABLE 16.1 Persons Living Alone and Lone Parent Households by Age

Age Group	*Below 35*	*35–49*	*50–64*	*Above 65*	*Total*
No of persons living alone	23,600	59,000	66,400	87,200	236,200
Lone parent households	2,200	18,500	34,800	18,500	74,000

16.1.1 Trends

Singapore became an aged society in 2017 and is set to attain "super-aged" status in 2026. By 2030, one in four citizens will be aged 65 and above, up from one in six in 2024 [1].

In 2024, total deaths reported were 26,442 [2], or on average, 72 people died daily. Life expectancy at birth is 83.5 years old with males at 81.2 years old and females at 85.6 years old [2].

About 77% [2] of the population resides in Housing and Development Board public housing, with the rest residing in private condominiums and apartments (17.7%) and private landed property (4.7%) in 2024. A total of 236,200 persons live alone [2] and 74,000 households are Lone Parent Households (a person is either never married, widowed, divorced, or separated and living with a child below 16 or never married children) (Table 16.1).

16.1.2 Geography

Singapore is zoned into two types of constituencies: Single Member Constituencies (SMCs) and Group Representation Constituencies (GRCs). A GRC is a larger electoral division serving a larger population and is sub-divided into four to five Divisions. Each SMC and Division is helmed by a Grassroots Adviser and served by volunteer community leaders. Each SMC and GRC Division is also served by several social service agencies (NGOs), active ageing centres, healthcare clusters, schools, and religious organisations.

As such, every SMC and GRC Division is well poised to become a compassionate community to provide care and support to the seriously ill, dying, caregivers, grieved, and bereaved.

16.1.3 Conviction of the leadership

The Singapore Hospice Council (SHC) partners its 26 Member Organisations [3] to lead the work in palliative and hospice care in Singapore. Its vision is to provide "quality palliative care for everyone" and is committed to improving the lives of patients with serious life-limiting illnesses and to empowering the journey towards the end-of-life for patients and their families, as well as caregiver support in Singapore. As an advocate for a good death, and the collective voice of the palliative care community, SHC raises public awareness and understanding of palliative care.

Many leaders, including both healthcare professionals and non-healthcare professionals, believe that dying is fundamentally not a medical event, but a social experience that happens in the family and the community. It is everyone's responsibility, not just healthcare or palliative professionals, and there have been active conversations over the years on de-medicalising death.

The SHC Board and Medical Leads of its 26 Member Organisations firmly believe that palliative care services should commence upstream as early as one can. This stems from data showing persistent late referrals, especially for non-cancer diagnosis. The overall median time from first palliative care assessment to death remained short at 21 days [4] with a marked contrast between cancer patients (31 days) and non-cancer patients (9 days). This lag may be attributed to the lack of awareness and knowledge of seriously ill patients and families to actively seek palliative care services, and non-palliative care healthcare professionals not providing that option to patients and families.

16.1.4 Laying the foundation

Laying the groundwork for *compassionate communities* is critical, as the concept is not always easily understood. At first glance, many may see it simply as a combination of an adjective and a noun—"compassionate" and "communities"—and associate it with general acts of kindness. Some reacted with "you mean Singaporeans are not compassionate enough?"

But in reality, it represents a deeper, more intentional movement that calls on all of us—individuals, organisations, and systems—to work together in supporting those facing serious illness, caregiving responsibilities, death, and grief. To bring this vision to life, we must first build awareness, foster understanding, and create platforms for meaningful engagement. Only then can we move forward to build a truly compassionate society where care at the end-of-life is not just a medical responsibility, but a shared community commitment.

The SHC has been instrumental in laying the foundation for the *Compassionate Communities Singapore* movement, a national effort to foster a more death- and grief-literate society. Through a strategic, multi-level engagement approach, SHC has rolled out a series of impactful initiatives designed to raise awareness, build capacity, and encourage collective responsibility in end-of-life care.

16.2 Strategic initiatives

16.2.1 Raising public awareness through accessible engagement platforms

At the foundation of SHC's efforts is the drive to normalise conversations around death, dying, and palliative care. SHC organises public roadshows and *Palliative Care 101* training sessions across Singapore. These initiatives provide approachable, jargon-free information to demystify palliative care, helping people understand how they can support loved ones through life-limiting illnesses and make informed decisions about their own care. These public engagements are held in heartland spaces such as malls, community centres, and libraries to meet people where they are, fostering grassroots-level awareness. The content is tailored for the target group vis-à-vis their language, culture nuances, and literacy level.

From July 2022 to June 2025, a total of 57 sessions of *Palliative Care 101* were conducted, reaching out to 3,323 persons. During these sessions, participants are asked to share how death looks like to them, their preferred place of death, challenges, and how to start a 'die-logue'.

> "The Palliative Care 101 was Hope Centre's first time organising a caregiver-focused programme. We wanted our caregivers to know how to have end-of-life conversations with their loved ones and be aware of the relevant community resources that are available," Ms Yeo Keng Suan of Hope Centre.
>
> As death is always being reminded in the Islamic faith, we hope that the course would help our community reflect on their attitudes towards death. They now understand the importance of preparing for death. With our members more willing to have end-of-life conversations, we can better assist them in planning for their end-of-life, in both physical and spiritual matters.
>
> Mr Muhammad Khidir Bin Haji Mohamed Ibrahim,
> Ustaz of Al-Muttaqin Mosque.

16.2.2 Engaging leaders and policy influencers

To create sustainable systemic change, SHC actively involves senior leadership in shaping a compassionate ecosystem. The *Leaders Forum* series targets C-suite executives and institutional leaders across healthcare, religious, cultural, social services, and education. These small-group forums provide a safe space to facilitate high-level conversations about end-of-life care as an organisation and societal priority. By highlighting the role that leaders can play, such as implementing compassionate workplace policies or supporting grief literacy, SHC ensures top-down support for broader cultural change from within an organisation. The Leaders Forum series also allowed for stakeholders in the same space to connect and form alliances.

> Initiatives such as today's initiation of Compassionate Communities Singapore, are powerful steps toward normalising grief support as a community-wide commitment. Community must be a place for not only the healthy. It must be where the seriously ill can enjoy support in the safety and protection of the familiar, a place that many would have lived at least

half their lives, if not more. Employers, neighbours, grassroots organisations, places of worship, schools, social service agencies or public service institutions, can and should take on stronger roles in the care of people at the end-of-life and their families through illness, dying, death, grief and bereavement.

Central District Mayor and Member of Parliament for Jalan Besar GRC, Ms Denise Phua.

16.2.3 Empowering the primary care sector

Recognising that primary care providers are often the closest touchpoint for individuals dealing with life-limiting illness, and for the aged frail residing in the community, SHC focuses on strengthening the capabilities and awareness of this sector. A primary care landscape scan was conducted in 2023/2024 to better understand the needs and challenges of general practitioners and polyclinic doctors (a polyclinic is a government-subsidised healthcare facility that provides a wide range of primary care services under one roof, larger than a typical clinic but smaller than a hospital). It identified a few challenges of primary care doctors: lack of confidence with prognosis, lack of confidence with administering controlled drugs, and lack of knowledge on palliative care referral processes. In response, SHC launched the SHC Primary Care Palliative Champions (PC2) Telegram Group in March 2025. The Group is only open to doctors and is backed by a multidisciplinary team of palliative care specialists. It provides access to a specialist palliative care team, including palliative care physicians, nurses, medical social workers, allied health staff, primary care doctors, and SHC administrative team. Primary care doctors are now only a text away to advice from palliative care specialists.

SHC also created the SHC Hospice Capacity Dashboard for any referring doctor to check capacity of hospices by just keying in the postal code of the patient's residence. This quick tool is to allow expeditious referrals. It works on a traffic light system: red meaning it is at full capacity and unable to receive patients; amber for referral of compassionate discharge patients (patients going home to die) only; and green means patients can be referred to them.

Dr Clare Tay, a General Practitioner, who has also had multiple referrals rejected previously because the home hospices were at maximum capacity, said the dashboard comes in handy during home visits.

> "When patients and families are agreeable, I access the hospice dashboard during the home visit and offer a suitable option based on availability of resources," she said.

Through training, resource sharing, and engagement platforms, SHC works with general practitioners, polyclinics, and community nurses to equip them with the knowledge and tools needed to have compassionate conversations and initiate timely referrals to palliative care services. This integration bridges the gap between clinical care and community support.

16.2.4 Building a credible, centralised resource hub

To support individuals, families, and professionals navigating end-of-life issues, SHC, together with its supporting clinicians, develops and continues to curate useful content regularly to build a trusted, comprehensive online resource hub. This e-library serves as a one-stop portal on palliative care resources, life stories, and research reports for the general public, patient, caregivers, and healthcare professionals. It is designed to be accessible to all levels of digital literacy, with multilingual resources and easy-to-navigate layouts. The hub also supports community champions and volunteers with ready-to-use educational materials.

SHC's webpage not only invites users to reflect on their end-of-life priorities but also provides practical tools to guide conversation and planning. The e-library hosts valuable content—from FAQs to self-assessment workbooks and caregiver fact sheets—making knowledge accessible anytime, anywhere. Our digital archives—newsletters, toolkits, and guides—empower audiences to explore at their own pace, with trust and intention.

Through this multi-channel approach, SHC ensures that its messages reach diverse audiences—families, working adults, youths, caregivers, and professionals—at times and on platforms most relevant and convenient to them. By combining authentic narrative storytelling with strategic platform use, SHC's campaigns do not just inform—they invite, comfort, and challenge (Figure 16.1).

FIGURE 16.1 QR Code to SHC e-Library

16.2.5 Establishing Community Signposts for ground-level support

To create a compassionate environment within neighbourhoods, SHC started with lower hanging fruits. On 1 October 2022, it piloted *Community Signposts*—touchpoints located in the community including active ageing centres, places of worship, nursing homes, community centres, general practitioners' clinics, and social service agencies. The initiative seeks to set up community-level voluntary support groups to provide signposting of palliative care resources to patients facing life-limiting illnesses, their families, and caregivers. (Figure 16.2)

The *Community Signpost* is not a physical counter or location. Instead, it is made up of a group of trained and committed volunteers. To start a Signpost, a team of at least eight volunteers will undergo a two-hour Palliative Care 101 training session. This equips them with the necessary information and resources to provide signposting. General palliative care knowledge such as the types of care services, service providers' directory, and referral process are also part of the course content.

Volunteers must be familiar with SHC's e-library where they can direct residents to online resources such as explainer videos and short films. Printed resources such as self-help books, brochures are given to each Community Signpost so that the community will have access to accurate resources.

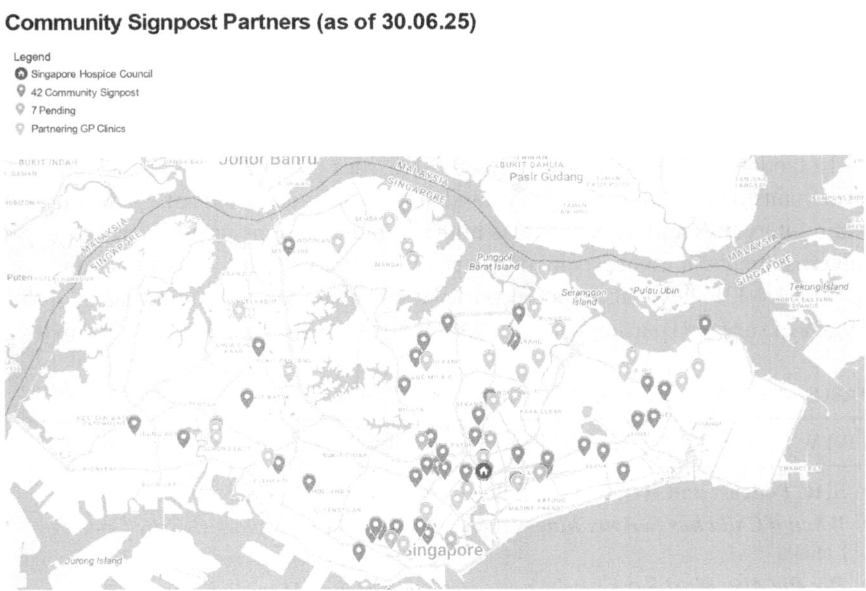

FIGURE 16.2 Community Signpost Map

Besides factual resources, volunteers are also given tips on communication skills to initiate conversations about end-of-life issues and why these conversations matter. Examples of SHC resources that are available at a Community Signpost:

1 "Palliative Care: What You Need to Know"—FAQ brochure
2 "The Hospice Link" newsletter—A thematic quarterly newsletter
3 "Nutrition in Advanced Illnesses"—Self-help booklet for caregivers
4 "Medications and How to Apply"—Self-help materials for caregivers
5 "Common Symptoms"—Self-help videos for caregivers, such as Common Functional Assessment Tools, Dyspnoea, and Pain Management.
6 "Final Hours"—Self-help booklet on death and dying
7 "Caring for Yourself After a Death"—Self-help booklet on grief and bereavement (Figure 16.2).

16.2.6 Creating signature events: Live Well. Leave Well. Festival

Amid past widespread efforts from various organisations to promote palliative care, SHC seeks to unify these diverse stakeholders into a cohesive advocacy platform. In line with the World Hospice and Palliative Care Day in October, SHC organises the annual Live Well. Leave Well. Festival (LWLW Festival) to foster collaboration and amplify impact through partnerships and a collective voice. The Festival aims to be a one-stop platform to raise awareness about hospice and palliative care, highlighting its multidisciplinary approach to providing relief, comfort, and support to individuals with life-limiting illnesses and their families. In 2023 and 2024, the LWLW Festival extended its reach, spanning into ten days to engage a broader audience (Table 16.2).

In tandem with the LWLW Festival, SHC runs a coordinated media campaign over mainstream media in Singapore and SHC social media platforms. These include radio interviews and trailers across multiple radio stations in different languages, advertisements in trains, social media stories, narratives, and calls-to-action.

The LWLW Festival garnered positive feedback. On a scale rating of 1 to 5, 89.5% of surveyed participants in 2023 and 2024 reported an increase of knowledge

TABLE 16.2 LWLW Festival Event Highlights for 2023 and 2024

LWLW Festival 2023 Event Highlights	LWLW Festival 2024 Event Highlights
• **SHC Podcast and Helpline Launch**	• ***Die Die Also Must Say*** Chatshow
• ***When a Child has Serious Illness*** Book Launch	• ***Voices for Hospices Charity*** Concert
• ***Die Die Also Must Say*** Chatshow	• ***Tree of Compassion*** Interactive Element
• ***You Light Up My Life*** Memorial Night	• ***Garden of Hope*** Exhibition Featuring "Legacy of Resilience" and "Renewal" Inspired by Patients' Artwork
• Movie Screening - ***Up***	• ***Live Well. Leave Well. Exhibition***
• **#SHCLiveWellChallenge** Fundraiser	• New Exhibit Launch
• **Nagomi Art** Interactive Element	

(4 or 5) in palliative care after attending the programmes. Common reasons for attending the festival programmes include relevance of topic to personal experience and to gain knowledge.

The LWLW Festival 2023 and 2024 attracted over 10,000 footfalls and featured a total of 52 talks, webinars, and workshops, with more than 1,200 participants. Publicity efforts achieved a social media reach of over 135,000 individuals, engaged over 2.5 million listeners through radio campaigns, and amassed over 2 million impressions for train advertisements. Notably, 60% of surveyed participants in 2024 were new to SHC's activities, highlighting its growing reach.

The LWLW Festival brings together the public, healthcare providers, allied health professionals, educators, and community organisations in a vibrant, reflective space. By focusing on living well and framing death as a natural part of life, the Festival helps reduce stigma and encourages open, culturally sensitive conversations.

16.2.7 Cultivating strategic partnerships

SHC understands that no single organisation can build a compassionate society alone. It actively cultivates partnerships across healthcare institutions, government agencies, NGOs, academia, the arts, and corporate sector. These collaborations amplify impact, enable resource-sharing, and create a united voice for compassionate care. SHC focuses on long-term relationships with partners who share aligned values and are willing to co-create solutions that are responsive to Singapore's evolving societal needs. In recent years, particularly from 2022 onwards, our work has focused on building a sustainable ecosystem of strategic partnerships—across sectors and communities—to catalyse the growth of compassionate communities throughout the country.

These partnerships include the following:

16.2.7.1 Healthcare sector: towards integrated and holistic palliative care

SHC partners with its 26 Member Organisations actively: encompassing being a collective voice, a capability builder, advocacy, production of resources, and quality improvements on service norms to research.

16.2.7.2 Government and grassroots: bringing compassion to the heartlands

A strategic partnership with government bodies and grassroots networks has enabled SHC to take palliative care into the everyday lives of Singaporeans. In 2022, we launched the Community Signposts initiative, in partnership with the People's Association and local grassroots organisations. These signposts serve as accessible touchpoints in neighbourhoods such as Kebun Baru, Yio Chu Kang, and Mountbatten, offering printed resources, volunteer support, and early signposting for caregivers and patients navigating end-of-life challenges.

16.2.7.3 Social Service Organisations and volunteers: extending reach through relationships

Volunteerism and civil society play a crucial role in SHC's compassionate community strategy. Social Service Organisations like Fei Yue Community Services, Dementia SG, and places of worship like Al-Muttaqin Mosque work closely with SHC for training and ensuring early conversations, care planning, and accessibility to those who need it in the community.

Complementing this is our volunteer Ambassador Programme, launched in 2022. SHC aims to recruit and train ambassadors annually to lead palliative care conversations in their circle of influence. Each ambassador is trained in *Palliative Care 101*, provided with an Ambassador Handbook on support resources and code of conduct, and outreach packs to speak to 20 friends and families over a two-year period.

16.2.7.4 Academia and research: building knowledge and shaping practice

Evidence and education are pillars of sustainable change. In 2023, SHC conducted Singapore's first national landscape scan on primary palliative care, aimed at understanding how doctors perceive and deliver end-of-life care in primary settings.

In 2024/2025, SHC worked with Temasek Polytechnic to conduct a population-wide survey on the Death Literacy Index to establish a baseline so as to measure improvements to Singapore's population death literacy over the years to come and to help shape immediate and mid-term community engagement and public education strategies.

SHC also maintains ongoing collaborations with institutions of higher learning such as the National University of Singapore, National Technological University, Temasek Polytechnic, Ngee Ann Polytechnic, and Nanyang Polytechnic to support curriculum development, training, industrial and internship placements, and research. These partnerships are vital to developing a future-ready palliative care workforce equipped not just with clinical knowledge, but with compassion and cultural competence.

SHC's journey towards a compassionate Singapore is neither linear nor owned by any single entity. Since 2022, its strategic partnerships have reflected a whole-of-society approach—deliberate, inclusive, and adaptive. These partnerships go beyond delivering programmes; they serve as a foundation for co-creating movements of care. By anchoring this work in trust, shared values, and long-term collaboration, SHC believes that a truly compassionate society is not only possible—but already emerging.

16.2.8 Maximising reach through media and campaigns

In our journey to cultivate a more compassionate and death-literate society, SHC embraces a multi-channel media strategy to reshape public perceptions around palliative and end-of-life care. From traditional outlets to digital campaigns, each medium is leveraged thoughtfully to tell real human stories that foster empathy, dismantle misconceptions, and extend a message of dignity, hope, and connection.

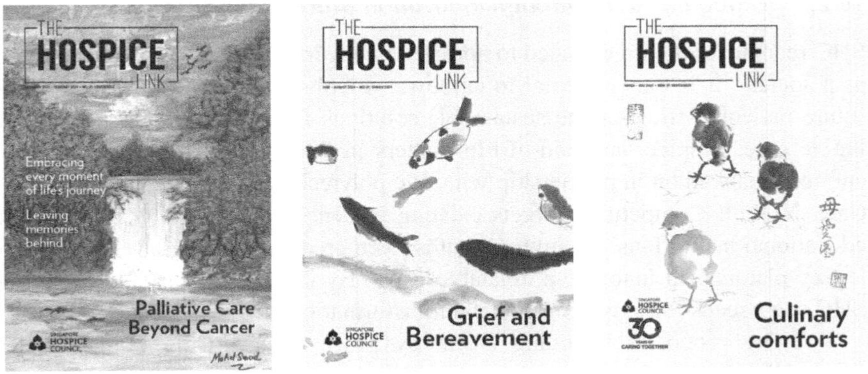

FIGURE 16.3 Covers of The Hospice Link Featuring Patients' Artwork

16.2.8.1 The Hospice Link newsletter

Every quarter, The Hospice Link offers heartfelt stories and practical guidance on palliative care. Popular editions include titles like "Culinary Comforts" and "Grief and Bereavement," "Palliative Care Beyond Cancer." These issues do more than inform—they bind readers across experience as caregivers, professionals, and members of the public, weaving narratives that encourage reflection and reassurance (Figure 16.3).

16.2.8.2 Social media: storytelling that connects and normalises

SHC leverages platforms such as Instagram, Facebook, LinkedIn, and YouTube to make palliative care visible and approachable for a broader audience, especially younger generations. Through caregiver stories, short videos from healthcare workers, myth-busting infographics, and culturally sensitive messaging, SHC normalises conversations around death, caregiving, and end-of-life planning. Regular posts tied to international events—like World Hospice and Palliative Care Day—highlight personal reflections, community initiatives, and volunteer voices, creating digital touchpoints that foster empathy and spark dialogue. Search Engine Optimisation (SEO) are actively adopted as strategies to increase the e-library's visibility in search engine results, ensuring that patients, families, general public, and healthcare professionals' access accurate knowledge and timely updates.

16.2.8.3 Podcast: conversations at a click

Understanding that audiences require new avenues for engagement that are convenient and easy to access, SHC launched the Live Well. Leave Well. podcast in 2023. The podcast now comes in English audio format (12 episodes), Chinese video format (4 episodes), and Malay audio format (5 episodes). The podcast enables sustained engagement and cultivates early conversation among a digitally savvy public.

16.2.9 Engaging youth through innovation: Hack Care:YOLO!

SHC recognises the urgent need to normalise conversations about death and dying as a society. It is thus essential to empower youths—tomorrow's caregivers and future patients—to co-create sustainable solutions for raising awareness for palliative care, hospice, and end-of-life matters in Singapore. This was how SHC curated a hackathon in partnership with five polytechnics in Singapore. The Hack Care: YOLO! Competition targets existing students aged 15–25 years old from educational institutions and invites youths to co-create solutions for eldercare and legacy planning in innovative, relatable ways. By involving the next generation, SHC sows seeds for long-term societal transformation.

Winning proposals including Death by Music (Death Café Using Music), Escape Room, and Legacy Fighters, were adapted and implemented during the LWLW Festival 2024 and 2025.

16.2.10 Grounding efforts in data and research

A data-driven approach underpins all SHC's work, guiding programme design, stakeholder engagement, and resource allocation. A key milestone was the release of Singapore's first Death Literacy Index (DLI) study in September 2025, which revealed a national score of 5.66 out of 10. This moderate rating indicates that while Singaporeans are somewhat aware of end-of-life issues, significant gaps remain in practical knowledge, confidence, and community support. This data is now used to tailor interventions by demographic group and measure progress over time, reinforcing accountability, and relevance.

16.3 Engagement of like-minded stakeholders

True to the nature of compassionate communities being bottom-up, a half-day Collaborative Dialogue was organised by SHC for like-minded stakeholders and individuals to Co-Create Compassionate Communities Singapore. About 50 participants attended.

A simple pre and post survey was conducted to gather feedback from participants and draw insights into the outcome of the dialogue and effect it had on participants. The survey showed that there was an increased in readiness of starting compassionate communities post survey. Facilitators familiar with the concept and approach helped moderate and guide the table discussions. Please see infographics for details: (Figures 16.4–16.6).

The Dialogue succeeded to define and co-create the vision and mission of Compassionate Communities SG, key factors for success, secure buy-ins and identified champions and drivers in different sectors, template charters by sector, and identified organisations ready to pilot Compassionate Communities within their respective organisations. It also established the roles that SHC takes in Compassionate Communities Singapore:

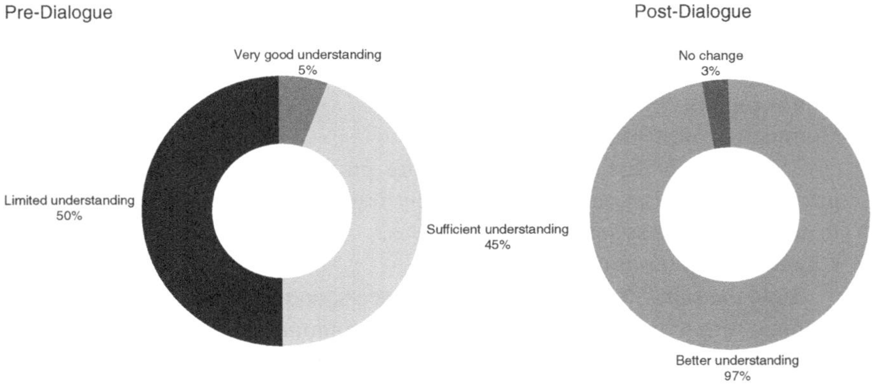

FIGURE 16.4 Level of Understanding of Compassionate Communities

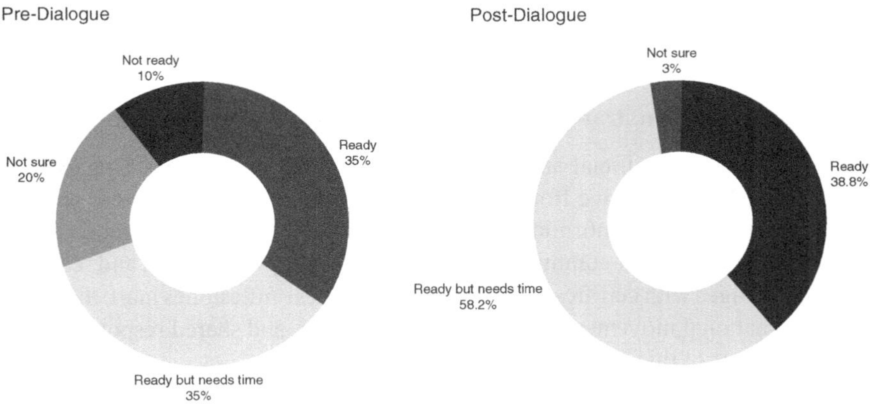

FIGURE 16.5 Organisations' Readiness to Start Compassionate Communities

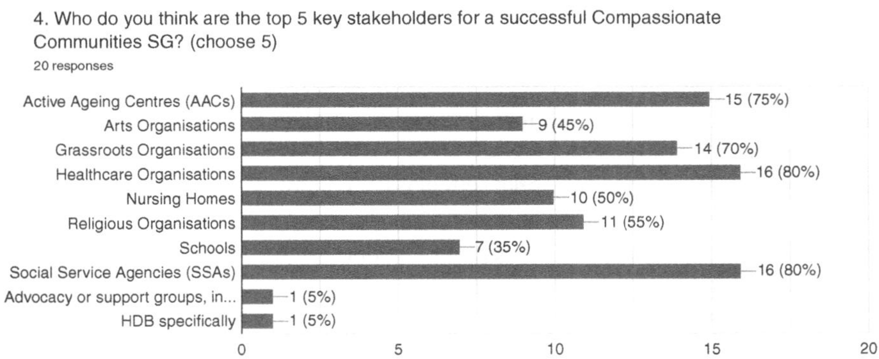

FIGURE 16.6 Top Five Key Stakeholders (Pre-Dialogue)

1 **Thought Leader and Advocate**
   Shape the national discourse on compassionate communities by advocating for policies, raising awareness, and promoting the integration of palliative care within community settings.
2 **Connector and Collaborator**
   Serve as a bridge between healthcare providers, social service agencies, grassroots organisations, and community organisations, fostering partnerships to co-create compassionate care initiatives.
3 **Capacity Builder and Educator**
   Build the capacity of individuals, volunteers, and organisations by providing training, resources, and toolkits to empower communities to care for those facing life-limiting illnesses and bereavement.
4 **Champion of community-led initiatives**
   Support and amplify community-driven projects that promote compassion, encouraging local ownership, and sustainable efforts to improve quality of life for the sick with life-limiting illness and their families, beyond the patient's passing

16.4 Conclusion: translating compassion into collective action

As we approach the official launch of Compassionate Communities Singapore on 12 October 2025, we move from intention to collective impact. The next phase of this journey includes confirming the participation of organisations that share our vision, formalising their commitment through the signing of charters, and recognising their pledges with certificates of participation. These milestones mark the beginning of a national movement rooted in care, inclusion, and shared responsibility.

At the heart of this initiative lies a powerful **vision**:

A compassionate and inclusive ecosystem where no one dies or grieves alone.

Our **mission** is equally clear:

Through education, advocacy, and sustainable partnerships, we unite to embrace, support, and honour both living and dying in Singapore.

Guided by the core values of **compassion** and **dignity**, and grounded in the principles of **empathy, inclusiveness**, and **collaboration**, we are working to:

1 Build an ecosystem of care that empowers individuals and communities with kindness.
2 Strengthen community networks so that no one journeys through illness, dying, or grief alone.
3 Honour dignity, personal choice, and cultural sensitivity in all aspects of end-of-life care.
4 Foster a spirit of shared responsibility—what we in Singapore refer to as the kampung spirit, a traditional ethos of neighbourliness and mutual care.

Our collective commitment as Compassionate Communities Singapore is to:

1. Improve health and death literacy across communities.
2. Create learning opportunities that nurture compassion and connectedness.
3. Share stories and lived experiences of people who are dying or grieving every day.
4. Nurture supportive relationships through neighbourhood and community-based networks.
5. Make visible the strengths and needs of informal caregivers—families, friends, and volunteers who provide essential emotional and practical care.

This initiative is not merely a programme; it is part of a wider global movement to de-medicalise care, recognise grief, and ensure that no one is left behind in life's most vulnerable moments. Compassionate Communities Singapore contributes to this global vision while remaining deeply rooted in our local context and cultural values.

As we move forward, the work begins not only with systems and structures, but also with each of us. With open hearts and a shared sense of purpose, we can embed compassion into everyday life—in homes, neighbourhoods, workplaces, and institutions. Together, we can build a future where compassion is a collective responsibility, and no one dies or grieves alone.

16.5 No one should die or grieve alone" — launch of Compassionate Communities Singapore and 'Winds of Compassion' community art installation

SINGAPORE, 12 October 2025—The Singapore Hospice Council (SHC) officially launched Compassionate Communities Singapore (CoCoSG), a national movement to build a compassionate and inclusive ecosystem where no one dies or grieves alone. The event was graced by Guest-of-Honour Ms Rahayu Mahzam, Minister of State, Ministry of Health and Ministry of Digital Development and Information, and Special Guest Ms Gho Sze Kee, Member of Parliament and Grassroots Adviser to Mountbatten GROs (Figure 16.7).

As part of the launch, SHC recognised more than 40 founding stakeholders who have pledged their commitment to this national movement. Representing healthcare, education, social service, community, ethnic, and faith-based organisations, these founding stakeholders embody the spirit of empathy, inclusiveness, and collaboration, working together to build an ecosystem of care that honours dignity, choice, and cultural sensitivity, while fostering a kampong spirit of togetherness, respect, and shared responsibility. Each founding stakeholder will also develop a Charter, outlining their commitment to CoCoSG and how they will strengthen community networks and foster meaningful connections that extend beyond institutional care (Figure 16.8).

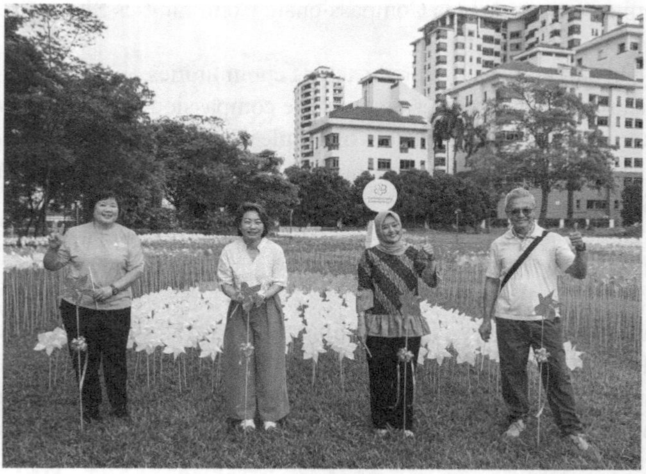

FIGURE 16.7 Launch of CoCoSG with Ms Sim Bee Hia, Executive Director of SHC, Special Guest, Ms Goh Sze Kee, Guest-of-Honour, Ms Rahayu Mahzam, and Dr Chong Poh Heng, Vice Chairman of SHC

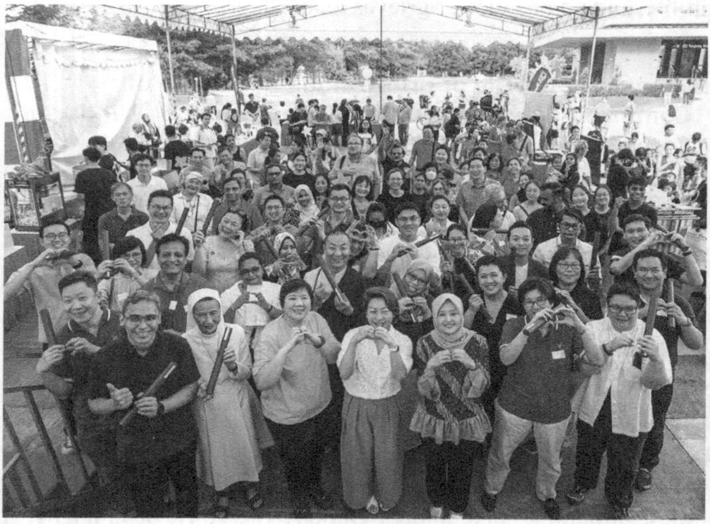

FIGURE 16.8 Group Photo with the CoCoSG Founding Stakeholders

As one of the founding stakeholders, Compassionate Communities Mountbatten was also launched as Singapore's first constituency-led compassionate community, embracing a whole-of-community approach. For caregivers, it is important to know they are not carrying their burdens alone. To further strengthen the spirit of care, a Mountbatten Compassionate Care Fund was also set up with a seed amount

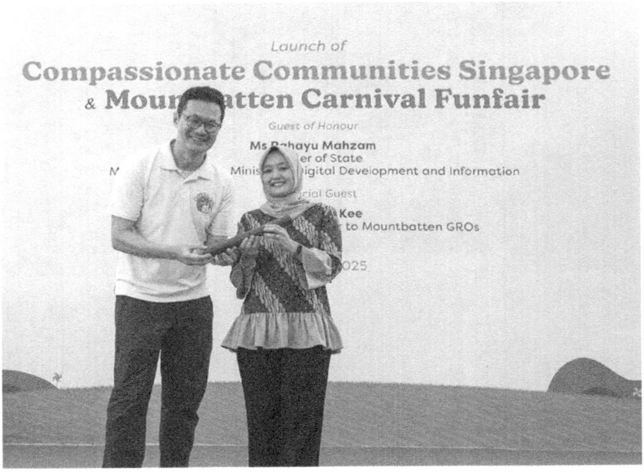

FIGURE 16.9 Presentation of CoCoSG Certificate to Mr Victor Lee, Mountbatten CCC

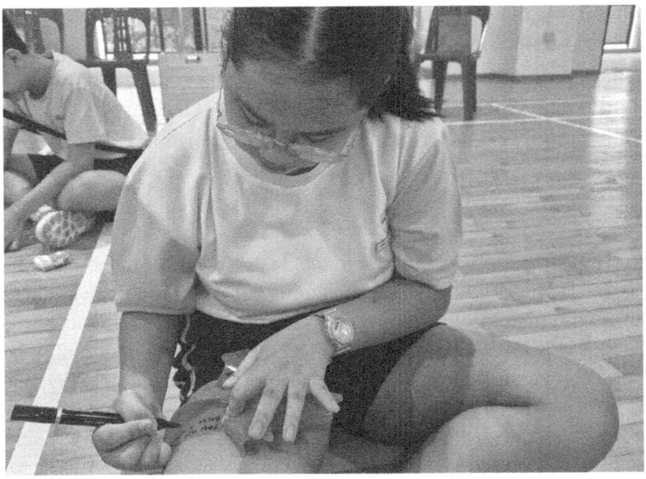

FIGURE 16.10 Student Making their Personalised Pinwheels

of SGD40,000 dedicated to supporting eligible Mountbatten caregivers, without any income requirements (Figure 16.9).

In conjunction with the launch, SHC unveiled the "Winds of Compassion" Community Art Installation, featuring 10,000 hand-decorated pinwheels, each adorned with a personal message co-created with 63 partners including SHC Member Organisations, schools, and community partners. Each pinwheel represents a small act of care—a symbol of how simple gestures, when multiplied across the community, can create a powerful ripple of compassion and connection. The installation serves as a visual

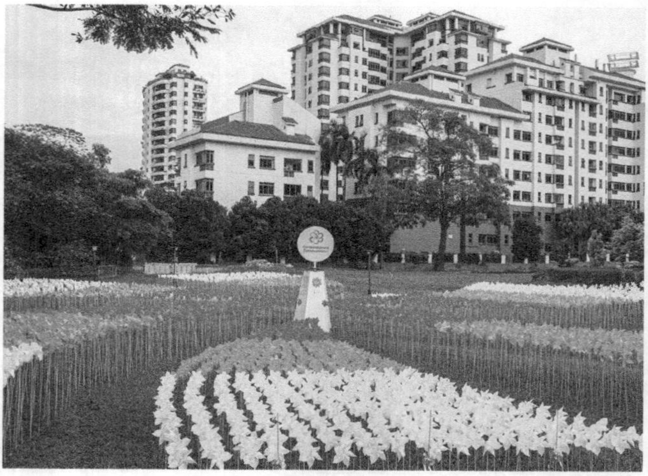

FIGURE 16.11 'Winds of Compassion' Community Art Installation

tribute to collective empathy and shared humanity, reflecting SHC's vision of a society where every life is valued, supported, and remembered (Figures 16.10 and 16.11).

The launch of CoCoSG marks a significant step forward in shaping a future where end-of-life and bereavement care are integrated within the fabric of society, supported by compassionate individuals, communities, and organisations working hand in hand.

References

1 The Straits Times, "Initiatives in place to tackle ageing issues as S'pore hits 'super-aged' status in 2026: Health Minister," 22 November 2024. [Online]. Available: https://www.straitstimes.com/singapore/initiatives-in-place-to-help-tackle-ageing-as-s-pore-nears-super-aged-status-in-2026-ong-ye-kung. [Accessed 19 September 2025].

2 Department of Statistics Singapore, "Department of Statistics Singapore," [Online]. [Accessed 2024].

3 Singapore Hospice Council, "Members," [Online]. Available: https://www.singaporehospice.org.sg/members/. [Accessed 19 September 2025].

4 Singapore Hospice Council, "National Quality Improvement Project - Minimum Data Set - FY2023," June 2025. [Online]. Available: https://www.singaporehospice.org.sg/e-library/docs/national-quality-improvement-project-summary-minimum-data-set-2023/. [Accessed 19 September 2025].

17

COMPASSIONATE COMMUNITIES

Up the East Coast

Hugh McElhinney and Joseph Sawyer

Abstract

This chapter tells the story of how a quiet, yet powerful movement is growing along the Suffolk coast, helping people talk about death, dying, and grief in more open and human ways. In a place shaped by rural living and an ageing population, loss is a familiar part of everyday life. Yet for many people, it is something carried in silence, without the words, confidence, or support to share it.

Compassionate communities up the East Coast began in 2020 with a simple idea: that care at the end of life is not only the job of professionals, but something communities can hold together. Working alongside local people, we describe how we have worked to create spaces where honest conversations can happen, in cafés, prisons, schools, libraries, workplaces, arts venues, and outdoor public spaces.

Through workshops, creative projects, book collections, benches, posters, and moments of shared reflection, people continue to find spaces to speak, listen, and support one another. The chapter weaves together these stories, from a man in prison speaking about his mother for the first time, to a child finding words for grief through a library book, to strangers pausing together at a public wall or bench.

Rather than offering a formula, this chapter shares what has been learned along the way: that small acts matter, that compassion spreads through relationships, and that when grief is shared, its weight becomes lighter, for individuals and for whole communities.

17.1 Introduction

With a population of around 400,000 people, Suffolk stretches across rural farming landscapes, picturesque coastal towns, and market villages interspersed with areas

DOI: 10.4324/9781003621348-18

of natural beauty. Life here is often shaped by the rhythms of farming, fishing, tourism, and local community. Yet the closeness this infers can also lie in tension with the realities of geographical isolation. There are large distances to travel between towns and villages, roads are subject to flooding, and public transport networks are not easily accessible. Connections with the rest of the UK are also not easy; many of the road and rail networks provide a flow from north to south and vice versa. With Suffolk being slightly out on a limb, transport inland can take a roundabout route. These factors can make the rurality of Suffolk both a treasure and a challenge.

Suffolk has one of the highest proportions of older people in the UK. At the same time, it is an area of significant social and economic deprivation. Whilst an ageing population brings wisdom and resilience, it also means illness, frailty, dying, and bereavement are everyday experiences. In rural communities, where health and social care services can be stretched, the task of navigating these experiences often falls on individuals and their families. This is particularly difficult in a state of socio-economic deprivation where people may struggle to make ends meet, even without the added responsibility of caregiving.

Within this context, conversations about death, dying, and grief have become increasingly hidden, whispered, or left until too late. This was the starting point for a programme of work that recognises the importance of these conversations and how they can breed relationships, which translate into meaningful actions of support and care. Where this happens at scale, entire communities begin to learn and develop. In Suffolk, this recognition became a movement: *Compassionate communities: up the East Coast*.

Since 2020, this initiative has aimed to build compassion into the fabric of community life. The vision is that there is a shared responsibility of a common resource in matters relating to death and dying. We tell the story of how the East Coast project has developed, the milestones achieved, the partnerships formed, and the lessons learned along the way.

17.2 The early days

Picking up on distant rumblings relating to what a compassionate community might be, St Elizabeth's hospice in Ipswich was fortunate to be able to employ a lead for this work. Establishing the role required support and belief from members of the senior leadership team who were able to recognise the limitations of the current approach to palliative and end-of-life care and the need to do things differently.

The organisation, along with other healthcare leaders, could see that philosophically, socially, and demographically there need to be a step change of cultural confidence. One where communities and individuals might grow confidence in the values associated with supporting one another through the experiences of death, dying, and loss. At the outset, there was not necessarily a clear plan, more a shared motivation and belief in the potential of what could and can still be achieved.

Shortly after the Hospice's commitment to employing a member of staff in this area, COVID-19 came into play. Whilst his provided challenges, it was also motivating and inspiring to see community initiatives flourish. Grasping the natural enthusiasm, we spent time making relationships and setting up working groups in communities across the Suffolk landscape.

Yet with burgeoning numbers, there was also a need to understand the essence of what we were trying to create. These early days were important in learning as much about what a compassionate community isn't as what it is. Increasingly large networks required orchestration, administration, and leadership, where this comes through an institutional lens, there is a risk that interventions are 'done to' rather than 'done with' the communities we were engaging with. These early days were therefore important in learning just how vulnerable new ideas that strive for cultural change can be. Our experience suggests that safeguarding the values and philosophy to which the movement adheres will breed long-term success, even if this feels challenging at the time.

17.3 Compassionate Conversations: planting the first seeds

Engagement with community groups highlighted the need for us to facilitate a ripple effect rather than be both creator and conductor. With this in mind, we set out on our Compassionate Conversations project in 2021. These two-hour workshops provide a safe, structured space for people to talk about death and dying, something many people had never done outside of moments of crisis.

The aim was to empower lay people with the confidence to offer support. We wanted people to feel confident that if they met someone affected by death, they could listen and share a space with them, no matter how fleeting. We wanted to dispel feelings of panic, where people might feel the need to cross the street, look at their phone or disengage. Participants learned that sometimes the most powerful thing they can do is simply to listen, to ask gentle questions, or to sit in silence with someone.

Workshops broke down myths ('talking about death makes it happen faster'), shared local resources, and showed how small acts of companionship ripple outwards, amplifying rather than dissipating. Our Compassionate Conversation programme has evolved over the last four years, people have signed up and now lead their own training or versions of it. Sessions have taken place in prisons, cafés, schools, creative hubs, community centres, and sporting clubs across Suffolk. To date, we have delivered over 112 sessions with 2090 participants in total.

17.3.1 Case study: a conversation in a prison

One of the first Compassionate Conversation workshops took place in a prison. This quote is from a man serving a long sentence.

> I've never told anyone this before. My mum died when I was inside. I didn't go to the funeral. I've carried that in silence for years. This is the first time I've been able to say it out loud.

That moment shifted the room. Others nodded, some shared their own stories, and the prison chaplain later remarked it was the most honest conversation he had witnessed in years.

17.3.2 Compassionate Workplaces: bringing empathy to the office

Using the compassionate communities charter as a blueprint for engagement, we extended our efforts to workplaces in 2023. The Compassionate Workplaces programme recognises employees who have experienced bereavement often feel isolated at work.

Workshops helped employers discuss what compassionate policies might look like and the effect allowing people adequate time off might have. We also discussed the ongoing nature of grief, how it is not something that you recover from but instead learn to accommodate as part of who you are.

17.3.2.1 Case study: a small business learns to respond

At a local café in the coastal town of Felixstowe, the owner admitted she had struggled when one of her young staff members lost her brother suddenly.

> I didn't know what to say. I gave her a few days off, but when she came back, I just expected her to get on with things. After the workshop, I realised I could have done more…even just saying, 'I'm here if you need to talk.' Now we've got a proper bereavement policy, and as a team, we've agreed we'll check in on each other, not just cover shifts.

For small workplaces without human resource departments, this was transformative whilst the effect can ripple out amongst the community rather than breed a dependency on services. Impact so far:

1. 19 sessions delivered
2. Over 70 workplaces engaged
3. At least two new bereavement policies introduced

17.4 Expanding into public spaces

As we developed, we continued to reinforce exactly what compassionate communities were by holding a greater understanding of what they were not. The success of ripple effect interventions led us to explore other community-oriented spaces. Around this time, we also looked to forge a closer working relationship with the clinical team, and they moved under the same management structure to allow for shared learning.

17.4.1 The 'Before I Die' wall: public reflections

In May 2023, the compassionate communities project moved into public spaces in a more visible way with the installation of a 'Before I Die' wall. The wall invited passers-by to write down something they hoped to do before they died. Responses ranged from the playful ('eat my body weight in ice cream') to the profound ('tell my sister I love her'). Each intervention focused on facilitating the ripple, providing a platform for engagement that would light the spark of conversation that might set fire through the community.

17.4.1.1 Quote from a passer-by in Lowestoft

> Writing down 'Before I die, I want to forgive my dad' felt scary. But seeing it there in chalk, next to strangers' dreams and wishes, made me realise I'm not alone in carrying unfinished business.

What mattered was not only the writing itself but the conversations that sprang up around it. Strangers stopped to talk, parents explained the wall to children, and the act of writing created a moment of reflection.

17.4.2 Awareness posters: support where you least expect it

Following on from the success of this initiative, we sought to place over 70 'awareness posters' in everyday settings: café toilets, community noticeboards, and General Practice (Family Doctor) waiting rooms. Each poster provided a gentle reminder that support was available, directing people to the Living Grief Hub, a free online resource offering bereavement counselling and local connections.

17.4.3 Case example: a sporting venue

At a community football club, posters were displayed in changing rooms. One young player later said:

> When my nan died, I didn't want to talk about it. But I kept seeing that poster in the locker room. Eventually I clicked on the QR code. That's how I found the Living Grief Hub.

17.5 Using the charter to identify collaborative partnerships

17.5.1 Bereavement Bookcases: libraries as safe havens

We constantly referred to the charter when considering our next moves. Sometimes a connection would form organically, sometimes this could be a dead-end but inevitably another connection would arise, and a door would open. Such a process led to our engagement with Suffolk Libraries. We became partners in 2023 through the installation of Bereavement Bookcases. Each bookcase was stocked with more than 50 titles for adults and children, exploring grief, resilience, and hope.

Installed in 14 libraries running up the coast from Ipswich to Lowestoft, the bookcases quickly became the most borrowed collection in the service. In just 15 months, 3,225 books were taken home.

17.5.2 Case study: a parent and child in Ipswich library

A librarian recalled a mother and her seven-year-old son sitting together in the children's corner:

> They borrowed a book about losing a pet. The boy had just lost his granddad, but he didn't have the words to talk about it. Through the book, they found a way to start the conversation.

17.5.3 Partnerships with the arts: Snape Maltings and The Red House

The arts have a unique power to express the inexpressible. This combined with their extended reach means they are an impactful collaborator when thinking about the dissemination of ideas that seek to bring cultural change. In 2024, a major partnership was formed with Snape Maltings and The Red House, home of the famous composers Benjamin Britten and Peter Pears. By identifying a champion within the organisation that understood the philosophy and felt motivated by the potential, we were able to embark on several collaborations that continue to yield significant outputs. The journey began with a 'think tank' hosted by Britten and Pears Arts. Researchers, activists, physicians, writers, and musicians collaborated to share ideas on the relationship between compassionate communities and music. This has generated several new initiatives including a commissioned play that has toured the UK, a choral ensemble performing at the hospice and engaging with creative health work in the context of grief, and a new venture 'music to die for', an online repository of pieces of music alongside their associated stories.

Following on from the think tank, Britten and Pears hosted a 'Spark Day' for generating ideas across six organisations, funding and owning the event themselves, it provided a powerful platform for collaboration across a host of local creatives and care providers.

Britten and Pears continue to lead their own projects whilst remaining connected to the compassionate community work done through the hospice. They host a Compassionate Café within their local grounds, offer a bereavement gardening group, and have expanded upon a 'walk on' service. This is an intervention set up by local bereaved people to simply walk and share stories of love, laughter, and loss with one another.

17.5.4 Bereavement benches: stillness in public places

In addition to creating experiences for people to engage with, we sought to establish more tangible entities that act as a more permanent representation and commitment to the work of a compassionate community.

In 2024, six bereavement benches were installed in Felixstowe and Woodbridge. Each bench provided a physical place to pause and remember. QR codes linked directly to support services, blending traditional memorial spaces with digital resources. One woman left flowers on a bereavement bench every month for a year. When asked why, she said:

> It's not for anyone in particular. It's for all of us who need somewhere to put our grief.

17.5.5 Schools and underrepresented groups

17.5.5.1 No Barriers Here: including every voice

Launched in 2025, *No Barriers Here* recognised that some voices are too often absent from end-of-life planning. Through art-based workshops, participants created visual advance care plans.

Case study: learning disability community

In one session, participants used art to show how they wanted to be cared for. A young man with a learning disability painted a bright red door. When asked what it meant, he said:

> It means I want people to knock before they come in. Even if I'm ill. It's my space.

For staff, this was a profound reminder that autonomy and dignity matter in every detail of care.

17.5.5.2 The Larch Project: intergenerational legacies

The Larch Project matched hospice patients with local students to co-create tributes celebrating the patient's life, through art, music, or storytelling. Each project culminated in a celebration involving families, volunteers, and staff.

Case study: a student and a patient

Ella, a 16-year-old student, was paired with Peter, a retired teacher receiving hospice care. Together they wrote a piece of music.

At the celebration event, Peter's daughter said:

> To see Dad come alive talking about music again was such a gift. Ella gave him something to focus on, and in return, she's got this memory of him that will last her whole life.

Ella later told her teacher:

> I used to be scared of death. Now I know it's sad, but it's not something to hide from.

17.5.5.3 Community connectors: reaching the margins

In 2023, St Elizabeth Hospice successfully applied for National Lottery funding for two 'community connectors'. These roles are dedicated to building relationships with underrepresented communities. Their conversations with local groups and communities, over 250 so far, have led to initiatives such as:

1. LGBTQ+ working groups to make hospice care more inclusive
2. Tours of the hospice for people with learning disabilities
3. Tours of the hospice for people with learning disabilities
4. A family day for Romanian families to visit and engage with hospice staff
5. Bespoke workplace sessions for underrepresented communities

Quote from a Romanian community leader

> We didn't think the hospice was for us. We thought it was only for English people, or only for the very end. But after the family day, we felt welcome. Now we know it's our hospice too.

Our connectors hold true to the principles of asset-based community development, they are allowed space and time to form relationships, supporting existing treasures to develop and ripple out to achieve their full potential.

17.6 Conclusion: a tapestry of compassion

Nearly five years on, Compassionate communities: up the East Coast has grown into a tapestry of projects, partnerships, and personal stories.

There are the big numbers, thousands of people engaged, hundreds of workshops, dozens of organisations. But the heart of the project is in the small things: the café conversation that eases loneliness, the book borrowed by a grieving parent, the student who carries the memory of a hospice patient into adulthood, and the employee who feels supported when returning to work after loss.

What makes this movement distinctive is not that it resides in one institution, but that it flows across many: prisons, pubs, cafés, schools, creative hubs, hospitals, community centres, sporting locations, and local government. Each has become a thread in the wider fabric of compassion.

Since the start of our journey, we have worked hard to learn what a compassionate community means in our local context. We have learnt to become comfortable that there is no set formula for success, that a community development approach needs to evolve organically which can mean you can be thrown off in unexpected and sometimes seemingly unwanted tangents. We have learnt that set metrics, outcomes, deadlines, and plans can sometimes conspire to conceal what is of true value, whilst we continue to work hard at the open endedness of this work, to be comfortable in the knowledge that it must take the shape and form it needs to rather than the one we might hold closest to our own personal or institutional ideals.

Ultimately, we have learnt that this is a lifelong process, without a specific end-point, a journey of partnerships, and connections that we trust will eventually breed a greater hospitality towards our inherent vulnerability, towards woundedness, failure, absence, loss, and all things imperfect.

17.6.1 Final reflection from a participant

> What I've learned is that grief isn't just something you carry alone. It belongs to all of us. And when a community shares it, the weight gets lighter.

Compassion is no longer only the role of the hospice or the specialist. It is the role of us all. And when communities embrace that role together, the result is resilience, humanity, and hope, even in the face of life's most difficult moments.

18

THE SOUTH WEST COMPASSIONATE COMMUNITIES NETWORK (SWCCN) IN WESTERN AUSTRALIA

A case study

Samar Aoun and Julieanne Hilbers

Abstract

The South West Compassionate Communities Network (SWCCN) was established in 2018 with the mission to build the capacity of the communities in the South West of Western Australia to be able to take a compassionate communities approach to dying, caring and grieving, guided by the Ottawa Charter principles for health promotion. This chapter gives examples of successes and challenges of two of the SWCCN key building blocks aimed at system changes in two settings, a health service and local government: The Compassionate Connector program, a partnership with a health service, involved volunteer Connectors supporting people living with chronic and advanced life-limiting illnesses by enhancing people's social connections and networks. The evaluation demonstrated a significant increase in social connectedness and a decrease in hospital usage.

The Compassionate Bunbury Charter, in partnership with the Bunbury City Council, has fostered community conversations and actions around caring, dying and grieving with ten guiding themes being identified by the community. The Charter is accompanied by a Toolkit of practical actions people can undertake individually and collectively. These two initiatives succeeded in creating supportive environments in the community, strengthened community action, developed personal skills in the community and attempted reorienting health services pending health system reform.

Public Health Palliative Care International endorsed SWCCN as a Compassionate Community in October 2025.

DOI: 10.4324/9781003621348-19

18.1 Introduction

18.1.1 Description of the community

The SWCCN is based in the South West of Western Australia, which covers 24,000 km^2 with a population of approximately 217,000 in 2021, with 2.6% being indigenous people. The area comprises one regional port town, Bunbury, and many smaller rural towns and communities. Based on the Accessibility/Remoteness Index of Australia, the South West is classified 48% outer regional, 42% inner regional and 10% remote [1]. The largest population growth is in older age groups. The leading causes of death in the South West region are: ischaemic heart diseases, lung cancer, cerebrovascular diseases, chronic obstructive pulmonary disease, dementia (including Alzheimer's disease), prostate cancer and intentional self-harm [2]. Coronary heart disease, Chronic Obstructive Pulmonary Disease (COPD) and dementia are among the leading causes of disease burden for people aged 65 and over.

According to the Australian Bureau of Statistics, Bunbury is Australia's regional centre for people living alone, having 34% of single-person household compared to 25% Australia wide [1]. Just over a third of the Australian population, whether rural or urban, reported loneliness [3].

18.1.2 Background of SWCCN

The SWCCN is a grassroots approach to mobilising the community. It began with a conversation between two people who understood how a population approach to palliative care could make a difference for their community [4]. These two co-founders (JH and SA) were population health professionals, living in the community, and who had both positive and negative personal experiences around care, death and grief.

JH and SA began talking to their personal and professional networks and soon two people became three, then four and then more. People quickly connected with the idea of a community-led approach to care, dying and grief. Soon, there was a core group of eight people who were keen to work together to launch a compassionate communities approach in the South West of Western Australia in 2018. This group was also keen to be part of a national conversation and successfully applied to be one of the eight National Compassionate Communities Forum Groundbreaker communities [4,5].

A social approach and improving community cohesion and resilience around care, death and loss are the primary goals of SWCCN. The mission is that "every person, every family and every community knows what to do when someone is caring, dying or grieving".

SWCCN is a registered charity and an incorporated organisation, managed by a committee of volunteers with representation from several sectors and may vary each year: members of the community along with people who have a professional role within community services including multicultural and community centres, health services, local government, aged care and business leaders.

SWCCN had no initial funding to get started as a network. Later on, it gained research funding to develop and evaluate the Compassionate Connector program and obtained philanthropic and government funding to support educational programs and community events such as community education associated with Dying to Know Day and advance care planning.

18.2 Part 1: Description of the Compassionate Connectors Program

The Compassionate Communities Connectors Program is a volunteer-led initiative designed to enhance the social networks of families living with chronic or life-limiting illnesses. The research trial, which consisted of the development, training, implementation and evaluation of the Compassionate Connectors Program, was undertaken in the South West of Western Australia, from 2019 to 2022, in partnership with the health service.

Specially trained volunteers (Connectors) supported existing members of the families' social networks and also enlisted the support of community members, Caring Helpers, to address the social and practical needs of these families. The Connectors were mainly retired community members with lived experience of caring for family members and many served as volunteers in a hospital or hospice but were looking for fresh ways of serving their community in ways they had more agency and autonomy than being a service provider volunteer [6].

The Connectors' role was about building the capacity of informal networks and circles of care around the person affected by advanced illness and their family by identifying the additional social and practical support they may require from within their local community and tap into formal and informal sources.

Caring Helpers could be members of the family, friends, neighbours or other people in the community who were willing and able to assist with activities such as: walking the dog, doing the shopping, collecting a prescription, going to the library, mowing the lawn, making a snack, tidying up or sitting with a person who needs a break.

The only paid position was that of the Coordinator but the role of Connectors was voluntary.

Promotional flyers were shared with the health service and community groups to recruit Connectors, as well as directly targeting the SWCCN membership base that was built up from awareness and educational events.

Promotional flyers to recruit patients were shared with the health service with a set of inclusion criteria. Palliative care, chronic disease and aged care health service teams referred patients/families to the program, and the Coordinator of Connectors matched these families with Connectors to ensure the fit was as good as possible.

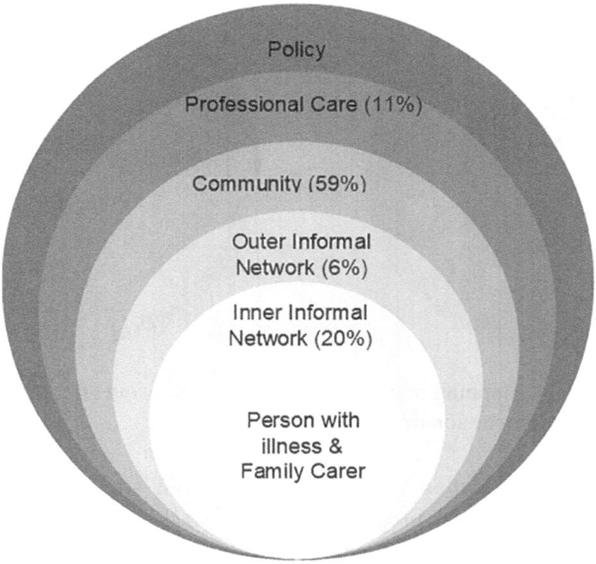

FIGURE 18.1 Percent of Help Provided to Person/Family with the Illness within the Circles of Care

Connectors attended a training course of two days' duration, initially, delivered by content experts. In further sessions, this was reduced to one day and a follow-up session a few weeks later. Sessions included information on public health palliative care, the importance of compassionate communities and how this project fits in, death literacy and advance care planning, grief literacy, communication skills, self-care, understanding advanced illness and the role of the palliative care and the chronic disease teams, and the volunteer processes and procedures adopted by the health service.

For the research trial, 20 Connectors were trained with 13 of them going on to support 43 referred patients with 30 of these completing the evaluation. Nearly 80% of patients' needs were in the social domain, and nearly half of the patients lived alone [7].

The majority of support sourced by Connectors to assist participants were drawn from the participants' 'outer' informal networks or the community at large (externally facilitated networks) rather than from within the inner informal networks of participants, as depicted in Figure 18.1. This reflected that over half of the patients participating in this study lived alone and hence did not have their own inner informal networks to support them.

18.2.1 Outcomes and impact

18.2.1.1 The Compassionate Communities Connectors Program

The primary outcome that was measured was the effect of the intervention on social connectedness. Secondary outcomes were the effect of the intervention

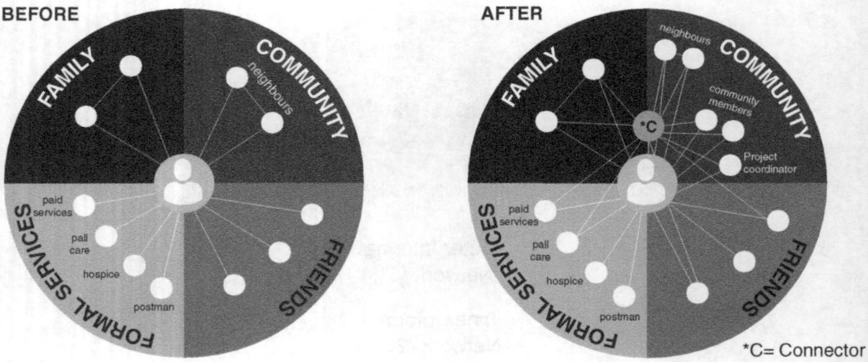

FIGURE 18.2 Social Mapping of a Family Network before and after the Intervention by the Compassionate Connectors

on unmet practical/social needs and support from social networks, and the self-reported impact of the program on social well-being such as coping with daily activities, access to formal services, community links, social activity and social isolation [8].

There were significant improvements in social connectedness, reflected in reduced social isolation, better coping with daily activities and a two-fold increase in supportive networks. The program was able to address gaps that formal services could not, particularly for people who lived alone, or were socially isolated in more rural communities that were out of the frequent reach of formal services [7]. Figure 18.2 demonstrates the difference in the connections for one family before and after the intervention by the Compassionate Connectors.

18.2.1.2 Feedback from Connectors

Volunteering as a Connector was viewed as a positive and feasible experience for fostering a sense of community among participants, developing relationships with other community members, seeing the difference that the Connector role made in the lives of those involved in the enhanced network and fostering growth in Connectors' emotional capacity and compassion. The Connectors felt the experience was personally rewarding for them to be able to make a difference and see the improvement in people's quality of life. While rewarding, the work was also challenging and differed in several respects from traditional volunteering, particularly in the agency Connectors can bring to their role [9].

> The more you give, the better it is for you. You know the reward is greater than the effort.
>
> *(C07)*

> Once people find out it's community helping community, there's an untapped resource out there'. (C31) and 'It's beneficial for everyone really, it's bringing back that sense of community and village that we've lost in society.
>
> *(C29)*

18.2.1.3 Feedback from families

Without exception, families reported positive feedback about their experiences with the largest impacts in increasing community links, increasing social activity and reducing social isolation [10].

> She wasn't there to tell me what to do. She was there to help me make sense of what was going on in my life.
>
> *(ID13)*

> One of the first things which was a catalyst for change was there's a level of accountability if somebody's coming to see you. You've got to get up, get dressed and you've got to face the world. You can't just lay curled up in your bed all day.
>
> *(ID13)*

18.2.1.4 Feedback from service providers

Service providers reported on their increased capacity to offer additional services where formal services were not available, particularly in remote/rural areas. They appreciated that Connectors went over and beyond what was expected of this role [10].

> I think it's a great service that's actually helping very socially isolated people realise that there are people out there that care about them but the social isolation side of things. So, I think it's terrific. I hope it continues. Just about every one of my clients could use one.
>
> *(HP046)*

> I think it's really bridged the gap; it goes beyond what a formal service can do and then it fills that gap of what family not able to do. So, it's that real. And I think they (Connectors) are a little bit more engaging. They are able to do a little bit more. It's a good thing.
>
> *(HP017)*

18.2.1.5 Cost-effectiveness

The combined healthcare usage and economic analyses of the Connector program demonstrated the benefits of using home-based and community-centred interventions, with gains for the health system through improved patient outcomes and reduced total healthcare costs, including fewer hospitalisations and readmissions, shorter lengths of hospital stay and an increase in outpatient contacts which are cheaper than hospital admissions. The results indicated that the Connector program may have shifted individuals away from the hospital system and towards community-based care. Estimated net savings of $AUD518,701 would be achieved from adopting the Connector program, assuming enrolment of 100 patients over an average six-month participation period [11].

18.2.2 Reflections

18.2.2.1 The role of the Coordinator of Connectors

The role of the Coordinator is vital to the success of the program. It became clear over the intervention that the Coordinator's role in taking ownership of implementation and seeing it through was the most significant predictor of success.

Key attributes of the Coordinator of Connectors that made a difference included organisational capacity and connectedness; the ability to recruit patients; volunteer preparation and mentorship; strong leadership skills, mentoring abilities and community connections. Identified key success factors included:

1. Leadership: Coordinators' leadership skills were the central strength and dynamism that maintained the network of participants and stakeholders. Their ability to raise awareness of the Connector program in the local community required that they be comfortable connecting with various stakeholders through presentations and networking.
2. Mentorship: Coordinators were required to be present for, and to support, Connectors. Feedback from Connectors suggested that the willingness and capacity of the Coordinator to support them was one of the most important aspects of their involvement. The ability to effectively match Connectors and people with chronic/terminal illness in terms of personality and approach was mentioned as a key skill of the Coordinator.
3. The ability of the Coordinator to help Connectors navigate unanticipated client situations or rapid decline.
4. Support from healthcare providers: Coordinators needed a strong, active relationship with healthcare partners. When this was not in place, it negatively impacted program progress and made the Coordinator's role more difficult.
5. Sufficient time: The time allocated for coordination influenced how Coordinators experienced their role. Once a program was established, less time would be required to keep it running smoothly.

18.2.2.2 Prerequisites and challenges

A public health program, such as the Compassionate Community Connectors program, links formal and informal networks of care that support chronically and terminally ill people and their families. When operating effectively, as shown in the Connector program, social connectedness and thus practical support of patients and families increases, and more appropriate health decisions are made, reducing costs in particular to acute and tertiary services. Such programs have five basic preconditions. They need:

1 A community with sufficient social capital to take up opportunities to support fellow citizens.
2 A community-organised group of volunteers (Connectors) with well-developed lay knowledge of health and community services, and of informal networks of care within their community.
3 Health service partners willing to build community partnerships with a Connector's group and negotiate risk in ways that allow reasonable autonomy for Connectors.
4 Opportunities to develop trust between participants in each element of the system.
5 Accountability that manages risk overall and nurtures trust, provided in this case by a salaried Coordinator working jointly with health services and community volunteers.

These conditions point to ways in which a Connector's program can struggle to commence or fail to be effective or sustainable.

1 Communities that are unwilling to offer support, such that Connectors cannot call upon caring helpers or formal supports but end up undertaking, rather than facilitating, the support tasks they identify.
2 Lack of leadership to establish a Community Connector's group and/or Connectors with insufficient knowledge of the caring resources of their community or lacking the skills to facilitate constructive connections drawing on a person's own social supports.
3 Health services that insist on directing Connectors' activities and treating them as extensions of the health service's work, not allowing reasonable autonomy for Connectors to enhance a client's social network and develop community-based support appropriate for the client's everyday needs.
4 A lack of trust between health service managers, and/or practitioners, and/or Connectors, and/or clients and/or caring helpers. (A lack of trust is implicit in some forms of risk management).
5 An absence of accountability that places some Connectors at risk and undermines possibilities for developing trust between participants. This can arise from a lack of skilled coordination trusted by both community Connectors and health services, preferably through a joint appointment; that is, accountability to both a recognised community group and a health service.

There can of course be overlap between groups. Healthcare practitioners as citizens can lead and participate in the Community Connectors program. But essential aspects are that the Connectors are volunteers with primary accountability to their community, not volunteers with primary accountability to a health service; and that professional coordination of Connectors is a joint appointment shared by community and health.

18.2.3 Future plans

There has been sound interest at the national and international levels with invitations to conferences to specifically explain the Compassionate Connector approach to care and its evaluation, including many requests for the training program. The Connector program is currently replicated in Sydney by a community-based aged care service. Further operationalisation of the concept includes the development of the Connector hubs and understanding how this approach can be adapted for culturally and linguistically diverse (CaLD) groups.

18.2.3.1 Connector hubs

Because of the success of the research trial, funding has been obtained to develop Connector Hubs in Western Australia, that incorporate in addition to the Compassionate Connectors another stream of Citizen Connectors whose role is about signposting people to get the practical and social support they need. The four aims of the Connector hub project are to:

1 Upscale the implementation and the translation of the Connectors Program in Bunbury and Kalamunda through two streams: Citizen Connectors and Compassionate Connectors. The focus of Citizen Connectors is to chat, listen and connect people through signpost conversations to the support they need. Compassionate Connectors focus on social connectedness and enhancing and mobilising caregiving networks in line with the original research project.
2 Update, expand and package the Connector training program to be delivered face to face and online.
3 Evaluate the impact of the two streams of the Connector Program in a community-based setting (Milligan in the Bunbury-Geographic regional area) and a local government setting (City of Kalamunda, an urban fringe area), by assessing the feasibility, acceptability and potential impact of the two Connector models, within the two mentioned settings.
4 Establish a Community of Practice to inform the development of an online learning hub where learnings can be shared with the broader community sector. This stage will focus on reflective evaluation practices to better understand the 'practice' of establishing and maintaining a Connector program in differing settings. Learnings from this project will inform the development of an online learning hub for others in the community sector to draw upon should they wish to implement a similar program.

There is interest from across the community sector in how some or all of these elements can be incorporated.

18.2.4 Cultural training

Australia is one of the most CaLD countries in the world. According to the latest census, three in ten people living in Australia were born overseas and one in four spoke a language other than English at home. Older CaLD populations are growing faster than older Australian-born, English-speaking population. Despite a rapidly changing demography, there is a lack of appropriate CaLD educational programs in death and grief literacy. CaLD migrants, especially elderly, risk becoming socially isolated due to lack of extended family networks and language barriers. They are also underrepresented in the use of palliative care services and grief counselling for reasons not limited to: availability and access of culturally, linguistically appropriate resources; cultural inclination to informally deal with such issues within own community networks as they did "back home". Needs and preferences of various programs focusing on death, dying and bereavement often exclude individuals who are not proficient in English, and/or those who require interpreter support.

Therefore, a second project that is underway is about capacity-building training workshops for cultural Connectors in partnership with the SWCCN and the Ethnic Communities Council of WA. This project aims to train individuals from several multicultural groups to become cultural Citizen Connectors in their communities, promoting effective communication and culturally appropriate support.

18.3 Part 2: Description of the Compassionate City Charter

Given their role in facilitating community engagement and well-being, local government is well-positioned to be an active player in supporting compassionate communities. The SWCCN has been working with the City of Bunbury (in Western Australia) over several years with an initial focus on community education (for example, death festival, compassionate communities forums). When it came to exploring the development of a Compassionate Bunbury Charter, these initiatives provided a good foundation for developing relationships and fostering an understanding of compassionate communities.

Compassionate City Charters are a useful tool for fostering community conversations and is a concise way of organising a purposeful program of civic action oriented towards end-of-life. [12]

The Compassionate Bunbury Charter is a whole of community responsibility; it contains aspirations that relate to community members, service providers, businesses, organisations, groups and clubs to pursue. It provides a pathway for Bunbury becoming a Compassionate City.

To develop the Charter, community consultations, via 12 workshops, took place over an eight-month period. Those who shared along the way included City of Bunbury Councillors and employees, chaplains, monks, new migrants, carers, retirees, people with life-limiting illnesses and Aboriginal members of the community. Input was also sought from the wider community online via the City of Bunbury Community engagement hub and social media. Interviews were subsequently undertaken with community leaders and presentations made at community forums. Ten themes were identified during community consultations (Figure 18.3).

1 Building capacity to give and receive.
2 Mobilising networks of care.
3 Supporting good communication.
4 Respecting people's wishes.
5 Fostering belonging and connectedness.
6 Providing opportunities to remember.
7 Nurturing creativity.
8 Leaders championing care and compassion.
9 Creating caring organisations.
10 Acknowledging compassionate acts.

What people shared and a review of what other compassionate communities around the world have done informed the development of the Charter, which can be accessed from https://comcomnetworksw.com/compassionate-bunbury-charter/.

What became evident during the conversations was that people were already doing things that aligned with a Compassionate Charter but for others they wanted to know more about what they could do. This led to the development

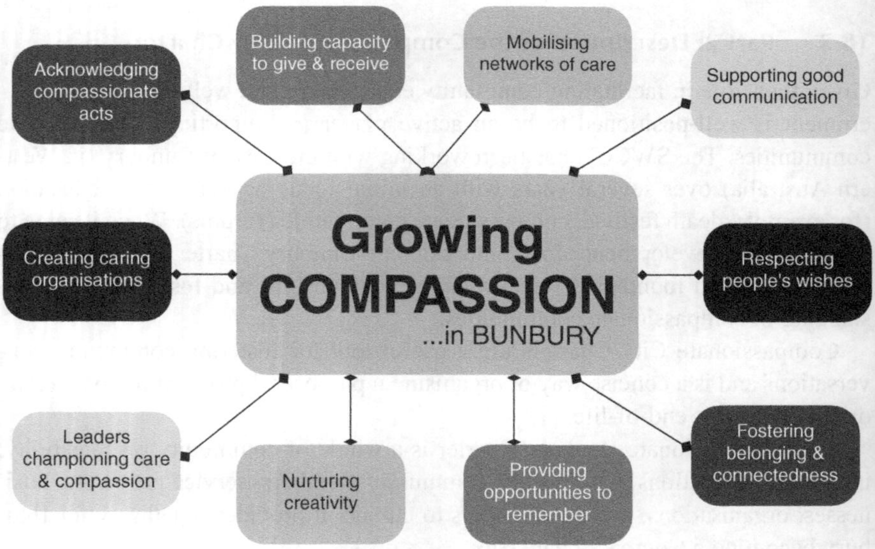

FIGURE 18.3 Ten Key Themes and Action Areas for the Compassionate Bunbury Charter

of a secondary document, a toolkit that focused on practical actions they can undertake individually and collectively to foster a compassionate community (Figure 18.4).

In June 2023, the City of Bunbury endorsed the Charter and offered to be the custodian, or holder of the Charter, on behalf of the community.

Acknowledging compassionate acts is one of the key themes of the Charter. The conversations leading to the Charter highlighted how the community already self-identified as a 'big hearted' community. SWCCN approached the Mayor to create the Compassionate Bunbury Mayoral Awards, which were presented to nominated community members on World Compassionate Communities Day (November 1). This is now an annual award and is open to people who live, work or volunteer in the City of Bunbury, who champion compassion and kindness within their family, neighbourhood, school, workplace or interest group (e.g., youth, sporting and craft). The ten themes identified in the Compassionate Bunbury Charter informed the development of the criteria to select how people will be acknowledged.

Community pledges were also made in support of the Charter, subsequent to its being accepted and included the development of educational material (How to be a compassionate friend in time of need). Further operationalising of the Charter included the implementation of workshops in partnership with local industry leaders focusing on Compassionate Workplaces and Understanding Grief. Furthermore, a

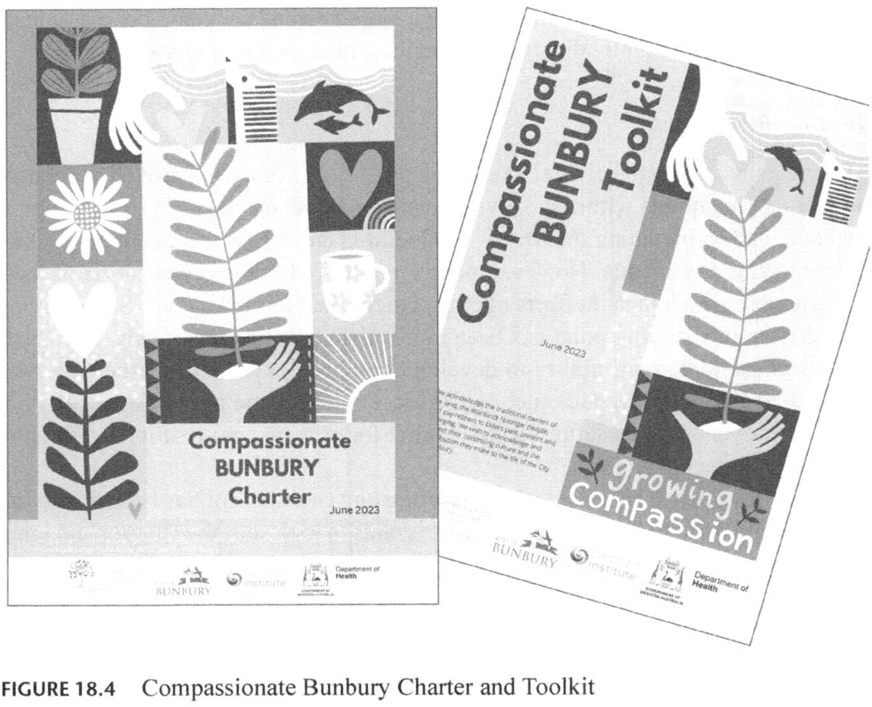

FIGURE 18.4 Compassionate Bunbury Charter and Toolkit

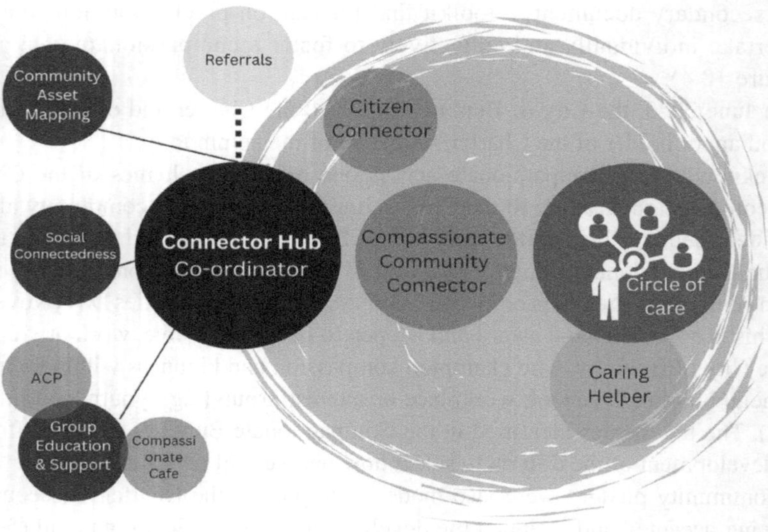

FIGURE 18.5 Aspects of Compassionate Communities Connector Hubs

partnership was formed between the SWCCN and Milligan, a local community centre, to support Milligan to become a Compassionate Connector hub (Figure 18.5). This 'Hub' draws together community education, citizen connector, compassionate connector and community directory strategies within a community setting.

18.3.1 Reflections

Making gains within the civic sector over a period of seven years proved dependent on having champions within the civic organisation. When champions were identified and leaders including the Mayor, Councillors and CEOs were supportive, significant gains were made. However, people regularly left the organisation of local government, which meant efforts of engagement 'had to start again'. Since having the Charter, this starting point has been more advanced than previously. The Charter has consolidated our ability to develop community events in partnership with the City of Bunbury's venues such as the local museum and regional art gallery. It has also proven to be a useful reference point for starting conversations with other local government agencies.

However, a pivotal activator for partnering and engagement has been the ability to 'bring money to the table' in the form of grants to kick start the Charter and other community events.

Along the way, presentations were made to Council and regular meetings undertaken with the leadership team within the organisation. This has been essential for them to develop a greater understanding of a compassionate communities approach.

18.3.2 Future plans

Future plans will focus on continuing to operationalise the ten themes within the Charter across civic settings.

18.4 Conclusions

Through these two initiatives, we have learnt a great deal about the value of a community development – building capacity – solution focused approaches within a public health model, the power of local champions and what sustains and challenges this work. The quantitative and qualitative findings suggest that investment in the Connector program has the capacity to reduce net health sector expenditure while also improving social connectedness and other outcomes for people with life-limiting illnesses.

A public health approach based on a close partnership between communities, health and civic institutions is the optimal practice model, as delineated by the palliative care New Essentials framework [13]. Through these two initiatives, we have demonstrated the possible partnerships between professional palliative care and other services, compassionate communities and the civic sector covered in the Compassionate City Charter.

Guided by the principles of the Ottawa Charter, these two initiatives succeeded in creating supportive environments in the community, strengthened community action, developed personal skills in the community and attempted to reorient healthcare services. However, adequate integration of a public health approach to end-of-life care with healthcare-based palliative care services awaits health system reform that can provide appropriate recognition and governance of collaborations between professionals and community-based volunteers.

We are very pleased to have been awarded by Public Health Palliative Care International Compassionate Community endorsement status in October 2025. It acknowledges our community sustained efforts since 2018 in leading and partnering for a public health palliative care approach in the south west of Western Australia, both in awareness raising and educational initiatives and a focus on systems change.

References

1. Australian Bureau of Statistics, *Population: Census*. ABS, Canberra, [Online] 2021. Available: https://www.abs.gov.au/statistics/people/population/population-census/latest-release
2. West Australian Department of Health. Data from HealthTracks, SW Health Region residents by condition 2014–2018. Accessed April 25 2025
3. M. Lim, B. Smith, K. Owen, L. Engel, P. Qualter and D Surkalim. *Social Connection in Australia 2023.* Sydney, Ending Loneliness Together, 2023.
4. J. Hilbers, H. Rankin-Smith, D. Horsfall and S. Aoun. "We are all in this together": building capacity for a community-centred approach to caring, dying and grieving in Australia. *European Journal for Person Centered Healthcare*, vol 6, issue 4, pp 685–692, 2018.

5. D. Horsfall, H. Psycholgios, H. Rankin-Smith, N. Read and K. Noonan. *Researching Compassionate Communities in Australia: A Short Term, Longitudinal Study.* Sydney, The GroundSwell Project, pp. 1–10, 2020.
6. K. Noonan, B. Rumbold and S. Aoun. Compassionate community connectors: a distinct form of end-of-life volunteering. *Progress in Palliative Care*, vol 31, 2022. doi: 10.1080/09699260.2022.2090051
7. S. Aoun, R. Richmond, K. Gunton, K. Noonan, J. Abel and B. Rumbold. The Compassionate Communities Connectors model for end-of-life care: implementation and evaluation. *Palliative Care and Social Practice*, vol 16, pp. 1–18, 2022. doi:10.1177/26323524221139655
8. S. Aoun, J. Abel, B. Rumbold, K. Cross, J. Moore, P. Skeers and L. Deliens. The Compassionate Communities Connectors model for end-of-life care: a community and health service partnership in Western Australia. *Palliative Care and Social Practice*, vol 14, pp. 1–9, 2020. doi:10.1177/2632352420935130
9. S. Aoun, R. Richmond, K. Noonan, K. Gunton and B. Rumbold. 'The more you give, the better it is for you. You know the reward is greater than the effort': the Compassionate Communities Connectors' experience. *Palliative Care and Social Practice*, vol 16, pp. 1–11, 2022. doi:10.1177/26323524221139874
10. S. Aoun, J. Rosenberg, R. Richmond and B. Rumbold. The Compassionate Communities Connectors programme: experiences of supported families and referring healthcare providers. *Palliative Care and Social Practice*, vol 17, pp. 1–12, 2023. doi:10.1177/26323524231173705
11. S. Aoun, N. Bear and B. Rumbold. The Compassionate Communities Connectors program: effect on healthcare usage. *Palliative Care and Social Practice*, vol 17, 1–11, 2023. doi:10.1177/26323524231205323
12. A. Kellehear. *The Compassionate City Charter*. 2015. Available: https://compassionate-communitiesuk.com/wp-content/uploads/2021/12/The-Compassionate-City-Charter.pdf
13. J. Abel, A. Kellehear and A. Karapliagou. Palliative care-the new essentials, In: J. Abel, A. Kellehear (eds) *Oxford Textbook of Public Health Palliative Care*. Oxford, Oxford University Press: 2022, pp. 30–37.

19

BUILDING A COMPASSIONATE COMMUNITY THROUGH A CULTURAL CARE PERSPECTIVE

Experience from Taipei City, Taiwan

Samuel Shih-Chih Wang, Chia-Jen Liu and Sheng-Jean Huang

Abstract

The global Compassionate Communities (CC) movement, inspired by Professor Allan Kellehear's health promotion framework, redefines the end-of-life (EoL) experience as a collective social responsibility rather than a clinical event. By decentralizing care from medical institutions to civic life, this approach integrates prevention and harm reduction into the fabric of schools, workplaces, and neighborhoods. This chapter explores the implementation of the CC model in Taipei, specifically within the Shilin Old Street pilot site, where municipal policy and grassroots engagement converge to facilitate aging-in-place. Central to this transition is the application of Madeleine Leininger's Culture Care Theory, which ensures that EoL support remains culturally congruent. In the context of Taiwan's traditional taboos regarding death, this dual framework transforms EoL dialogue into a form of "life wisdom." Through culturally resonant interventions like temple gatherings and life story cafés, the Taipei model demonstrates a sustainable, inclusive synthesis of global health strategy and local cultural heritage.

19.1 Introduction

The global Compassionate Communities (CC) movement has emerged as a public health response to the growing need for end-of-life (EoL) support and community-based care [1–5]. Pioneered by Professor Allan Kellehear and rooted in the principles of health promotion outlined in the Ottawa Charter, the CC approach positions health, death, dying, caregiving, and grief as shared social responsibilities, not solely medical matters [6]. It emphasises prevention, harm

DOI: 10.4324/9781003621348-20

reduction, and early intervention while encouraging citizens, schools, workplaces, and institutions to create caring environments that foster dignity at the EoL [7,8].

In Taipei, this global vision has been contexualised through culturally grounded practices and partnerships. The Shilin Old Street neighborhood was selected as the pilot site for CC Taipei, combining municipal leadership, community engagement, and cultural wisdom to support aging-in-place and palliative care. The model integrates home medical services, social support, and public education, demonstrating the glocalization of compassionate care [9,10].

Complementing this is Madeleine Leininger's Culture Care Theory, which advocates for culturally congruent care that respects individuals' values, beliefs, and lifeways [11–13]. This framework is particularly relevant in Taiwan, where traditional Chinese beliefs often discourage open conversations about death. By applying the Culture Care lens, Taipei's initiative reframes EoL dialogue as part of life wisdom, using culturally resonant strategies, such as temple-based gatherings, life story cafés, and ancestral festivals, to encourage participation while honoring tradition.

Together, the CC model and Culture Care Theory offer a synergistic framework that informs both policy and practice. In Taipei, they form the basis of a sustainable, inclusive approach to EoL care, one that acknowledges death as a communal experience and promotes compassion as a civic value.

19.2 Cultural context of the community

Understanding the cultural context of a community is vital for building a sustainable and culturally sensitive CC [14–20]. In Taipei's Shilin Old Street neighborhood, the development of community-based palliative and EoL care was shaped by deep historical, demographic, and cultural factors that made it a compelling location for piloting Taiwan's first CC initiative.

19.2.1 Historical and cultural heritage

Shilin Old Street is located in the Jiujia Village of Shilin District and is recognised as one of the oldest developed areas in Taipei City. At the heart of the community stands the Shennong Temple, established in 1812, which serves not only as a site of religious practice but also as a civic and cultural gathering space. This temple honors Shennong, a mythological figure known as the "Divine Farmer," revered as the originator of Chinese medicine. The temple's presence makes it a natural anchor for initiatives focused on health and well-being.

The area also includes heritage sites such as the Guo Yuanyi Cake Museum, representing long-standing traditions in Taiwanese culinary arts. These cultural symbols evoke a strong sense of local identity, continuity, and belonging—values crucial for mobilizing community action. The proximity of the community to the Taipei Metro system adds a modern and accessible dimension to the otherwise traditional setting, facilitating participation by both residents and external partners such as university students and NGOs.

19.2.2 Demographic characteristics

According to 2021 statistics, Shilin Old Street is home to 6,201 residents, with 33.29% of the population aged 65 or older. This figure is significantly higher than Taipei City's overall average of 19.22% and the national average of 14.05% [21]. The aging population structure highlights a growing need for age-friendly health and social services, particularly those focused on long-term care, palliative support, and aging-in-place initiatives.

The neighborhood's relatively stable population, comprising mainly multigenerational families who have lived in the area for decades, further reinforces social cohesion. Such cohesion is a key asset in community health promotion and an essential condition for the successful implementation of a CC. Residents often share similar values, rituals, and social expectations, creating a high potential for shared initiatives and mutual support.

19.2.3 Religious and social norms

Traditional Taiwanese beliefs and Confucian ethics play a major role in shaping the community's attitudes toward aging, illness, and death. Concepts such as filial piety (孝), ancestor worship, and the maintenance of family honor deeply influence how people approach EoL matters. Openly discussing death, especially with elders, is commonly perceived as taboo and even disrespectful. As such, any community initiative touching on issues of dying, grief, or terminal illness must be framed with cultural sensitivity.

To navigate these cultural norms, the CC initiative in Shilin Old Street employed indirect yet effective communication strategies. Instead of using terms like "death" or "palliative care," the initiative adopted the language of "life issues" (生命議題), "life aesthetics" (生命美學), and "mutual support" (互助關懷). These terms align with culturally accepted ways of discussing mortality by emphasizing continuity, legacy, and emotional connection, rather than finality or loss.

Religious institutions like the Shennong Temple were instrumental in building community trust. The temple not only hosted events such as health talks and ancestral exhibitions but also helped legitimise the program in the eyes of local residents. By integrating health promotion activities with religious festivals and lunar calendar events, the initiative ensured a culturally congruent rhythm of engagement (Figure 19.1).

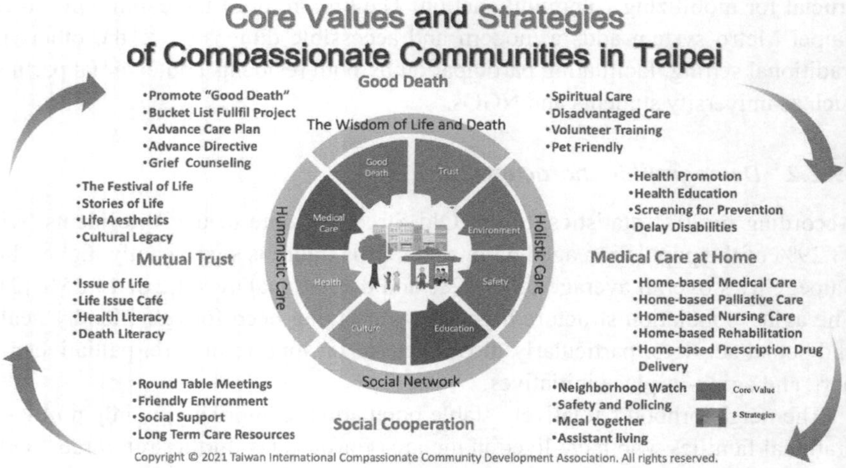

FIGURE 19.1 Core values and strategies of compassionate communities in Taipei

19.2.4 Community dynamics and social capital

Shilin Old Street is characterised by strong interpersonal networks and an ingrained culture of neighborly interaction. Daily life often includes visits to the temple, participation in communal meals, and engagement in local rituals. These routines provide natural opportunities for the dissemination of health information and the cultivation of social support networks.

The community's rich social capital was further strengthened by collaborations with educational institutions such as the University of Taipei. Students engaged in intergenerational learning projects, such as the Life Issue Café and home visits to older adults, which fostered mutual respect, reduced age-related stereotypes, and deepened social ties.

Community leaders, including the village head and temple caretakers, were deeply involved in the planning and implementation of CC activities. Their leadership provided continuity, credibility, and cultural insight, ensuring that the project was not perceived as an external imposition but as an extension of community values (Figure 19.2).

19.2.5 Structural support and accessibility

One unique feature of the Shilin Old Street community is the integration of cultural tradition with modern public health infrastructure. The Taipei City Hospital Yangming Branch, located nearby, played a critical role in delivering home-based medical care and coordinating outreach services. Through its collaboration with local NGOs and volunteers, the hospital extended its reach into the community without undermining its informal social systems [22].

The establishment of the Shennong LOHAS Station exemplifies this integration. Situated within the temple grounds, the station offers health screenings, meals, and

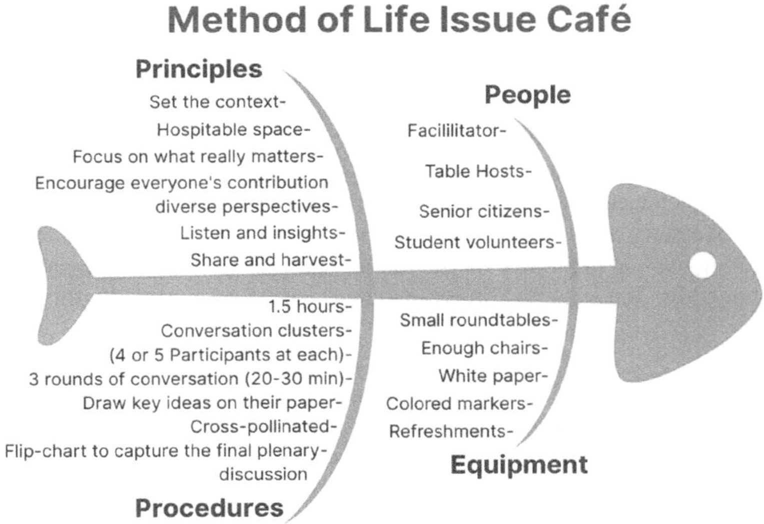

FIGURE 19.2 Design model of a life issue cafe

educational seminars twice a month, timed with religious observance days. This model leverages existing community routines to introduce healthcare services in a familiar and non-intrusive manner.

19.3 Culturally sensitive practices in CC: activities and innovations

Implementing a CC in Taipei required careful consideration of cultural norms, community dynamics, and the social stigma surrounding EoL discussions. The success of the Shilin Old Street CC initiative was largely due to its ability to design and deliver activities that were not only innovative but also culturally sensitive and aligned with the lived realities of its residents. This section outlines the key practices and innovations that allowed the Taipei CC to thrive within a traditional East Asian cultural context.

19.3.1 The Life Issue Café: a redefinition of dialogue

One of the most notable innovations of the Taipei CC is the Life Issue Café—a culturally adapted version of the "Death Café" concept. In Taiwanese society, direct discussion of death is often seen as taboo, particularly among older generations. To overcome this barrier, organisers reframed the discourse by emphasizing "life issues" rather than "death" only.

The Life Issue Café created a structured, safe space where elders and young university students could engage in intergenerational conversations about health, life goals, legacy, and caregiving. Rather than focusing on the fear and finality of death, participants reflected on the meaning of a good life, personal values, and what it means to live with dignity until the end. Activities typically included guided small-group discussions, collective visual recording of reflections, and sharing sessions. This respectful and life-affirming approach reduced resistance while promoting death literacy through culturally acceptable pathways [23].

Surveys conducted during these events revealed a shift in attitudes: a large percentage of elderly participants reported greater comfort in discussing EoL issues and stronger motivation to prepare for the future. Students also gained valuable insights into aging, loss, and empathy—deepening their sense of social responsibility [23].

19.3.2 The Festival of Life and Life Aesthetics Exhibitions

Cultural sensitivity was further embedded through community rituals and exhibitions that connected EoL themes with traditional practices. The Festival of Life is an annual event modeled after ancestral remembrance days and temple festivals. It encourages storytelling, reflection, and celebration of life achievements, enabling participants to confront mortality through a familiar and emotionally resonant format.

The Life Aesthetics Exhibitions showcased artifacts, photos, and creative works related to deceased community members. These exhibitions served multiple purposes: they honored memory, fostered healing, and educated the public about the emotional and spiritual dimensions of loss. By integrating art and memory within culturally significant venues—such as the Shennong Temple and the Guo Yuanyi Cake Museum—these programs successfully normalise public engagement with themes of death, dying, and grief.

Such cultural interventions not only promoted social cohesion but also reclaimed death as a communal, rather than purely medical, experience. These practices made it possible to speak about the EoL while upholding the values of reverence, legacy, and ancestral continuity.

19.3.3 Shennong LOHAS Station: health services in a spiritual setting

The establishment of the Shennong LOHAS Station within the temple grounds represents a pioneering model of culturally embedded healthcare. The station operates twice a month, coinciding with lunar calendar holy days, when community members naturally gather for worship. Services include meal sharing, health consultations, basic screenings, and seminars on both traditional and modern medicine.

The strategic use of religious space enhances legitimacy and participation, especially among elders who are more likely to trust familiar institutions. Health education topics are carefully chosen to avoid conflict with cultural taboos. Instead of lectures about death, the focus is on "living well," healthy aging, and "preparing for peace." Through this approach, the station subtly introduces palliative and EoL concepts under the broader umbrella of life care. This model demonstrates how physical and symbolic space can be co-occupied by healthcare and tradition to create a welcoming, stigma-free environment for community care.

19.3.4 Bucket List Fulfillment and Advance Care Planning

A deeply human and innovative practice in the Taipei CC is the Bucket List Fulfillment Project. Elders were invited to express life goals or unresolved wishes, which were then supported by volunteers and care providers. Whether visiting a childhood home, reconnecting with a long-lost friend, or completing a craft, these acts of closure fostered emotional peace and affirmed personhood.

In tandem, Advance Care Planning (ACP) sessions were offered through the hospital's home care team. These sessions provided information on legal and medical rights, explained Do-Not-Resuscitate choices, and facilitated documentation of personal EoL wishes. Conducted with empathy and cultural sensitivity, ACP helped normalise proactive planning and encouraged family discussions that would otherwise be difficult to initiate.

19.3.5 Pet Grief Support and intergenerational learning

Recognizing that pets are deeply integrated into family life in modern Taiwan, the Taipei CC also developed Pet Grief Support activities. Memorial events, photo exhibitions, and reunion gatherings allowed individuals to grieve pet losses in a socially supported setting. This inclusive approach addressed a commonly overlooked form of grief and expanded the definition of compassionate care.

Meanwhile, intergenerational learning formed the foundation of youth engagement. Students participated in life story recordings, home visits, and caregiving exercises. These interactions nurtured empathy, challenged stereotypes, and equipped young people with the tools to become future community leaders in compassionate care.

In summary, the Taipei CC succeeded not merely because it followed a set of international guidelines, but because it embedded those principles in the everyday cultural life of its people. Through a mosaic of spiritually rooted gatherings, intergenerational engagement, symbolic rituals, and nonthreatening discourse, the community redefined what it means to live, and die, with dignity in a Taiwanese context.

19.4 Culturally based leadership and participation

One of the most defining features of Taipei's CC initiative, particularly in the Shilin Old Street neighborhood, is its grounding in culturally embedded leadership and broad-based community participation. Rather than imposing a top-down medical model, the initiative cultivated leadership from within the community and established partnerships that reflected existing social hierarchies, religious structures, and civic practices. This culturally attuned leadership model contributed significantly to the legitimacy, accessibility, and sustainability of the program.

19.4.1 Community-led design and public–private partnership

The initiative was catalyzed by a collaboration between the Taipei City Hospital Yangming Branch and the Jiujia Village administration, supported by the broader Taipei municipal government. However, its implementation was carefully co-designed with community stakeholders. The project embraced a public–private–community partnership model, inviting participation from neighborhood leaders, local businesses, social welfare institutions, cultural organisations, and religious representatives.

The formation of a promotion committee comprising professionals, scholars, religious figures, and community elders was instrumental in ensuring that decision-making reflected diverse community voices. This committee provided advice on culturally appropriate messaging, designed community events, and mobilised volunteers. Their involvement helped root the program within familiar institutions and practices, making it more acceptable to residents who might otherwise be hesitant to engage with topics of death and dying.

The Shennong Temple, a long-standing spiritual and cultural anchor in the community, played a key leadership role. The temple's leadership opened its doors to health activities, lent spiritual credibility to the initiative, and served as a gateway to engaging the older population—many of whom regularly attend religious events but would not otherwise participate in health-related programming.

19.4.2 Empowering local leaders and volunteers

Culturally based leadership also meant recognizing and empowering informal leaders within the community. This included shop owners, long-time residents, neighborhood watch captains, and retired elders who held respect and influence. These individuals became important messengers and mobilisers, helping to share information about the initiative in casual, trustworthy ways. Word-of-mouth communication, community bulletin boards, and temple announcements were utilised to invite participation in activities like the Life Issue Café and health seminars.

The program also emphasised volunteer empowerment as a leadership pathway. Local residents were recruited and trained to provide peer support, assist with logistics, and facilitate group discussions. Training sessions focused not only on knowledge about palliative care but also on cultural humility, empathetic communication, and emotional support [24].

This decentralised leadership model allowed the initiative to take root in daily life. Volunteers led neighborhood visits, organised group meals for elders, and helped coordinate cultural events, embodying a grassroots form of compassionate action that was both sustainable and culturally resonant.

19.4.3 *Intergenerational engagement as leadership practice*

A particularly innovative aspect of the Taipei CC initiative was the incorporation of university and high school students into the leadership structure. Young people were not just observers but active contributors, participating in home visits, oral history projects, creative exhibitions, and the facilitation of Life Issue Cafés. These interactions allowed for the exchange of life experiences and wisdom, and students gained hands-on experience in leadership through empathy and service.

By encouraging intergenerational collaboration, the project reframed leadership as a shared responsibility across age groups. Elders offered their stories and values; students contributed energy, technical skills, and creativity. The result was a dynamic leadership ecosystem where tradition and innovation coexisted.

19.4.4 *Cultural legitimacy and civic pride*

Crucially, the leadership and participation model strengthened the cultural legitimacy of the CC initiative. When Taipei Mayor Dr. Ko Wen-je personally unveiled the Shilin Old Street CC plaque in 2018 and declared April 6 as Taipei International Compassionate Community Day, it marked an important moment of institutional validation. This ceremonial endorsement resonated with traditional values of authority and public recognition.

Moreover, community members expressed a growing sense of ownership and pride in their collective achievements. Residents were no longer passive recipients of care but active co-creators of a compassionate social environment. This transformation of identity, from "patients" to "participants," was perhaps the most enduring outcome of culturally-based leadership in action.

19.5 Current developments and outcomes

The CC initiative in Taipei, launched first in the Shilin Old Street neighborhood, has evolved into a robust, city-wide model of culturally embedded, community-driven palliative and EoL care. Its development reflects both a deep respect for local traditions and a commitment to health innovation. This section summarises the key developments since its inception and the outcomes observed in both quantitative and qualitative terms.

19.5.1 *From pilot to city-wide expansion*

Following its formal establishment in April 2018, the Shilin Old Street CC became the prototype for a broader municipal strategy. Taipei City's government, in collaboration with Taipei City Hospital and community partners, replicated the model across other administrative districts. As of the time of reporting, 20 villages across 12 districts in Taipei have formally established CC.

Each local CC was designed with unique thematic characteristics based on its population and cultural traits. For example, Huxing Village in Neihu District emphasised faith-based aging support, Hulu Village adopted a pet-friendly grief model, and Changchun Village focused on building intergenerational friendship networks. This diversity showcases how the flexible Taipei CC model accommodates the distinct needs and assets of each neighborhood while maintaining core values of humanistic care, community participation, and cultural sensitivity.

19.5.2 Key service components and infrastructure

Throughout these communities, several key service components have become standardised:

1 Shennong LOHAS Stations offer periodic health consultations, meals, and education within culturally familiar spaces like temples or community centers.
2 Home-based medical care is delivered by Taipei City Hospital in collaboration with local volunteers and NGOs, ensuring continuity of care, especially for elderly or socially isolated individuals.
3 ACP workshops and documentation support are provided in nonthreatening, community-based formats to encourage proactive decision-making around EoL wishes.
4 Life Issue Cafés foster reflective, intergenerational dialogue on life and death, reshaping attitudes toward mortality and aging.

These services are integrated under a community-healthcare partnership framework, where health professionals work in tandem with trained volunteers, cultural leaders, and students to address medical, psychosocial, and spiritual dimensions of care.

19.5.3 Participation and engagement outcomes

Community engagement has increased substantially since the launch of the program. In 2018, pilot data from four Life Issue Cafés showed that 27 senior participants and 60 university students took part in structured dialogues around life and death. Survey data revealed that 84.2% of seniors and 90.9% of students agreed it was important to talk about life and death issues, although many still found it emotionally difficult. Notably, nearly 79% of seniors and 91% of students reported they felt more capable of facing death calmly following the experience [24].

These findings suggest that culturally sensitive formats like the Life Issue Café have measurable impacts on death literacy, emotional resilience, and intergenerational understanding. Participants also report an increased willingness to engage in ACP discussions, reach out for emotional support, and participate in public health activities.

19.5.4 Shifts in community perceptions and behavior

A major qualitative outcome of the initiative is the transformation in how community members perceive death and caregiving. Where EoL matters were once avoided due to cultural taboos, there is now greater openness, normalization, and agency. Elders speak more freely about their values and wishes, while family members and volunteers feel more confident initiating conversations about illness, grief, and remembrance [25,26].

This shift is particularly evident in the context of grief support, where the inclusion of pet memorial activities and public storytelling events has expanded the social space for mourning. By incorporating these rituals into everyday community life, the initiative has destigamtised expressions of loss and created an emotionally supportive environment for healing.

Furthermore, community members now perceive themselves not as passive recipients of services but as active contributors to a compassionate, aging-friendly society. This evolving identity fosters a sense of belonging and civic pride that sustains participation even beyond formal project timelines.

19.5.5 System-level recognition and institutionalization

The successes of Taipei's CC model have gained recognition at both national and international levels. Professor Allan Kellehear, founder of the International Compassionate City Charter, officially invited the Shilin Old Street initiative to join the Public Health Palliative Care International network. In 2018, Taipei Mayor Dr. Ko Wen-je unveiled the official CC plaque at a public ceremony and declared April 6 as Taipei International Compassionate Community Day, marking institutional endorsement of the city's commitment to community-based palliative care.

To consolidate and expand these efforts, the Taiwan International Compassionate Community Development Association was formed. This organisation supports replication in other cities, facilitates knowledge-sharing, and builds cross-sector alliances for compassionate policymaking.

19.5.6 Resilience during COVID-19

The outbreak of the COVID-19 pandemic tested the resilience of the CC model [27]. Despite restrictions on face-to-face gatherings, Taipei's CC adapted quickly. Life Issue Cafés were moved online, volunteers made check-in phone calls, and digital legacy projects allowed continued reflection and connection. These responses demonstrated the flexibility and sustainability of the community-based model, even under crisis conditions. The initiative's ability to maintain operations and continue supporting socially vulnerable groups during the pandemic highlighted its role not only as a health strategy but also as a social resilience mechanism.

In conclusion, Taipei's CCs have transitioned from a single neighborhood pilot to a dynamic, city-wide movement. Through culturally grounded practices, collaborative leadership, and flexible service delivery, these communities have made significant progress in changing public attitudes, improving quality of life, and fostering a culture of compassion across generations. Their outcomes offer both a model and an inspiration for similar efforts around the world.

19.6 Reflections on challenges and successes

The implementation of Taipei's CC has illuminated both the potential and complexity of embedding EoL care within community life. Several successes stand out as important achievements, while key challenges offer critical lessons for future development.

19.6.1 Key successes

One of the most significant successes of the Taipei model is its ability to integrate culturally sensitive practices into everyday community structures. Through partnerships with temples, schools, and neighborhood leaders, CC activities became part of the community's natural rhythm. Programs such as the Life Issue Café, Festival of Life, and Shennong LOHAS Station were received positively because they honored local traditions and offered nonthreatening entry points to topics like aging, loss, and dying.

Another major success is the intergenerational learning fostered through collaboration with university students. These interactions not only improved youth understanding of aging and mortality but also revitalised older participants through mutual respect and emotional exchange. The initiative also succeeded in mobilizing diverse sectors, including government agencies, healthcare providers, NGOs, and religious institutions, under a shared vision of compassionate care.

Finally, the city's formal endorsement, evidenced by the declaration of April 6 as Taipei International Compassionate Community Day, helped legitimise and institutionalise the CC approach. This balance of grassroots energy and municipal support has been essential to the program's growth and sustainability.

19.6.2 Challenges and lessons learned

Despite these achievements, several challenges emerged. Cultural taboos surrounding death made it initially difficult to engage community members in conversations about EoL planning. Organisers had to invest time in reframing the narrative, using terms like "life issues" and focusing on legacy, love, and gratitude to ease resistance.

Sustaining volunteer participation posed another challenge. Many volunteers were enthusiastic initially but required ongoing support, recognition, and training to remain engaged over the long term. Finally, building cross-sector collaboration required significant effort to align diverse perspectives, particularly when bridging the gaps between medical, religious, and civic institutions.

Overall, the Taipei experience demonstrates that culturally grounded leadership, patient engagement strategies, and flexible partnerships are vital for overcoming barriers and building lasting CC.

19.7 Future directions for our Compassionate Communities

Building on the success of the Shilin Old Street initiative and the broader implementation of CC across Taipei, the future development of the movement in Taiwan points toward deeper integration, greater inclusivity, and long-term sustainability.

One primary direction is the nationwide expansion of the CC model. The establishment of the Taiwan International CC Development Association reflects a commitment to scaling up the initiative beyond Taipei. This includes adapting the model to different local cultures, community capacities, and geographic contexts—from urban centers to rural townships.

Another priority is embedding death literacy and life education into formal education systems. By introducing these topics in high schools and universities, future generations can develop a healthier relationship with aging, caregiving, and grief. Encouraging cross-generational dialogue through academic and community partnerships will remain a core strategy to sustain community participation and intergenerational empathy.

The use of digital technologies is also being explored to expand access and engagement. Virtual Life Issue Cafés, mobile platforms for ACP, and online memorial spaces can help reach populations that are homebound or socially isolated. The COVID-19 pandemic highlighted the importance of flexible, hybrid models that blend digital and in-person engagement.

Additionally, a key focus moving forward is on evidence-building and policy alignment. Developing standardised evaluation tools and engaging in longitudinal studies will help quantify impact and inform policymaking. Continued collaboration with public health agencies and social service sectors is vital for integrating CC values into broader healthcare and welfare systems.

Ultimately, the future of Taiwan's CC lies in sustaining a shared civic culture where compassion is not only practiced but also institutionalised and celebrated as a vital element of community well-being.

References

1. Brito, G.; Flores, S. Compassion in palliative care: A review. *Curr. Opin. Support. Palliat. Care* 2018, 12, 472–479.
2. Kellehear, A. Compassionate cities: Global significance and meaning for palliative care. *Prog. Palliat. Care* 2020, 28, 115–119.
3. Pfaff, K.; Markaki, A. Compassionate collaborative care: An integrative review of quality indicators in end-of-life care. *BMC Palliat. Care* 2017, 16, 65.
4. Abel, J.; Kingston, H.; Scally, A.; Hartnoll, J.; Hannam, G.; Thomson-Moore, A.; Kellehear, A. Reducing emergency hospital admissions: A population health complex

intervention of an enhanced model of primary care and compassionate communities. *Br. J. Gen. Pract*. 2018, 68, e803–e810.
5. Sallnow, L.; Richardson, H.; Murray, S.A.; Kellehear, A. The impact of a new public health approach to end-of-life care: A systematic review. *Palliat. Med* 2016, 30, 200–211.
6. Kellehear, A. *Compassionate Cities*. Routledge: London, 2012.
7. Tsouros, A.D. The who healthy cities project: State of the art and future plans. *Health Promot. Int*. 1995, 10, 133–141.
8. Aicher, J. *Designing Healthy Cities: Prescriptions, Principles, and Practice*. Krieger Publishing Company: Malabar, FL, 1998.
9. Roudometof, V. Theorizing glocalization: Three interpretations. *Eur. J. Soc. Theory* 2016, 19, 391–408.
10. Robertson, R. Glocalization. *Int. Encycl. Anthropol* 2018.
11. Leininger MM. *The theory of Culture Care Diversity and Universality*. NLN Publ. 1991 Nov; (15-2402): 5–68. PMID: 1795998.
12. Leininger, M.M. Culture care theory: A major contribution to advance transcultural nursing knowledge and practices. *J. Transcult Nurs* 2002, 11(3), 189–192. https://doi.org/10.1177/10459602013003005
13. McFarland, M.R.; Wehbe-Alamah, H.B. *Leininger's Culture Care Diversity and Universality: A Worldwide Nursing Theory* (3rd ed.). Jones & Bartlett Learning, 2018. Burlington, Massachusetts.
14. Kellehear, A.; O'Connor, D. Health-promoting palliative care: A practice example. *Crit. Public Health* 2008, 18, 111–115.
15. WHO. Palliative Care. Available online: https://www.who.int/health-topics/palliative-care (accessed on 26 November 2021).
16. Kellehear, A. Compassionate communities: End-of-life care as everyone's responsibility. *QJM Int. J. Med*. 2013, 106, 1071–1075.
17. Bomba, P.A.; Orem, K. Lessons learned from New York's community approach to advance care planning and MOLST. *Ann. Palliat. Med*. 2015, 4, 10–21.
18. Gómez-Batiste, X.; Mateu, S.; Serra-Jofre, S.; Molas, M.; Mir-Roca, S.; Amblàs, J.; Costa, X.; Lasmarías, C.; Serrarols, M.; Solà-Serrabou, A. Compassionate Communities: Design and preliminary results of the experience of Vic (Barcelona, Spain) Caring City. *Ann. Palliat. Med*. 2018, 7 (Suppl. 2), S32–S41.
19. Kelley, M.L.; Prince, H.; Nadin, S.; Brazil, K.; Crow, M.; Hanson, G.; Maki, L.; Monture, L.; Mushquash, C.J.; O'Brien, V. Developing palliative care programs in Indigenous communities using participatory action research: A Canadian application of the public health approach to palliative care. *Ann. Palliat. Med*. 2018, 7, S52–S72.
20. Tompkins, B. Compassionate communities in Canada: It is everyone's responsibility. *Ann. Palliat. Med*. 2018, 7, S118–S129.
21. Department of Budget, Accounting and Statistics, Taipei City Government. The Dependency Ratio and Aging Index. Available online: https://www-ws.gov.taipei/Download.ashx?u=LzAwMS9VcGxvYWQvMzY3L3JlbGZpbGUvMC82NDg5NC9iMjM3NmY3My1lMGQ1LTRkMGYtOTRkZS02OTAwZTE4NWFkMjcucGRm&n=MTA56Ie65YyX5biC6auY6b2h57Wx6KiI6aCF55uuLnBkZg%3d%3d&icon=..pdf (accessed on 20 November 2021).
22. Chao, K.-I.; Wang, S.-C.; Huang, T.-C.; Woung, L.-C.; Lee, O.K.; Chu, D.; Chu, C.-M.; Liu, C.-J.; Huang, S.-J. The current status of health literacy promotion in Taipei City hospital. *Taipei City Med. J*. 2017, 14, 224–233.

23. Huang, C.-Y.; Hsu, S.-H.; Wen-Jung, S.; Lee, Y.-H.; Ueng, R.-S.; Wu, M.-P.; Shih, C.-Y.; Huang, S.-J. Promoting death literacy—A high value health care for good death at home. *Taipei City Med. J.* 2017, 14, 269–278.
24. Liu, C.-J.; Yeh, T.-C.; Wu, S.-W.; Chen, T.-H.; Hsieh, M.-H.; Wang, S.-C.; Huang, S.-J.; Woung, L.-C. Cross generation shared learning in Compassionate Community. *Taipei City Med. J.* 2019, 16, 145–152.
25. Miles, L.; Corr, C.A. Death cafe: What is it and what we can learn from it. *OMEGA-J. Death Dying* 2017, 75, 151–165.
26. McLoughlin, K.; McGilloway, S.; Lloyd, R.; O'Connor, M.; Rhatigan, J.; Shanahan, M.; Richardson, M.; Keevey, A. Walls, wisdom, worries, and wishes: Engaging communities in discussion about death, dying, loss, and care using Café Conversation. *Prog. Palliat. Care* 2016, 24, 9–14.
27. Public Health Palliative Care International and Dr Julian Abel. Developing Compassionate Streets and Neighbourhoods during COVID-19. Compassionate Communities UK. Available online: https://static1.squarespace.com/static/57f61928d2b857de53f3b0a6/t/5e8a5ff9e8170a5ffa3a6a66/1586126851603/ComComCovidPHPCI.pdf (accessed on 20 November 2021).

20

BRIDGING THE GAP IN ACCESS TO PALLIATIVE CARE SERVICES THROUGH THE COMPASSIONATE COMMUNITIES FOR UGANDA INITIATIVE (CCUI)

Mark Mwesiga, Lacey Ahern, Teresa Majkut, Saphrah Amumpaire, Rosemary Kiwanuka and Paul Mwambi

Abstract

The Palliative Care Association of Uganda (PCAU) have embraced a compassionate community model within the context of Ugandan's cultural community norms around death, dying and loss. PCAU partner with healthcare professionals in different areas to initiate compassionate communities and involve local communities including schools. They recruit and rely on Village Health Team volunteers, who are trained in a community-centred, public health-supported palliative care method. They have found the involvement of school students and the experience they have gained valuable. It is hoped they will take with them into the adult life and be the bridge from one generation to another, enabling compassionate communities to be a cultural norm.

20.1 Introduction

Community is an integral part of all tribes of the Ugandan people. It is a common occurrence in all parts of Uganda that neighbours share in each other's lives, often eating, working, worshipping, and celebrating together. The Palliative Care Association of Uganda (PCAU) is working to leverage the existing strength of communities in Uganda to support people in their most vulnerable moments: when grieving the death of a loved one, navigating a new diagnosis, and facing the end-of-life. By partnering with local professional palliative care or hospice teams, PCAU collaborates with community members to train volunteers in community-centred, public health-supported palliative care methods, acknowledging the unique needs of each setting.

This grassroots approach empowers community members to care for one another and fosters youth involvement, allowing for multi-generational collaboration that

DOI: 10.4324/9781003621348-21

enriches both the young and the old. PCAU's Compassionate Communities model emphasises the needs of individuals whilst rooting care in the collective strength, resilience, and compassion of Ugandan community life and ultimately generates a cyclical model sustainable for generations to come, ensuring that care, dignity, and compassion remain central at every stage of life.

20.2 The aspects and context of our community

Winston Churchill famously referred to Uganda as the "Pearl of Africa" in his 1908 book *My African Journey* [1]. Located on the equator, Uganda is home to warm, friendly people and offers a variety of tropical fruits, stunning scenery, and a rich biodiversity [2]. Uganda is popularly believed to have some of the best weather in Africa and is home to the world's largest population of gorillas [3].

Uganda is in sub-Saharan Africa, where many of the world's poorest people live. According to the World Bank, in 2024, sub-Saharan Africa accounted for 16% of the world's population, but 67% of the people living in extreme poverty [4]. With high levels of poverty, countries like Uganda have the lowest healthcare expenditures per capita [5], low life expectancy, and inadequate access to healthcare services, safe water, education, and sanitation facilities [6].

In Uganda, the burden of disease is characterised by communicable diseases, childhood illnesses, and an increasing prevalence of non-communicable diseases (NCDs). Studies indicate that in 2016, NCDs accounted for 1 in 3 deaths, with an estimated mortality risk of 22% [7]. This burden is primarily due to cardiovascular disease and cancer, exacerbated by underlying risk factors like hypertension, tobacco use, and alcohol use [7]. According to the 2024 Uganda National Population and Housing Census, individuals aged 60 years and above account for 5% of the total population. Whilst this figure may seem modest at first glance, its implications for the country's healthcare systems and broader socio-economic structures are profound, as this ageing population will bring demand for age-related healthcare services and social support.

As healthcare needs expand, challenges such as poor-quality health services, limited hospital coverage, inadequate infrastructure in rural areas, and a 30–60% shortage of health workers and medicines hinder Uganda's health services' ability to meet the growing needs of its citizens. Moreover, Uganda's Ministry of Health found that households' out-of-pocket expenditure on healthcare exceeds 40%, a staggering cost given that over 41% of Uganda's population lives below the international poverty line [8]. These challenges affect several social and economic aspects of everyday life and significantly impact the well-being and care that Ugandans receive. Amidst challenges of scarcity and deprivation, the need for palliative care continues to grow with the increased incidence of NCDs and an ageing population.

> Let us touch the dying, the poor, the lonely, and the unwanted according to the graces we have received and let us not be ashamed or slow to do the humble work.
>
> *Mother Teresa*

To combat the stressors that NCDs and an ageing population pose to the existing healthcare systems, PCAU is pioneering initiatives to rebuild Compassionate Communities in Uganda. The initiatives are rooted in a health-promoting approach to palliative care, aiming to support solidarity among community members.

The World Health Organisation (WHO), in its new conceptual development model for palliative care worldwide, has emphasised the need for empowered people and communities. According to the WHO, individuals, families, and communities must play their role as partners in the development of health and social services, as well as in the engagement in shared decision-making about their health. It is this background that necessitates such an initiative, which involves nonprofessional palliative care actors to help address health and suffering in the community.

20.3 Do Ugandans generally discuss death, dying, and bereavement?

Uganda has many tribes that speak different languages. There are 65 Indigenous communities, as outlined in the country's constitution. The number of tribes can vary based on various classifications, cultural beliefs, norms, values, and practices. Several published studies, especially on the concept of advance care directives of the African people, tend to generalise norms, beliefs, values, and customs about death, dying, and bereavement. For example, a 2016 study by Rabi Ekore and Bolatito Lanre-Abass published by the *Indian Journal of Palliative Care* 2016 stated that "Africans ordinarily do not encourage the contemplation of death or any discussion about their own or their loved ones' death" [9]. However, due to the existence of various tribes, religious beliefs, and cultural practices among Africans, death rituals, including discussions and mourning practices, are varied. For example, how a given group of people "celebrate" the death of a person talks much about the society's philosophy and attitude towards life and death [10]. Vicky Wadawa, in a 2012 New Vision article titled "Sending off loved ones the Ugandan way," offers key insights into experiences of death among different tribes in Uganda, including the Bankanyole, Bagisu, Acholi, and Baganda [11]. What is not in doubt is the fact that death has long been viewed as a part of life within African society and that death is approached and rationalised through various means. Death is spoken about by the old to the young, death and burial are celebrated in multiple ways by different societies, and the practices surrounding dying and death are communal in many African cultures. The Bakonzo and Banyankole tribes, for example, bury the dead near the homestead. This is premised on the cultural belief that the dead are still part of the family. Burying near the homestead is to "send a message" to the dead and ancestors that they are still considered to be part of the family [10]. Genuine discussions about sickness, care, and support are held among the Banyankole. The same tribe has several proverbs about death and dying. In many African societies, the information about death and dying is passed on through generations in fireplace stories, folk tales, rituals, and family group discussions, among others. Indeed, in many African societies, funerals are not just a time of mourning; they are a deeply emotional, spiritual, and community-focused event. They offer a way to honour the dead, comfort the grieving, and unite extended families and neighbours in a show of solidarity [12]. In most societies, extended families and neighbours share funeral costs to ease the financial burden. Village burials often involve committees, structures, and resources. Family and neighbours gather at the deceased's house, bringing food from their homes [13].

20.4 Rooted in African Heritage, where the old pass on positive values to the young

As the lead organisation advocating for the integration of palliative care into Uganda's social services, the PCAU recognises that all community members have a role in alleviating the pain and suffering caused by life-limiting illnesses. PCAU has therefore initiated a Compassionate Community programme that seeks to reawaken neighbours in communities to mind the plight of the sick, frail, and older persons around them. The initiatives by PCAU are culturally appropriate and deeply rooted in our African heritage. The African context highlights the vital roles family members, neighbours, and the local community play during times of sickness, suffering, death, dying, bereavement, and in caring for older or frail individuals. However, as we continue to evolve as a society, experiencing migration, urbanisation, and population growth, the support of extended families and immediate neighbours gradually diminishes.

Through a public-health-focused palliative care approach, PCAU is empowering communities in Uganda to foster a sense of community and support for one another by harnessing individual acts of kindness by ordinary people. This way, communities are not only supporting their own but also standing firmly together to advocate for their rights. There are more opportunities for education, awareness, information sharing, and improved referrals for individuals with health issues, older persons in need of support, and those living with disabilities.

20.4.1 Social support and informal caregivers in Uganda

Several studies have demonstrated that a strong family and neighbourhood environment, combined with support from our social networks, is essential for maintaining good health. The opposite of good social support is loneliness, isolation, and exclusion. First and foremost, it appears that social support encompasses emotional support, a sense of belonging within a family and community, feeling valued, practical assistance, and information and guidance [14]. In Uganda, like in the rest of sub-Saharan Africa, informal care is a vital part of care for many people with chronic diseases. Informal carers are individuals (relatives and non-relatives) who support patients and often provide unpaid assistance with activities of daily living for chronically ill patients [15]. Females are typically the majority of informal caregivers for their care recipients [16]. The non-formal caregivers will start at the nuclear family level, then move to the neighbourhood, local religious group or church, and community volunteer, before transitioning to professional caregivers at hospitals. It is therefore essential that all these are involved in the patient and caregiver education if care is to be enriched. Informal care is involved not only in the care of patients during the diagnosis and treatment stages but also at the end-of-life, due to the high variability of palliative care services in Africa [17].

20.5 The approach by the Palliative Care Association of Uganda

At the heart of efforts to build Compassionate Communities in Uganda is the acknowledgement that sickness, death, dying, loss, ageing, and caregiving are contextual, social experiences that affect all human beings without exception. They are inherently universal. PCAU recognises that having strong social relationships with individuals and institutions within one's community facilitates better life choices and helps alleviate pain and suffering during times of need. Conversely, loneliness, exclusion, discrimination, and stigma exacerbate the pain and suffering of individuals with illness and their families.

20.5.1 Restoring communities: the journey to compassion and connection

When initiating the programme in a new location, the first step for PCAU is to enter a partnership with a stand-alone hospice or palliative care team at the local hospital. Together with the local palliative care team, PCAU identifies a parish or ward as the area for implementation. The target population for a mapped Compassionate Community is between 2,500 and 3,800 individuals in a specific location. A detailed assessment of the population in the region follows, including the mapping of key health-focused partners, resources, and institutions. The implementation of the initiative relies heavily on compassionate volunteers from the Village Health Team, who are carefully selected and trained.

Based on the findings of the baseline assessment, the programme team collaborates with volunteers to develop interventions with clear, measurable outcomes. To inspire younger generations to sustain these Compassionate Communities, each implementing palliative care team collaborates with primary or secondary schools in their vicinity to establish children's and youth palliative care clubs. PCAU's experience has shown that children and youth clubs in schools are key catalysts of change in communities. The palliative care team members become key mentors to the palliative care clubs. The clubs conduct various activities, including essay competitions on acts of kindness, community awareness outreach, fundraising events, home visits to the sick and elderly, radio and TV talk shows, music and theatre competitions themed around palliative care and compassionate messages, and more. In all they do, the professional palliative care team members and trained volunteers are always available to guide and support students in their integral roles.

20.5.2 Case study: Palliative Care Club at the Taibah International School

Interview with Saphrah Amumpaire, Teacher of English Language and Patron of the Palliative Care Club at the Taibah International School. So far, four schools across Uganda have formed partnerships with PCAU and local palliative care organisations to integrate students into the Compassionate Communities for Uganda Initiative (CCUI). Taibah International School, in Central Uganda, has run a successful Palliative Care Club since 2023, with student involvement exceeding 120 members. Amumpaire, the patron of the club, noted that her students' involvement in palliative care has made them kinder, more considerate, and more compassionate to the less privileged, as they witness the struggles and suffering people endure. She believes that "school is well-designed for compassion to thrive," and granting students the opportunity to care for the ill and dying in their community unlocks that compassion.

Through their involvement with the club, students participate in writing competitions focused on palliative care and perform community outreach. Last year, students partnered with a local doctor whose child had sickle cell disease. By organising a fundraiser called African Day and Night, the students were able to raise enough money for the child to receive treatment. During the event, the doctor provided free sickle cell testing kits, and over 300 children and staff were genetically screened for the disease. Thanks to the dedication of the students and the doctor, the child is now recovering well, and people in the community gained valuable awareness of their sickle cell status.

The benefits of the club extend beyond just students and the ill. As a result of her involvement with palliative care, Amumpaire was one of 25 people accepted into the Ubuntu Institute of South Africa. *Ubuntu* is an African word that means humanity – it seeks to encapsulate the universal bond common to all humans. Amumpaire shared that *ubuntu* is what separates us from animals and makes us human, which, according to her, is the *kindness, patience, and compassion* so crucial to palliative care.

The Palliative Care Club has trained dozens of students in compassionate treatment and inspired many to continue in this line of work. As a direct result of their involvement with the club, some students have decided to pursue a career in palliative care and have even engaged in short-term work experiences with PCAU. This partnership did just as it was intended to bridge the gap in palliative care access and train the next generation of compassionate care professionals (Figure 20.1).

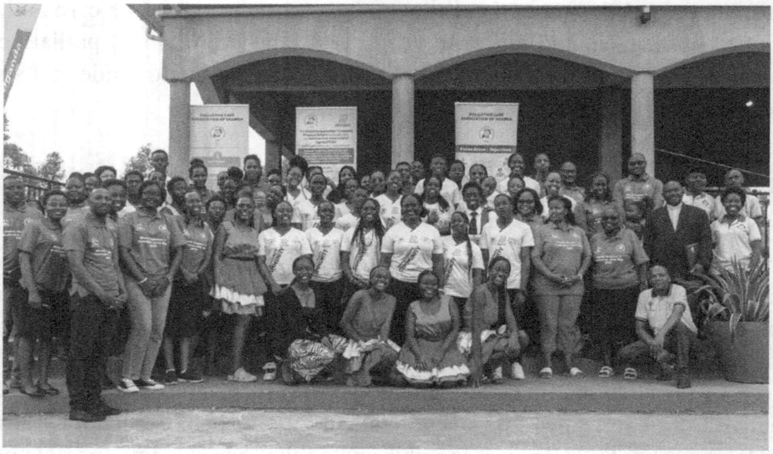

FIGURE 20.1 The Initiative to Build the First School Compassionate Community in Uganda was Launched in October 2023 at Taibah International School by the Palliative Care Association of Uganda (PCAU), Working with the Ministry of Health and the Professional Palliative Care Team of Lweza Community Health Program

PCAU's Compassionate Communities model involves multiple generations, ensuring its continuation for years to come. The elderly patients greatly enjoy the happiness and companionship these students bring into their lives, finding comfort in these interactions and a renewed sense of connection and engagement with others. In turn, the students gain valuable insights, learn from the wisdom and life experiences of the elderly, and develop empathy, patience, and a deeper appreciation for intergenerational relationships.

> Taking care of others, helping others, ultimately is the way to discover your joy and to have a happy life.
>
> *- Archbishop Desmond Tutu*

Therefore, PCAU's Compassionate Community approach enhances existing practical models of palliative care service delivery by focusing not only on the individual with an illness and their family but also by significantly strengthening the care networks surrounding them.

In doing so, the approach helps to improve the conditions in which people with life-limiting illnesses live and increase their access to resources. PCAU also aims to enhance the social determinants of health [18], which includes economic stability, social and community context, neighbourhood and environment, and access to and quality of healthcare and education (Figure 20.2).

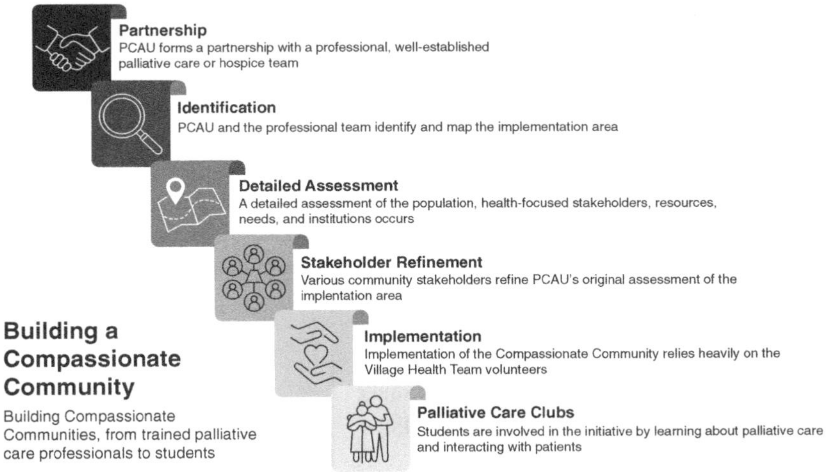

FIGURE 20.2 Palliative Care Association of Uganda Compassionate Community Initiative Summarised

20.6 Healing sound, healing words: creative arts at the centre of Compassionate Community work in Uganda

In many parts of Africa, music is a fundamental part of daily life, woven into social rituals, celebrations, and storytelling. Music plays a vital role in African people's cultures, serving not just as entertainment but as a powerful medium for communication, expression, and cultural identity.

A 2023 article by Rafael Campo highlights that poetry plays a crucial role in palliative care, as patients, families, and end-of-life professionals face the limitations of allopathic treatments. Several studies also show that incorporating poetry into palliative care provides a unique and powerful way to deliver emotional relief, express unspoken emotions, and create a sense of closure [19].

What is important to note is that the caregiving role in long-term care, including palliative care, can be a demanding and emotionally draining journey. Families and caregivers, therefore, need therapy, and creative arts such as music and poetry are beneficial. This extends to loss and grief. In Ugandan communities, when death occurs, it causes an emotional outburst, which family members and close relatives express in forms of chants, recitations, and songs. In most parts of Uganda, death is accompanied by songs and contemplation during the funeral.

A key interest of palliative care clubs at primary and high schools in Uganda, under the PCAU Compassionate Community initiative, is the use of creative arts. During the launch of the first palliative care club in Uganda in 2023, the students of Taibah International School sang songs of celebration, recited poems reflecting on kindness and compassion, and performed plays. Other schools participating in the programme have poems, composed songs, and are developing and utilising drama series. All these are not only for therapy but also for amplifying voices and information dissemination.

The Ishaka Adventist College Palliative Care Club, in partnership with the Ishaka Adventist College Palliative Care Unit in Southwestern Uganda, recites several poems during community outreach and palliative care awareness activities. They came together to create a poem that showcases their commitment to palliative care and their selfless dedication to improving the lives of those around them. An excerpt from the poem, which was written and performed entirely by the students, is transcribed below.

A community delighted to serve one another

Written by: Promise Ampumuza
Student Ishaka Adventist College

In every hand that reaches wide
In every voice that stands with pride
We build a home, not made of stone.
but of compassion, fully grown.

A compassionate community
A compassionate community

We gather not for fame or gain,
But to ease others' pain.
To listen when the rest of the world is aloud
To lift those who walk, bowed

A compassionate community
A compassionate community

Our mission breathes in all we do
In healing touch and follow-through.
With every meal, with every smile,
we walk with others
Every mile.

A compassionate community
A compassionate community

No need too small,
no soul unseen
In every act, our hearts stay keen.

From young to old, from lost to found
We sow our care in common ground

20.7 Lessons learned from building Compassionate Communities in Uganda

PCAU's journey to initiate the CCUI has been thriving. Through practical community training, PCAU and partner palliative and hospice care teams are implementing community programmes in four separate and distant districts. In each of the communities, there is a palliative care school club, which is a catalyst for change. The students teach their parents and families about the concept of kindness when they go back home from school. The students who participate in the palliative care clubs have shown great interest in learning from older people. One of the great lessons PCAU has learned is that for a Compassionate Community to thrive, there must be knowledge and affirmation from community elders, opinion leaders, and volunteers. These must be positioned and empowered to be the champions of the initiative in each of the communities. They therefore act as agents of change.

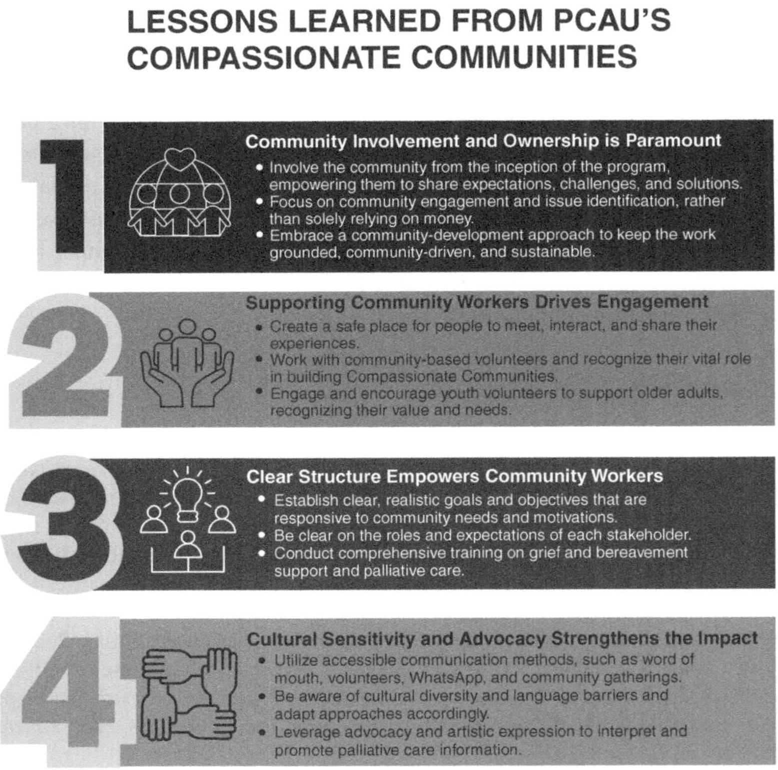

FIGURE 20.3 Lessons Learned

Each specific Compassionate Community area is unique, providing its own lessons. Compassionate Communities across Uganda are leveraging existing community strengths and building upon African cultural attitudes towards care. Communities are not hesitant to utilise their own resources. Once they are fully sensitised to their roles in palliative care, neighbours reach out to the sick, visit, collect food items, and give them to the hungry. Some are starting village and loan savings schemes to challenge the dire poverty they face. But the community leaders of the initiative, especially volunteers, need periodic refresher training on their roles and opportunities to provide feedback. Compassion fatigue is also real among volunteers because they want to do so much, yet the needs are enormous – weekly, monthly. And quality follow-ups are essential.

Though specific to Uganda, PCAU's model of Compassionate Community implementation can serve as a foundation for other countries to adapt to their own cultural context. The fundamental aspects of PCAU's model are highly applicable to a variety of settings, and countries around the world can benefit by focusing palliative care initiatives on the communities they aim to serve (Figure 20.3).

20.8 Conclusion

The PCAU created a method to bridge the gap in access to palliative care services through the CCUI. By partnering with local, professional palliative and hospice care teams, PCAU trains community volunteers in public health-informed care practices. The local teams also partner with primary and secondary schools to create Palliative Care Clubs, aiming to equip the next generation of palliative care leaders with the skills they need to care for their fellow community members effectively. Overall, PCAU's CCUI creates a sustainable, intergenerational model of continued care by harnessing the compassion of individuals and reinforcing the culture of care within communities.

References

1. W. Churchill, *My African Journey,* Hodder and Stoughton, 1908.
2. The Africa Channel, "Why is Uganda called the pearl of Africa," *The Africa Channel*, 13 June 2020. [Online]. Available: https://www.theafricachannel.co.uk/why-is-uganda-the-pearl-of-africa/. [Accessed 11 October 2025].
3. Standard Safaris, "Which African country has the biggest number of gorillas?" [Online]. Available: https://www.standardgorillasafaris.com/blog/which-african-country-has-the-biggest-number-of-gorillas/. [Accessed 22 October 2025].
4. World Bank Group, "Pathways out of the polycrisis," World Bank Group, 2024.
5. A. Y. Chang, K. Cowling, J. L. Dieleman and A. E. Micah, "Past, present, and future of global health financing: A review of development assistance, government, out-of-pocket and other private spending on health for 195 countries, 1995–2050," *The Lancet,* vol. 393, pp. 2233–2260, 2019.
6. A. Addae-Korankye, "Causes of poverty in Africa: A review of literature," *American International Journal of Social Science,* vol. 3, no. 7, pp. 147–153, 2014.

7. A. Meghani, C. Ssemugabo, G. Pariyo, A. Hyder, E. Rutebemberwa and D. Gibson, "Curbing the rise of noncommunicable diseases in Uganda: Perspectives of policy actors," *Global Health Science Practice,* vol. 9, no. 1, pp. 149–159, 2021.
8. Ministry of Health, "A roadmap towards universal health coverage in Uganda 2020/21 to 2029/30," *Ministry of Health,* p. 6, 2020.
9. I. Ekore R and B. Lanre-Abass, "African cultural concept of death and the idea of advance care directives," *Indian Journal of Palliative Care,* vol. 22, no. 4, pp. 369–372, 2016.
10. I. A. Paul and M. Yakobo, "Socio-cultural perspectives of the Bakonzo of Uganda about death," *IOSR Journal of Humanities and Social Science,* vol. 24, no. 4, pp. 57–68, 2019.
11. NewVision, "Sending off loved ones, the Ugandan way," 14 January 2012. [Online]. Available: https://www.newvision.co.ug/news/1298949/sending-loved-ones-ugandan. [Accessed 22 October 2025].
12. J. A. Obika and P. W. Otim, "Returning to the world of ancestors': Death and dying among the Acholi of Northern Uganda, 1900s–1980s," *Journal of Eastern African Studies,* vol. 16, no. 3, pp. 375–394, 2022.
13. Monitor, "How burial associations have helped Ugandans during funerals," 2 April 2025. [Online]. Available: https://www.monitor.co.ug/uganda/news/national/how-burial-associations-have-helped-ugandans-during-funerals-4987338. [Accessed 22 October 2025].
14. J. Drageset, G. Haugan and M. Eriksson (Eds.), "Social support," in *Health Promotion in Health Care – Vital Theories and Research,* Springer, pp. 137–144, 2021.
15. P. A. Akpan-Idiok, I. O. Ehiemere, E. F. Asuquo, J. A. Chabo and E. C. Osuchukwu, "Assessment of burden and coping strategies among caregivers of cancer patients in sub-Saharan Africa," *World Journal of Clinical Oncology,* vol. 11, pp. 1045–1063, 2020.
16. E. Kisangala, M. Heslin and E. J. Webb, "My husband is my responsibility: Motivations and activities of informal caregiving for patients with chronic diseases in Uganda," *Discover Public Health,* vol. 22, p. 217, 2025.
17. R. G. Gambe, J. Clark, S. A. Meddick-Dyson, B. O. Ukoha-Kalu, G. N. Nyaaba and F. E. M. Murtagh, "The roles and experiences of informal carers providing care to people with advanced cancer in Africa-A systematic review and critical interpretive analysis," *PLOS Global Public Health,* vol. 3, 2023.
18. World Health Organisation, "Social determinants of health," [Online]. Available: https://www.who.int/health-topics/social-determinants-of-health#tab=tab_1. [Accessed 26 October 2025].
19. R. Campo, "'I wonder'— The role of poetry in palliative care," *JAMA,* vol. 329, p. 329, 2023.

21

A DEEP DIVE INTO COMMUNITY CONNECTORS

Julian Abel and Rachael Basak

Abstract

In this chapter, we will discuss the opportunity that connector programmes provide, starting with Luis Enrique's story of grief and loss, and then continue with the role of social capital and infrastructure known as treasure mapping. We will go on to write about the role of connectors from Frome in Somerset and the biological impact of compassion. The chapter concludes by examining an example from Princess Alice Hospice in Surrey, UK and how they introduced a connector programme into their hospice.

21.1 Introduction – Luis Enrique – a story

A European Champions League Final in Munich is not the obvious place to start a chapter on the role of connectors in a community, but an extraordinary event happened there on 31st May 2025. The Champions League is the culmination of European club football competition. The highest placed teams in the top leagues across Europe meet each other in a rather prolonged knockout competition that runs from September through to the next May. In 2025, the final was contested between the French team Paris St German (PSG) and the Italian Club Inter Milan. As it turned out, PSG won in an overwhelming fashion but that is not the main point of our story. At the end of the match, after PSG had won, their fans unfurled a large flag, covering the heads of about 100 fans, depicting the PSG manager Luis Enrique planting the team flag in the centre circle with his daughter Xana. The background to this story is that Luis Enrique had won the Champions League final with a previous team, Barcelona in 2015. At that time, Xana, aged 6, joined him in the centre circle wearing the Barcelona team football strip. Together, they planted the team flag in the centre circle.

DOI: 10.4324/9781003621348-22

Sadly, in 2019, Xana died from a rare bone cancer. Luis Enrique, for a while, gave up his job as a football manager. He often spoke openly and movingly about the gratitude he had for the short time he spent with Xana. In preparation for the 2025 Champions League Final, the PSG Ultra fans had made the large banner of their manager and his daughter planting the flag in the centre circle. The banner would have been displayed whether PSG had won or not. The Ultras are the most fervent fans, not known for their sensitivity and caring attitude, certainly not known for their grief literacy. Yet at that moment, in front of a television audience of 100 million people across the globe, they revealed an enormous act of compassion, appreciation and community over the unfortunate death of a child from cancer.

This story illustrates three very important principles in relation to community and connection. The first is the availability of social capital. This term refers to the availability of supportive relationships between individuals in a community setting. The greater the availability of social capital, the greater a sense of belonging exists in a community. The second point concerns social infrastructure. This describes the spaces in which social capital flourishes. The third is the glue, or the fuel that makes social capital and social infrastructure function, which is compassion. When these three meet, community forms.

Football stadiums and football fans are not the most obvious place for the development of social capital. Having lived through supporting a football team in London in the early 1970s, it was the opposite. Aggressive football fans called skinheads ruled the roost, creating intimidation, violence, racism and fear not just in the football stadiums but on the streets as well. Yet the PSG event turns this whole story on its head. The football stadium became a symbol of compassion, with the fans using both social capital and infrastructure to broadcast their message of sympathy and support for their manager, in a stadium of 75,000 fans. This was an enormous demonstration of grief literacy publicised across the world. Afterwards, Luis Enrique said, 'Xana is always in my heart' [1].

This chapter discusses how a deep dive into community can be achieved through the role of the connector, making use of social capital and social infrastructure to support people going through the experiences of death, dying, loss and caregiving. As this story illustrates, support can be found in everyday places, often surprising to the untrained eye, and understanding how to see and make use of this is the key to building compassionate communities.

21.2 Maps of misery or treasure maps?

Social capital and social infrastructure combine to create a community environment. These precious resources often remain hidden and unconnected. This is because when services, whether they are state, businesses or third sector, are supporting communities, they paint a map of misery. A map of misery is everything that is wrong with a community, including phrases such as social deprivation, hard-pressed communities, lack of infrastructure and others. This misery map creates a reason for a service going into that community to sort out the problems. Proof of effectiveness is then assessed by how many items on the map of misery are addressed. However, community priorities are very different from those of outside organisations. In addition, maps of misery ignore community strengths.

Treasure maps offer a very different starting point for both communities and services. This can be conceptualised as social capital being the treasures of the people in a community, and social infrastructure, the places in which those treasures flourish. John McKnight and Cormac Russell, leaders of Asset Based Community Development, talk about treasures of the individual being gifts, skills and passions [2]. Gifts are the things we are born with, the natural talents that seem to be a quirk of nature. These include athletic and sporting ability, singing, a natural affinity for playing a musical instrument, having a very forgiving social nature and many others. Skills are things we learn along the way and can be anything from music making, creativity, sporting achievement or academic skill. They also include the things we learn from our work, whether this is administration, a practical skill of building or anything that can be of use in a community. Passions are the things we feel very strongly about and are motivated to take action. These passions can be environmental activism, artistic expression, community activities, educating children and many, many others. McKnight and Russell estimate that every person has about 12 of these treasures. Sadly, people often do not realise they have these talents, and they can go unnoticed and unused.

Gifts, skills and passions are not much use from a community perspective when someone keeps them to themselves. However, sharing them in community magnifies them enormously. Cormac Russell recounts a story about a neighbour as an example.

> OK, so maybe you're a singer. Beautiful. We hear you every morning singing in the shower. You know, that's wonderful. You clearly have a gift. But, you know, we've got a choir. And I don't know if you've heard it recently, but it's awful. It needs you. We can't do without you. So that's a compelling call, by the way. I didn't say come be a volunteer. I don't really care whether you believe in God or not. It's your voice I'm after, you know.
>
> *[3]*

Mapping treasures of people in a community must be done from within. Community members can come together to create a map of who is able to do what in a neighbourhood, who to turn to in a moment of need. The Aboriginal Australian expression 'who's your mob?' captures it perfectly. When your car breaks down, or the washing machine empties itself all over the floor, who do you turn to for help? Knowing your neighbourhood, your neighbours and other community members is a way of developing the map. It also includes groups and activities in your area such as a choir.

Mapping out where community groups are held, and how they can be accessed, forms the basis of a treasure map. Community electronic resource directories are a good way of compiling this. Many already exist. If anyone wants to know about community activities, whether this is groups, sports, interests, hobbies or any other kind of community activity, they can look it up on the resource directory. The directory requires constant updating, and we will discuss this in the context of community connectors. Services and charities can go on the directory, but this is not the main point. If the directory is mainly about services, there is no space for community and the discovery of bringing to light what already is in a community and connecting it together is lost.

21.3 Connectors! A deep dive into community

Electronic resource directories of community activity are all very well, but on their own they are often poorly updated and consequently poorly used. Areas may have multiple directories which add to the confusion of which one to choose. Some are dominated by services and barely tell the story of what is going on in a community. So, directories alone are not much use.

The solution to this problem is to have people talk about the directories and their content. This is the role of the connector.

Connectors are people who know what is going on in their community and how to chat, often fuelled by tea and cake. Knowing about what is happening in community can be simply through chatting with people, participating in community activities or knowing how to access a user-friendly resource directory. Community connectors are activated citizens who understand the value of chatting. This role was developed by Jenny Hartnoll, lead of the community development service Health Connections Mendip in Frome, a town of 28,000 people in the county of Somerset, in the west of England. Jenny had created a resource directory so that when she saw people referred to her by the primary care team at the medical practice, she could direct people to community activities should they be interested. She realised quite quickly that having people talking about what goes on in a community, and how community members can support people in their community, would be a great way of linking resources with community by talking about it. In addition, people can find out and be connected to community without having to go through the medical practice or see social prescribers. What happened next was surprising.

Jenny designed a short training of between 1 hour and 90 minutes. She invited community members to this training, which consisted of letting them know what was going on in their community, how to access the resource directory and to encourage people to talk about it in appropriate moments in their daily life. This was not trying to solve people's problems, but rather if something came up in a conversation such as an interest in a particular hobby, or feeling isolated, or knowing where to access advice, then the community connector could say, 'I don't know the answer to your problem but I know where you might be able to find it.' Passing on the web address of the resource directory is an option or suggesting attending a talking café – another of Jenny's developments – just to meet people and chat to other connectors. The community connector is not a volunteer. People are not stepping forward to do something on behalf of an organisation. Rather, they are activated citizens who contribute to the overall social capital of a community.

And this is where the surprise happened. Bit by bit, over a period of four years, Jenny and her team trained over a thousand Frome residents. After a year of training connectors, Jenny sent out a survey to find out how many times a year people were having conversations about how the community can support community. Connectors reported back that they had, on average, 20 conversations a year. This meant that 20,000 conversations a year were taking place about community support in a town of 28,000 people [4].

It is difficult to think of another way of getting such a deep dive into community, connecting with such a large proportion of community members. Electronic communication will not do this because many people will not access it or are excluded from it for several reasons. Local news helps but not everyone reads local papers or watches local TV. The more people who are trained as community connectors, the more the conversations will take place, and the more community becomes connected.

The next issue to address is who can be a community connector, and the answer is almost anyone. It is helpful to consider people who are natural connectors as a starting point. The list is extensive. Hairdressers are a prime example. They chat all day with their clients, who naturally tell the hairdresser about what is happening in their lives. Problems often appear and having a knowledge of community resources means that signposting to help can be a natural part of the conversation. The list explodes from there, because taxi drivers, receptionists, bar staff, librarians, café staff, community police support officers and many, many others are included.

There is a special place for connectors when it comes to diversity. One of the big problems often associated with any organisation, including charities, is that they cater for a particular kind of clientele, even if the doors are open to everyone. It is impossible to design something that suits all the different kinds of people and cultures. This means people are excluded and this is often those who are already excluded in a variety of ways, mainly for reasons of diversity. The consequence is that services may not be of interest to diverse communities and may isolate even further those who have already been isolated. Treasure maps are very particular to each community. Different cultures, ethnic and others have different interests, meeting places and activities. The only way of understanding this and forming a treasure map that is useful for that particular community is when this is done by the community itself. One of the enormous strengths about community connectors is that they can be from any and every type of background. Particularly important from a service delivery perspective, who attends community connector training can be monitored.

If there is a group that is missing out and not represented, then whoever is running the training can build relationships with those people and groups and invite them to become connectors. What a resource directory will look like in one town or village will be different from others.

These principles of how to develop a deep reach into communities can be extended even further. For example, people who use or work in homeless shelters, drug and alcohol services or dementia carers can all be included, because particular groups or services are relevant to these people and may not be so for others. Simply keeping an eye on where connectors come from is a significant way of overcoming traditional service and organisational discrimination and provides some evidence that active participation is happening in a wide variety of backgrounds.

21.4 The biology of community – survival of the kindest

To people who have little contact with communities and not much faith in human nature, this may all sound like a pipe dream and could be a place where people can be exploited. However, there is a very different lens on the role of community connectors which comes from a new look at the biology of communities, and this throws a light on human potential.

Human beings got up on their hind legs about 2 million years ago. Our ancestors survived in small groups of between 25 and 200 people. We did not just survive during our precarious evolution, we flourished. This is especially the case for Homo sapiens, our current version of humanity, which spread all over the world in the most inhospitable of climates. The traditional biological version used to explain this success is survival of the fittest, in which the biggest, most violent, most powerful and most aggressive people took control and led everything. Our modern world is built on the premise that the people who are leaders deserve to be so because they are 'the best.' The term survival of the fittest was coined by the British philosopher Herbert Spencer, not Charles Darwin, who was the father of evolutionary theory. In fact, Darwin's last book was called The Expression of Emotion in Man and Animals, and he was really interested in our social nature.

Over the last 20–30 years, this view has been challenged. There has been increasing interest in the evolutionary benefit of sociality. Human beings are social by nature. We are not sloths, snow leopards or polar bears who live alone and shun company. We like to hang out in groups. We have done so because this helped us to survive. The essential drive that impels us in this direction is the need to have a strong sense of belonging, where people are valued for who they are, and they value others in the same way. The characteristics of kindness, care and compassion function as the glue that binds communities together. What has changed over the last 30 years from the perspective of academic studies is that the evidence for the mechanisms of how this happens has been uncovered. When looking for evidence of the biological impact of community, it is discovered everywhere. It is seen through hormonal, neurological and genomic pathways. It is also found in behaviour, emotions, cultural practices, rituals, love and friendship. And the roots of this are found throughout the animal kingdom, in 600 million years of evolution. Friendship between animals and humans, as well as between different species of animals, is evident and if you want to see what a really good hug looks like, have a look on YouTube for lions reunited with the people who nurtured them after being rescued as a cub [5].

This is not suggesting that you go and hug a lion, because the likelihood is that they will either see you as food or a threat, and the outcome will be the exact opposite of a hug! The point is that care, compassion and kindness are the root of sociality and this has helped us to survive. A much better description of our biology is survival of the kindest.

'Oh' you may say, 'survival of the fittest refers to life that most fits into an environment.' This is unhelpful for two reasons. First, when Herbert Spencer used the phrase survival of the fittest, he was not referring to fit into an environment but to the most powerful deserving their privilege. This was at the time of the British Empire and the domination of the large proportions of the world by the most powerful, the most heavily armed. The second reason is that using the phrase fittest does not capture the social nature of animals, especially humans, where care and compassion bind communities together.

An objection to using the phrase survival of the kindest is that, looking around the current world, the opposite is highly visible. We do not need to look far to see evidence of violence, exploitation, anger, lack of care and inequality. However, this is looking at maps of misery rather than treasure maps. Understanding the detail of how our social nature flourishes is critical to understanding how and why community connectors work and is so successful in transforming the environment of fear to one of belonging.

In the hunter-gather setting, surviving together in a community was vital. If an individual was separated from their tribe, then their life was at risk, both in the short term and the long term. Up until about 15,000 years ago, megafauna, large animals, roamed the Earth. They disappeared when we ate them all through hunting in groups. Prior to this point, and for some time afterwards as well, we were at risk from predation, whether this was sabre-tooth tigers, lions or other large flesh-eating beasts. In addition, if we fell and injured ourselves, the ability to get food alone was severely compromised and starvation in an already precarious situation was a big risk. Furthermore, without others we could not bring up children and find warmth and friendship. So, isolation increased our risk of dying.

In immediately dangerous situations such as a sabre-tooth tiger rampaging through a community group, then we needed a biological response to getting us out of danger as quickly as possible. People may be familiar with the fright, flight, fight and freeze reflexes. In these moments, our bodies prioritise individual safety and prime our reflexes for getting out of danger. Thinking about what to do in life-threatening situations is not a priority and might delay a crucial response to flee. Our brain has a coordinating centre called the amygdala which monitors activity from sense organs, eyes, ears, nose, touch etc. for danger. If this is detected, the pathways to the thinking part of our brain are dampened down and safety becomes the main activity. Access to this thinking part of the brain, particularly the prefrontal cortex, is shut down. The prefrontal cortex is critical to organising our higher human social functions. It regulates emotions, makes sense of memories, is responsible for both logical thinking and creativity and moderates social behaviour. These are not relevant in a moment of high danger. In other words, when there is a sense of threat, the ability to think is shut down [4].

The implications are profound for communities. For humans to access their incredible potential of kindness and compassion, there must be a sense of belonging. When this happens, the amygdala quietens down and access to the prefrontal cortex is free flowing. This opens a wide variety of friendliness pathways, from body language, tone of voice, care and concern and having a welcoming environment. People, through social connection, have a deep impact on biology. Community matters a lot, and good social relationships are more effective at reducing our risk of dying than giving up drinking excessively or smoking 15 cigarettes a day, more effective than dieting and exercise.

This is highly relevant to the role of the community connector. If you walk into a café in Frome, you are likely to be served by someone who is a community connector. When you walk through the door, they might look up and greet you with a friendly smile, or just a welcoming glance. Your level of threat in an unfamiliar environment goes down a few notches and when they come over and talk to you in a friendly way, it goes down even further. You feel at home, like you belong and this is where all our health biology kicks in. We seek these places of belonging, in our home, work and public spaces.

What this means is that every human being, without exception, has the potential for care and compassion. Connectors use this potential to help create environments of safety, so the ripple effect of waves of belonging happens across neighbourhoods. This is so effective that Frome is now known as a friendly town. People are moving there because of this, and it has created a housing problem. Connectors are purveyors of waves of belonging. It is not just their individual action that makes a difference, it is the sea of connection and belonging that happens in a wide variety of environments.

21.5 Talk Listen Connect training

Compassionate Communities UK designed a training that takes about 90 minutes. It covers much of the material in this chapter. It is divided into two parts. The first part is about talk listen connect (TLC) and the second is learning a bit about grief literacy. The sessions are interactive and cover what TLCs are, why they are important and how the whole programme makes use of the natural drive of survival of the kindest that impels humans to form communities, to create a village wherever we live. Learning about survival of the kindest is often met with a big sense of relief. People know in their hearts that relationships are important and saying that science agrees strikes an emotional chord. The session then introduces the concepts of treasure mapping and maps of misery, and participants uncover the treasures in their own community. This is gratifying as people discover treasures they did not even know were there, such as a favourite shop, a park where people gather of any kind of group in the community and even a football stadium! The first part finishes with an interactive session on listening skills.

We decided to add in about 20–30 minutes on grief literacy. This is because if you are a community connector, you are inevitably going to have conversations about the experiences of death, dying, loss and caregiving. One in a hundred people die each year and, on average, nine people are directly affected and involved in this. This means that 10% of the population go through the experiences involved with death, dying, loss and care giving every year, and yet two thirds of people are not confident in talking about it and worry that they will say the wrong thing. There are some simple rules which are easy to follow which make it easier. Statements that are sympathetic and do not minimise or fix grief work well, such as 'I am sorry for your loss' or 'I don't know what to say to comfort you, but I am here for you.' Statements that fix or minimise can be upsetting, such as 'you should be over it by now' or 'they are in a better place.'

Community connectors are active citizens who live in and learn about their community. How they do this, and what they talk about, is individual to them and being an activated citizen means that people go about their daily lives with a good heart, helping when they can, not interfering, not fixing and not counselling. It is about being a good neighbour and community member. Everyone will do this in their own way, and this is the beauty of it. It is not for services to tell people how to behave to transform communities, it is for people to work out how to do this themselves, in ways that suit each community.

Compassionate Communities UK also has a train the trainer programme so that if areas would like to role TLC training out to large numbers of people, they can train trainers who can then run regular TLC sessions.

21.1 TLC CASE STUDY – WITH PRINCESS ALICE HOSPICE, SURREY

In 2024, Compassionate Communities UK (CCUK) launched TLC to grow a national network inspired by the compassionate community work in Frome, Somerset.

Princess Alice Hospice was the first organisation to partner with CCUK and pilot a 'train the trainer' model. Their team has embraced TLC to empower local people to support one another through life's challenges, while also raising awareness of hospice care in the community.

For over 40 years, Princess Alice Hospice has provided free, outstanding and compassionate care for people living with life-limiting illness, and those close to them. Their care area straddles Southwest London (the London Boroughs of Kingston and Richmond) and part of Surrey a large county in the UK. As the world changes, they stay focused on that commitment acknowledging that with care and support that is right, more people can live well, die well and grieve well.

The Talk Listen Connect focus on grief, connection and reducing loneliness aligns strongly with their work as well as the emphasis on empowering citizens to support each other. This is just the beginning, and we're excited to see the programme grow.

So far:

1 235 people have taken part in a TLC session delivered by Princess Alice Hospice (as of 27th February 2026)
2 6 of them have gone on to become TLC trainers

The 90–120 minute session helps people feel more confident listening and being there for others in their neighbourhoods, connecting them with community offers.

Sessions have been delivered to:

1 People with learning disability and neurodiversity
2 People living and working in hostels and care homes
3 Homecare and leisure centre staff
4 Local voluntary and health sector teams
5 Hospice staff, volunteers and members of the public

From 51 feedback responses:

Overall, 76% felt more confident connecting with others afterwards.

Many said they felt inspired to use what they learned in everyday life with an average rating of 8.8 out of 10 and a median of 9, indicating that most participants felt strongly motivated to apply the learning in their daily lives.

Here's what some participants shared:

> It reminded me how much we all share as humans – and how powerful it is to connect with intention.
>
> A great initiative in these busy, more selfish times.
>
> The session felt safe and meaningful – thank you.
>
> The session reminded me "of the impact that little everyday kindnesses can have on someone and that TLC can be practiced every day and everywhere"

21.6 Summary

Connection and belonging have a dramatic impact on health and well-being. This is true in general and at end-of-life as well, not just for the person with the illness but those who surround them. Belonging is not something manufactured by services. It must come from the community itself and making use of our most ancient, most primal asset is how communities are transformed. Central to achieving this is to move from a place of fear to one of belonging. Activating citizens to fulfil this human potential is our greatest hope for humanity and we should all strive to accomplish this aim, for we are all in this together.

References

1. Sky Sports, "PSG win Champions League: Luis Enrique 'emotional' after supporters unveil banner in tribute to late daughter," *Sky Sports*, 2 June 2025. [Online]. Available: https://www.skysports.com/football/news/11095/13377557/psg-win-champions-league-luis-enrique-emotional-after-supporters-unveil-banner-in-tribute-to-late-daughter. [Accessed 3 October 2025].
2. Nurture Development, "Touchstone Eight: Celebrate every step of the way," 9 March 2018. [Online]. Available: https://www.nurturedevelopment.org/blog/abcd-practice/touchstone-eight-celebrate-every-step-of-the-way/. [Accessed 23 October 2025].
3. Compassionate Communities UK, "Survival of the Kindest: Cormac Russell – De-centering the Professional, Re-centering the Citizen," 2021. https://www.nurturedevelopment.org/uncategorized/survival-of-the-kindest-podcast-decentering-the-professional-with-cormac-russell/.
4. A. M. Kredlow, R. J. Fenster, E. S. Laurent, K. J. Ressler and E. A. Phelps, "Pre frontal corex, amygdala and threat processing: Implications for PTSD," *Neuropsychopharmacology,* vol. 47, no. 1, pp. 247–259, 2022.
5. H. C. Mendip, "Annual Report," 2016.

22

REORIENTATION OF HEALTHCARE VIA COMMUNITY-FOCUSED SERVICE REDESIGN

Emma Hodges and Katie Burbridge

Abstract

The purpose of this chapter is to offer a practical, low-cost and participatory tool to support the reorientation of health services, one of the six statements from the Ottawa Charter for Health Promotion.

There are many different approaches and models to health service design. Services can be designed by a specific organisation for their team to deliver and may or may not involve 'patients.' Some focus on a care pathway design across partner organisations, again this may or may not have involved the people the services are designed for. In the UK context, healthcare service design often starts with data to be improved, costs to reduce or a workforce capacity challenge to manage.

Bate and Robert state, "there is also the issue of the gap between the rhetoric or ideology and the practice. In most countries, despite the longevity of the 'patient involvement' concept, healthcare systems are still not putting patients first. A recent report [The State of Healthcare 2005, Healthcare Commission] suggests that the health service in England could often seem to be designed around the needs of healthcare staff rather than patients".

The model advocated by this chapter is inspired by Cormac Russell, Director of Nurture Development, and starts by finding out what resources and skills the community already has. It follows an asset-based community development methodology. Building trust and working together to decide what services can add to a community, is a different approach and one that should become increasingly relevant if the new NHS plan for neighbourhood health is an authentic approach to truly understand the power of communities.

DOI: 10.4324/9781003621348-23

22.1 Introduction

Healthcare professionals are often engaged in leading compassionate communities and city programmes rather than residents or community leaders [1]. This is not surprising given the medicalisation of death, dying, loss and caregiving; however, it creates a risk that activities are not truly following the principles of health promotion. Dumont et al. (2022) found from a literature search that most of the activities associated with compassionate communities relate to education and awareness e.g. professionals skilling up lay people [1] rather than a mutual learning exchange and reorientation of healthcare to society.

Russell (2020) describes the difference between a democratic and a technocratic way of government organisations behaving. In a democracy, statutory service providers and charities are an extension of civic life; however, when these providers start to replace civic life with more services – doing things for residents – then this technocratic approach "relegates citizens to second place; it turns them into clients and consumers" this positions health and care professionals as 'experts.' This creates issues of power, some communities become marginalised, citizens retreat, funding goes on the costs of institutions and we start to use language such as 'deprived communities' creating division rather than a truly collaborative approach [2].

Service providers, even those that start off as social and community organisations, become increasingly institutionalised with organisational and professional identities, ways of working and a way of being that becomes 'stuck' and harder to change [3].

Challenging traditional, technocratic models of service design requires new ways of thinking and working. It should not be assumed, certainly in the UK context, that all health and care professionals have the confidence to move from a consulting room or conversations with a 'patient' and their family to sitting with resident groups in community venues and exploring the barriers and challenges they are experiencing with the very area of care the professionals are trying their best to deliver.

Of course, there are many health and care professionals who do have the skills and emotional intelligence needed for community development and are doing wonderful work in the field of palliative and end-of-life care. Like anything, community development is a skill that can be taught, although some people are more naturally gifted at it than others, and that is ok. It is more important that it happens than who does it. Whilst there is benefit to health and care professionals spending time with communities, in a world with significant skill shortages in the sector, there is a balance to be considered. We still need doctors to be doctors and nurses to nurse.

There are many organisational and professional barriers to using community development tools in practice, but these can be overcome with appropriate support, organisational flexibility and commitment.

Models of healthcare service redesign often include process mapping, reviewing existing services or imagining new ones. This method does not enable a stepping back from the focus on a service mindset to enable a community mindset to evolve. In a service mindset, the following phrases dominate:

1 We are too busy
2 There are not enough staff
3 There is not enough money
4 We cannot do any more
5 We have no capacity
6 We are worried about our waiting list size
7 We need to see these 'patients'
8 What about the risk
9 We have specialist skills

When focusing on a community mindset, there is a shift in language and approach:

1 What is already happening out there?
2 Is there anyone or a group with the skills to do this already?
3 Is there anyone or a group who could do this with a little more training?
4 Have communities been involved with or designed changes themselves?
5 Do we have to do this – is it wanted/needed?
6 Does this matter to the community/communities?
7 How do people want to get involved?
8 How can we help the existing skills and 'grass roots' infrastructure?

Examples of how this relates in practice are:

Bereavement – a service mindset will be concerned about increasing demand, and seek funding for more services, trying to combat waiting lists. A community mindset will find out about all the existing clubs and groups that are already in the neighbourhood the walking groups, men-sheds, knit and natters etc. and chat with them to find out about how they support people who are grieving. A community mindset will explore whether providing some training to all those existing community groups would help them feel more able to support people who are grieving, if they do not already. A community mindset then might look for where there are gaps and find people interested in partnering to set up relevant groups. All these activities focus on capacity building rather than service provision.

Day Centres – A service mindset might go and collect people from their houses to take them several miles away to a 'day centre' or 'day hospice' – creating temporary social connections with other people who are also collected and taken several miles away from their home. A community mindset might focus on where there are already groups that meet, find out if the groups are accessible to people with a serious illness, consider how to support these groups to enable people to stay with the social connections they already have or build these locally when they are absent. Any clinical component of a day centre approach can be supported differently, rather than compromise social connectedness.

22.2 The model

The model of community-focused service redesign described in this chapter, designed by Dr Emma Hodges, emerged from various practice experiences over several years, including integrated neighbourhood team development, increasing inclusivity in social care and how to reimagine services to fit with the new essentials of palliative care model [4]. Cormac Russell describes a 'three-lane' approach:

1 Where institutions should consider first what communities can do for themselves,
2 Second, what communities can do with a little help and
3 Third, what communities need from outside organisations.

Russell states that "following this sequence is critical but is a rarity in the practice of institutional professionals" [5]. In practice, taking a community development approach to service redesign, it felt necessary to break these three lanes into four stages as per Figure 22.1.

The first and fourth stages align with Russell's three lanes; however, this model splits the second lane into two distinct steps. There is a difference between providing a little bit of support or training to an existing community resource and working in partnership. Splitting out the second lane has created more discussion and creativity in practice than the three-lane model.

In the model 'community-focused service redesign,' there is a central ethos of belonging. This ethos includes asking who is missing – if the service redesign is engaging with a particular community, do they feel like they belong or have they

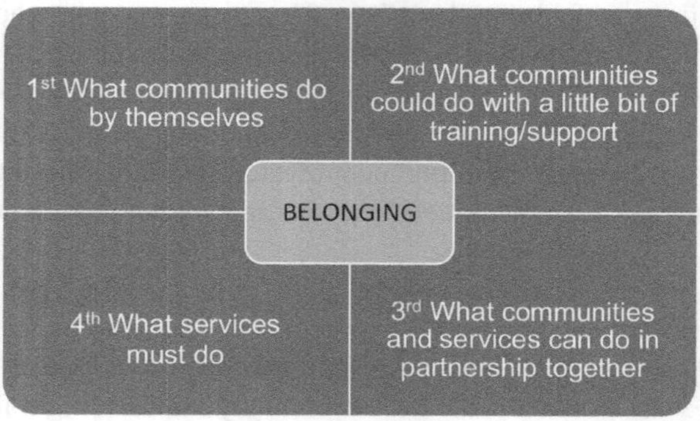

FIGURE 22.1 Community-Focused Service Redesign Model Developed by Dr E Hodges (2023)

been included because it suits the healthcare system for them to do so? Are there members of the community missing in the discussions and engagement? It is critical to ensure that in taking a community development approach, it isn't assumed that 'one size will fit all' and that a solution co-designed with a dominant group may well lack some of the nuances needed for other members of the community.

The aim of this model is to enable members of the community and practitioners to explore together what is needed to reduce health inequities. The inclusion of the word belonging reminds us that one model or approach is unlikely to meet suit the varying strengths and challenges within diverse communities. It is important to consider language and definitions when using the model to ensure that there is a shared understanding before starting any workshops or to modify the language to a local context.

The community-focused service redesign model has been tested in several settings with two case studies presented below:

22.3 Case study one

22.1 COMPASSIONATE COMMUNITIES AND ACORNS CHILDREN'S HOSPICE

Acorns Children's Hospice covers a large part of the West Midlands, approximately 19.8% of the population is aged 18 and under, which equates to approximately 1,193,000 individuals.

The national prevalence of life-limiting conditions (LLCs) in children (aged 0–19 years) in England had increased over 17 years from 26.7 per 10,000 in 2001/2002 to 66.4 per 10,000 in 2017/2018. Excluding some diagnoses which may not be considered LLC reduced this prevalence only slightly to 63.2 per 10,000 in 2017/2018 [6]

Across the West Midlands, working with partners, the purpose of Acorns Children's Hospice is to positively impact children with short lives, and Acorns Vision is to provide outstanding specialist care to every child and their family who need them now and in the future.

Palliative care for children represents a small and highly specialised field of healthcare that is different from, albeit closely related to, adult palliative care. Ideally, support for children with palliative care needs starts at diagnosis, and for many children with LLCs, this can be at birth.

The WHO defines children's palliative care as "the active total care of the child's body, mind and spirit, and also involves giving support to the family. It begins when illness is diagnosed and continues regardless of whether a child receives treatment directed at the disease" [7]. Health providers must evaluate and alleviate a child's physical, psychological and social distress. Effective palliative care requires a broad multi-disciplinary approach that includes the family and makes use of available community resources; it can be successfully implemented even if resources are limited. It can be provided in tertiary care facilities, in community health centres and even in children's homes [7].

The constant financial challenge for children's hospices means that fulfilling this vision is difficult. Adopting a public health palliative and end-of-life care approach is a potential solution; however, most work in this field has been for adults rather than children and young people with life-limiting and life-threatening conditions.

Integrating children's palliative care into the public health domain represents a transformative shift in how care is conceptualised and delivered. This approach places the child, their experience of childhood and their caregivers at the centre, not only within healthcare systems but also within communities and society at large. Whilst access to medical services is essential, so too is the right to a meaningful childhood, one that affirms children's human rights and recognises their identity as children, regardless of whether their life course is brief, prolonged or continues into adulthood.

This model is not merely an adjustment to existing systems; it is a radical reimagining. It calls for a fundamental change in how Acorns designs, delivers and evaluates care, aiming to improve the lives of children with palliative care needs and their families across the West Midlands.

As a starting point, given there were very few examples to learn from, Acorns partnered with Compassionate Communities UK (CCUK) and agreed on three key areas of action:

1 Think Tanks
2 Webinars
3 Service redesign workshops

CCUK established a series of Think Tanks to link together other areas and organisations interested in public health palliative and end-of-life care for children and young people. These sessions included a general discussion about the issues faced by children, young people and their families, a presentation by the team at Hummingbird House in Queensland and a presentation by the Childhood Dementia Initiative, also based in Australia, staff from across the three Acorns Hospices had the opportunity to attend and participate in discussions.

The key themes that came out of the Think Tanks were:

1 Acorns provides support for parents and the family whose child has died. Albeit there is low confidence in the wider community in knowing how best to support someone who is grieving the death of a child.

2 Parents often feel isolated and experience negative and intolerance due to the physical and behavioural aspects of many LLCs.
3 The public does not understand the range of conditions and associated symptoms that children, young people and their families experience and that titles such as Childhood Dementia may help improve understanding.
4 Policies and systems designed to support children, young people and families are sometimes lacking in detail and understanding of children's conditions, leading to inequalities.

In addition to the Think Tanks, the Children, Young Persons and Family Team at Acorns attended a series of webinars to help increase knowledge of what a public health palliative and end-of-life care approach is, how it links to compassionate communities and what it might mean for practice.

The webinars were well attended and were sometimes challenging in trying to show the difference between a holistic approach for an individual family that includes community facilities such as schools and identifying an approach to capacity building in a community for all families.

The third element of this preliminary work included a series of redesign workshops, using the community-focused service redesign tool, focusing on six different elements of Acorns' care, such as transition, bereavement and sibling support.

The workshops were held with Children, Young Persons and Family services team members to show the use of the tool and build confidence to then use the tool with external stakeholders and families.

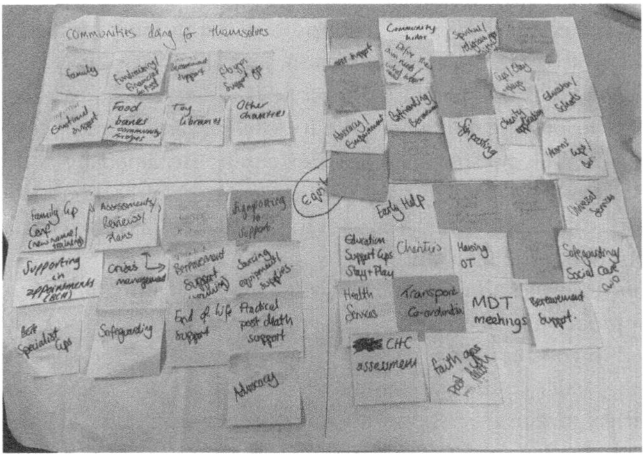

FIGURE 22.2 Flipchart with Post it Notes Using the Community-Focused Service Redesign Model

The workshops used flip chart paper and post it notes to consider the strengths that children, young people, their families and communities already have, what they provide for each other without any professional input. By using the tool and looking at each section in order, a range of opportunities, improvements and actions emerged.

The insight helped further focus Acorn's strategy for the development of a compassionate community approach.

As a result of the three areas of work, several actions have been agreed upon. There has been a restructure of the Children, Young Persons and Family team with the introduction of a community engagement and participation post for each of the three hospices and its surrounding areas. Several projects have been identified, including co-design of resources with young people and families to support transition from childhood to adulthood from a community and social perspective, co-design with parents, resources for employers to help build confidence in how to support employees who are living with or grieving a child with a life-limiting and life-threatening illness, a project to build knowledge and capacity in the community to reduce the judgement and isolation felt by families.

Acorns has joined the Compassionate Birmingham network given that this is one of the areas covered by the hospice and is engaging in several projects as part of the city's commitment to public health palliative and end-of-life care. This work is reflected through Acorns Children's Hospice Strategy 2025–2028 and the children's palliative care and public health position statement 2025 [8].

Children's palliative care, when viewed through a public health framework, offers a transformative approach to care and service delivery. It places the child and their carers at the heart of a supportive community and acknowledges their place within the broader population. This aligns with the NHS England's guidance on children's neighbourhood MDT's, a team of professionals who collaborate to provide integrated care for children and young people in their local area [9]. This perspective promotes equity, sustainability and collective responsibility. The following principles underpin neighbourhood MDT's and the public health approach, outlined in the Children's palliative care and public health position statement [8].

In conclusion, children's palliative care providers must embrace a public health approach and adopt innovative ways of working. Care provision should be rooted in co-production, ensuring that the voices of the child, their family and the wider community are heard and valued. By understanding what truly matters to those we support, we can deliver care that is compassionate, responsive and meaningful. This participatory model is essential for the successful and sustainable implementation of children's palliative care.

The community-focused service redesign tool has provided Acorns with a simple model that can be utilised with any community and services to ensure that Acorns is building on the strengths already existing in the areas served.

Acorns Children's Hospice, remain committed to supporting the development of this approach.

22.4 Case study two

22.2 ADULT SOCIAL CARE TEAM

The model was tested with a local authority's adult social care team. The local authority covers a truly diverse geography, and the team wanted to improve their equity of access for people needing care and support.

In considering how to best support the local authority, it made sense to focus the use of the model on specific communities to understand their common experiences. The team chose the Somali community and as for the children's hospice case study, the aim was to both demonstrate the tool and give the team confidence to use it going forward.

The session was conducted online with a range of organisations and some members of the Somali community. Each of the quadrants was completed by sharing a Microsoft PowerPoint presentation online and typing into the slide live.

Feedback on the session was positive, the support within the Somali community was very clear, as were the possible areas where statutory and voluntary sector organisations could provide more support and training to enable the community to develop more knowledge and understanding around how the health and care system works.

Figures 22.3–22.6 show the discussion on each of the elements of the model at the online workshop.

Discussion 1 - What is the community doing

- Connected by language. Understand the needs of the community due to cultural understanding.
- Knowledge of different generations, history of being connected to the first wave of refugees.
- Understand changes in the education / economics of transitioning from Somalia to the UK
- Understand the local issues such as welfare, housing, supporting people through education, domestic violence
- The mosque as a central focus, seeing people regularly, spotting who isn't attending, marriages, naming ceremonies and funerals being opportunities for people to gather.
- Share information on a Friday when someone doesn't attend and when it is spotted that someone is sick so that hospital visiting is arranged
- Food is brought to create togetherness for example for new mums
- Yoga and other community activities.
- Parties, Eid and Ramadan
- Everyone knows each other
- Family orientated, form small communities that look out for each other
- By the time they seek support they have already utilised what is around them.

FIGURE 22.3 Quadrant 1 Discussion

Discussion 2 - What could the community do with a little bit of help/training

- Raise confidence, trust and connections within communities about what different services can offer
- Advisors in the community support each other on a wide range of issues to help understand and navigate the support needed, supporting these community advisors would help
- Support 'word of mouth' networks in the community by raising awareness on key health and care issues such as cancer screening, menopause awareness, mental health and domestic violence e.g. support the informal support networks
- Raising awareness within the community support building confidence to seek help
- Raise awareness about what support is available and how to access it e.g. support for neurodiversity
- Connecting – enhancing the bridge between community, charity and statutory provision
- More awareness of the issues and support around carers to avoid crisis
- Improve confidence to access culturally appropriate support
- Improve accessibility of information
- Multi-cultural understanding for young people who are querying identity and traditions
- Better support for new arrivals trying to navigate establishing themselves in the UK and in the community
- Have informal health champions from within the community on a range of issues demonstrating the benefit for the community not just for service providers

FIGURE 22.4 Quadrant 2 Discussion

Discussion 3 - What could we do in partnership with the community

- For community coordinators (both informal and formal) to be able to create the connections with the local authority to avoid crisis
- Spend more time together to proactively resolve barriers and challenges collaboratively
- Taking time to assess strength, weakness, opportunities and threats together
- Health and care staff spending more time with the community to create connections, build trust and reduce barriers out in the communities
- Explore with communities how to break down some of the barriers and understandings re available services
- Build the trust together than enables communities to be honest about how they feel about services provided
- Ensuring capacity building is done together
- Engage closely on any digital developments
- Ensure services don't take over in order to enable communities to keep the connections

FIGURE 22.5 Quadrant 3 Discussion

Discussion 4 - what must we as service providers do

- Provision of social work statutory services and care assessments
- Delivery of the care act provisions
- Crisis management
- Create more joint working and shared support
- Create a clearer breakdown of who is who to improve communication
- Clear contact directory for key issues
- Commission care packages
- Provide training on adult social care provision and statutory requirements
- Create clarity on who is who, what to expect from adult social care, what some of the pitfalls are and how to avoid them in accessible ways designed with the community e.g. spending direct payments
- Carer assessments
- Case management
- Targeted recruitment to bridge the gap between the community and council
- Ensure directory of services is up to date, meaningful and accessible
- Provide training on safeguarding to community groups

FIGURE 22.6 Quadrant 4 Discussion

> The richness of support within the Somali community and the engagement in the workshops showed the richness of culture and natural compassion, skills and resources that are often overlooked by statutory providers. In the exercise with adult social care, by the time the discussion moved to services, many of the things 'services must do' related to capacity building and sharing of skills with the community, as well as the recognition of the importance of building trust. The transition from a service delivery mindset to a health promotion approach happened during the workshop.

22.5 Conclusion

Public Health Palliative Care is interested in service design as a key area of practice for change. This requires different models of service redesign that are more participatory and encourage building on community strengths rather than more traditional models of the deficit approach of health service design.

The community-focused service redesign model is a practical tool that supports engagement and discussions to reorientate healthcare services and work alongside community members and other stakeholders.

The tool can be used online or face to face and can generate a series of actions and improvements that are co-designed and can be co-delivered. There are distinct advantages to using the tool face to face as part of a public participation approach, as this can deepen understanding and create connections that cannot be achieved online.

Testing the usefulness of the tool is low cost and offers the opportunity for a different conversation with community members and stakeholders. Using the tool with an internal audience can help practitioners understand the shift in the model towards community strengths ahead of using it with different external groups. The tool is adaptable across different cultural settings. Whilst the questions are the same, the answers are derived from individual communities and are community specific. Flexibility of design is critical to being able to develop services using a ground-up participatory methodology.

There are limitations in the use of the tool based on the confidence of institutional professionals, capacity, organisational culture and operating practices. However, these can be overcome, and the simplicity of the community-focused service redesign tool enables anyone to facilitate discussions and workshops using it.

One of the strengths of the tool being used with a range of stakeholders is that the shift from service to community mindset can happen organically within the discussion and workshop.

References

1. K. Dumont, I. Marcoux, E. Warren, F. Alem, B. Alvar, G. Ballu, A. Bostock, S. R. Cohen, S. Daneault, V. Dube, J. Houle, A. Minyaoui, G. Rouly, D. Weil, A. Kellehear and A. Boivin, "How compassionate communities are implemented and evaluated in practice: A scoping review," *BMC Palliative Care*, vol. 21, 2022.
2. C. Russell, *Rekindling Democracy*, Wipf & Stock Publishers, 2020.
3. R. Greenwood, C. Oliver, T. Lawrence and R. Meyer, *The Sage Handbook of Organisational Institutionalism*, Sage Publications, 2017.
4. J. Abel, A. Kellehear and A. Karapliagou, "Palliative Care – the new essentials," *Ann Palliat Med*, vol. 7, 2018.
5. C. Russell, "From what's wront to what's strong: A guide to community-driven development," [Online]. Available: https://researchoutreach.org/articles/whats-wrong-whats-strong-guide-community-driven-development/. [Accessed 27 October 2025].
6. L. K. Fraser, D. Gibson-Smith, S. Jarvis, P. Norman and R. Parslow, *Make Every Child Count – Estimating Current and Future Prevalance of Children and Young People with Life Limiting-Conditions in the United Kingdom*, Martin House Research Centre, 2020.
7. World Health Organisation, *Palliative Care for Children*, WHO, 2023.
8. J. Downing, D. Randall, K. Mcnamara-Goodger, P. Ellis, G. Palat, Z. Ali, J. Hunt, R. Kiman, M. Friedel and S. Neilson, "Children's palliative care and public health: Position statement," *BMC Palliat Care*, vol. 24, pp. 24–89, 2025.
9. NHS England, *Guidance on Neighbourhood Multidisciplinary Teams for Children and Young People*, NHS England, 2025.

23

DEATH LITERACY AS COMMUNITY PRACTICE

Learning through Skills, Experience, Action, and Knowledge

Kerrie Noonan and Niki Read

Abstract

This chapter outlines a community-based approach to building death literacy grounded in research and practice and designed to support public health, palliative care, and compassionate communities' initiatives. It draws on the Death Literacy Index (DLI) as well as practical resources and methods for delivering community education. The DLI has been used to identify existing strengths, highlight gaps in knowledge and skills, and evaluate the impact of programs over time. This chapter introduces the SEAK model (Skills, Experience, Action, Knowledge) as an accessible and engaging way to bring death literacy concepts to life in community settings. Drawing on practice-based experience, this chapter provides a guide to engaging people in death literacy conversations, learn from their community and taking action. The DLI can be used both as an evaluation tool and as a way to strengthen community capacity by re-socialising conversations about death, dying, and grief.

23.1 Introduction

Death literacy refers to the knowledge and skills that people and communities' access to understand and make informed decisions about end-of-life and death care [1]. The concept was developed from a body of interdisciplinary, mixed methods research on the role of care networks at the end-of-life [2]. This research employed creative methods, such as photovoice and social network analysis, which illuminated aspects of the care experience that are often hidden or unacknowledged [3,4]. Themes such as the functions, barriers, and capacities of care networks, lack of access to information and difficulties navigating services were identified, along with everyday learning, knowledge, and skills about end-of-life caring, all of

DOI: 10.4324/9781003621348-24

which was ultimately labelled "death Literacy" and led to the development of the Death Literacy Index (DLI) [5,6]. The DLI has provided another layer of insight by providing a validated tool to measure change and understand community capacity in relation to death, dying, and bereavement. As a public health tool, it supports benchmarking across settings and populations, helping to identify strengths and gaps of knowledge and skills in populations. The DLI can also be used as a tool that measures change, and the effectiveness of education and engagement efforts over time, for example, in compassionate communities' projects [54].

In addition to their research efforts, the authors of this chapter have been actively involved in developing community-based education, training, and community development programs related to death, dying loss, and grief. This chapter draws on this practical experience, and it aims to provide both a written and visual guidance on using the death literacy concept and the DLI in community settings. Illustrations are intentional and are included for enhanced comprehension, diverse engagement, and conceptual clarity, which aids modelling of behaviours that can help build confidence and be a powerful catalyst for action [7,8]. You will notice the illustrations are evocative and demonstrate how practices can look and feel in a community setting.

23.2 The SEAK model

In our project development, we have utilised the concept of death literacy as a practical way to frame community education, develop resources, and provide a framework for evaluation. To introduce death literacy into communities in an accessible way, we developed the SEAK Model of Death Literacy – Skills, Experience, Action, and Knowledge (SEAK) (see Box 23.1).

The content and learning styles of the workshop are heavily influenced by the research evidence and the DLI; however, using SEAK provides a more accessible way to introduce the topic of death literacy. Using everyday language, the SEAK model focuses on how people can "talk, care, learn, and act" as a response to understanding their own death literacy experiences for increased engagement. The following section provides two examples of the SEAK model in action in education programs and evaluation:

1 Community education and workshops
   - Film viewing, engaging with *death literacy* and *end-of-life planning* card decks, and discussions
   - Modular workshop delivery formats
   - Settings and case studies
2 Workshop evaluation
   - Using the DLI for Benchmarking and pre/post/follow-up evaluation
   - Strength's analysis and/intervention design

BOX 23.1 DESCRIPTION OF THE SEAK MODEL OF DEATH LITERACY

SEAK model of death literacy

Skills (practical knowledge)

Feeling equipped to have conversations and do "hands-on" support.

Experience (experiential knowledge)

Wisdom is gained from life experiences with loss and grief. Ability to use that wisdom to understand my own experiences and draw upon them.

Actions (and attitudes) (community knowledge)

Connecting with supporters who can support you through caregiving, dying and grieving.

Knowledge (factual knowledge)

Knowledge about the death system and how it impacts people grieving, dying, and caregiving and death practices. Working through the facts about your options and the choices available in your region.

23.3 Community education and workshops

A descriptive outline of multi-modal workshop methodology (suggested option 1- complete modular package)

When a group of people come together for death literacy workshops in a community setting (named to suit your own intervention), they are often uncertain of what to expect, and curious. Once conversations get started, the group often become animated and lively, opening up to the topic and each other and held by the material and the tools, as illustrated in Figure 23.1.

Explaining what death literacy is and how it came to be is important for setting up expectations and trust, as is outlining the SEAK model for greater context (Box 23.1). After talking about why death literacy is important, as outlined in Box 23.2, the workshop moves into engaging with the deck of Death Literacy cards every participant has been provided with. Each person, using the card sorting template (Figure 23.2), is invited to sort their own deck of Death Literacy cards into *yes*, *no* or *not important* piles, and then to select the top two *yes* and *no* cards. This is a spontaneous and informal exercise for the purpose of entering the conversations. The exercise brings an immediacy to the workshop, participants start to have a sense of their strengths in the area of death literacy, and an understanding of what is important to them to think about or take action with next. The steps for sorting the Death Literacy cards are listed in Table 23.1.

BOX 23.2 WHY DEATH LITERACY IS IMPORTANT

Death literacy is important because:

- Talking about death and dying brings us to our shared humanity
- It helps us navigate future encounters
- It helps us remember what is important to us
- It helps us plan for the best quality of life and reduce stress
- It can positively impact grief and loss

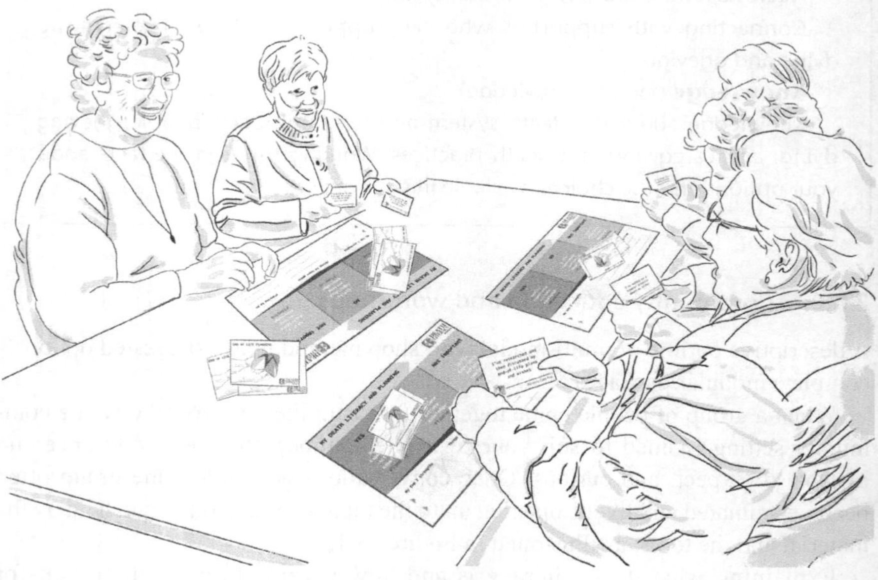

FIGURE 23.1 Community Members Engaging with *Death Literacy* and *End-of-Life Planning* Card Decks. Illustration by Niki Read

The short explainer video (Figure 23.5) is then viewed to support integration of the content with their discoveries. Participants are then invited to select their top two *yes's* and *no's* and discuss them first in pairs, and then as a group, as seen in Figure 23.3. We ask them to consider questions like "where did you get this skill or strength from, how did you develop this, and why is this important to you"? This illuminates the "what we know, and what we now know we don't know," which helps us to take consider actions for planning for the end-of-life we, or someone in our lives, might want.

We then take these discussions further and invite people to stand up in the room with their top two yes cards. Each card has a SEAK identifier on it, and participants are asked to sort themselves into four corners of the room (Figure 23.4), with SEAK each in a separate corner. We get to see and experience a general sense of

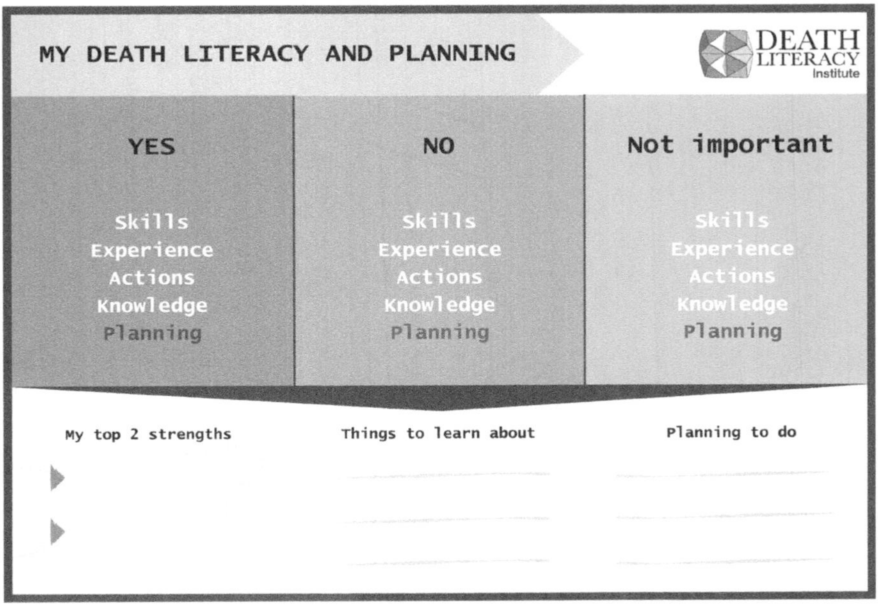

FIGURE 23.2 Sorting and Discussing Death Literacy Cards. Illustration by Niki Read

TABLE 23.1 Instructions for using the Death Literacy Cards

The Death Literacy cards are organised into four categories:

- Skills
- Experience
- Actions
- Knowledge

Using the cards during workshops:

- Each participant receives one deck of Death Literacy cards.
- Participants are invited to go through the cards one by one and place each card in either the *yes, no, not important* section of the card sorter template; where; – *yes* = I have this skill, experience etc. or have done this action, – *no* = I have not "got" this skill, experience etc. or done this action, and – *not important* means not important at this stage or not important to me.
- Don't overthink this, and feel free to discuss with your table as you go.
- Then sort your top 2 *yes* cards and top two no cards.
- Write down your top 2 *yes* cards in the "my top 2 strengths" section.
- Write down your top 2 *no* cards in the "things to learn about" section

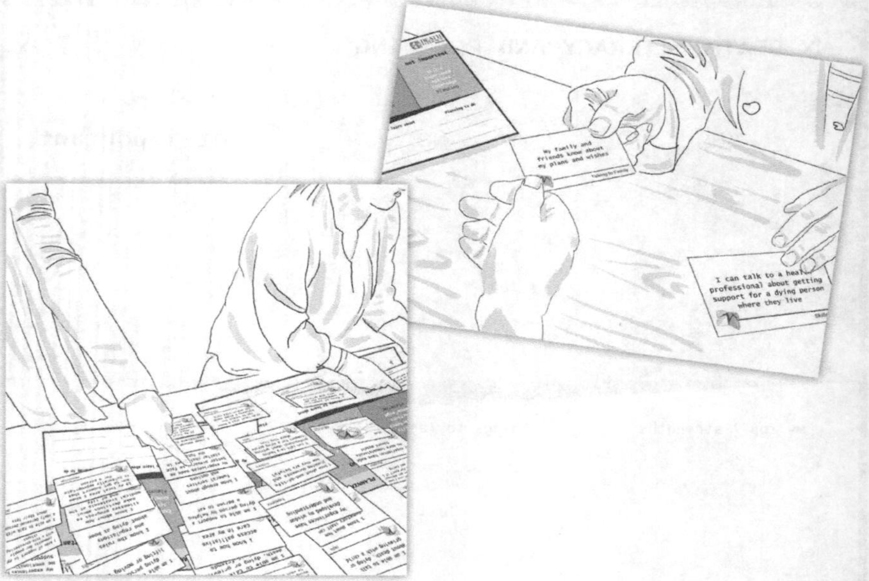

FIGURE 23.3 Death Literacy and End-of-Life Planning Cards Sorting Template

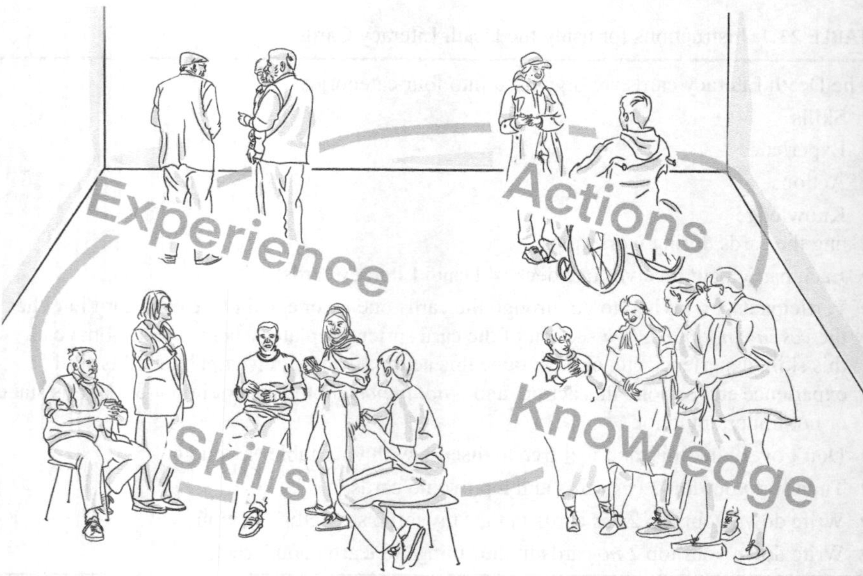

FIGURE 23.4 Experiencing the Death Literacy in the Room. Illustration by Niki Read

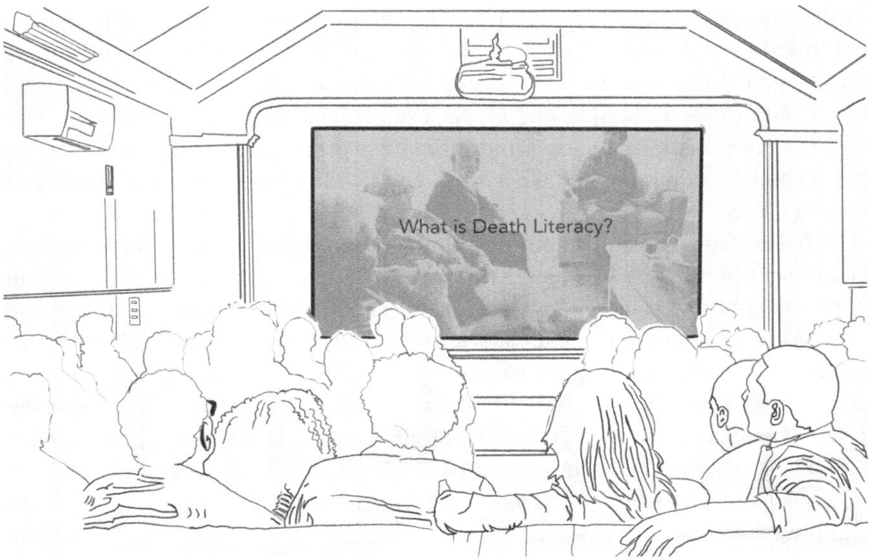

FIGURE 23.5 People in Community Setting Watching the Death Literacy Video That Encourages People to See Themselves through the SEAK Framework. Illustration by Niki Read

TABLE 23.2 Instructions for using the End-of-life Planning cards

The End-of-life Planning cards include some the many actions you can take to prepare for end-of-life. There are also "wild" cards where you can create and add your own planning actions.
Using the cards during workshops:
• Each participant receives one deck of End-of-life Planning cards (Go to www.deathliteracy.institute for more information).
• Participants are invited to go through the cards one by one and place each card in either the *yes*, *no* or *not important* section of the card sorter template, based on what planning they have done.
• A "wild card" can be used to add any other planning that is important to you but not listed.
• From your *no* pile, write down the three planning actions that are most important to you that you will do soon in the "planning" section.
• Discuss what is in your *no* pile, what reasons are there in your group for not doing some of these?

the death literacy in the room today. Some groups might have, for example, most people in the "experience" corner, a few in "skills" and "action," and barely any in "knowledge." This is discussed as a group and is often marvelled at.

Leaning into this, participants are then invited into a speed learning exercise, where they are asked to seek out someone in the room who has a *yes* card to one of their *no* cards and ask them the similar questions as earlier – "where did you get this skill or strength from, how did you develop this, and why is this important to you"? Discussions go for a few minutes and then are repeated multiple times with different people finding each other. This activity is often energising and the conversations focused and intimate – participants rarely want to stop, but it can be a good time to take a break and let the conversations continue in an informal way.

What follows is a collection of information modules based on the knowledge component of the SEAK model. Knowledge of issues related to death, dying, and bereavement is often scored low in a DLI survey [6]. Information modules include end-of-life planning documents and legalities, information about palliative care, lesser-known facts, social network activation and tools, and details about funerals and bereavement. After this more traditional education segment, participants then follow a similar process to that of the Death Literacy cards, sorting their deck of end-of-life planning cards, as outlined in Table 23.2.

Participants are then invited to discuss in pairs what is in their *no* piles, and to explore their reasons for not having undertaken some of this planning. Planning, which they may now choose to take action on, following the workshop, is listed on the card sorting template. The workshop, which, as described, takes four hours, ends in a group conversation, where we ask participants to reflect on:

1 What struck a chord with you today?
2 Did anything surprise you?
3 Has today inspired you to do anything?

This blend of educative, participatory and action-oriented learning allows participants to "talk, learn and act" in a multi-modal manner; there is an opportunity to connect and learn from the material, the reflective exercises and from each other in a very pragmatic way. One palliative care volunteer workshop participant reported that the experience was a "…good mix of doing, listening and reflecting." Each element is vital for people to walk away with a more embodied sense of death literacy. The objectives, content, and experience of the workshop are what makes the program a very useful tool for compassionate community settings, where the goal is to shift the experience of dying, caregiving, loss, and grief from being solely health and medical or private issue to one that can be shared. By improving personal understanding of end-of-life matters, participants can become more informed and proactive in their personal and professional lives, supporting themselves and others through the complexities of death and bereavement.

The primary objectives of the workshops are:

1 To normalise death, dying, and grief as a part of life
2 To reflect upon our own knowledge and actions
3 To encourage death literacy in everyday life
4 To learn from and share with each other

BOX 23.3 PC VOLS CASE STUDY

"I didn't expect to learn as much about creatively thinking through how to be more death literate."

In 2024, a group of palliative care volunteers attended a four-hour death literacy workshop with the authors. The volunteers were invited to reflect on their own death literacy and that of the group so that they may be better placed to support their palliative clients and each other in the future. The workshop helped them not only to identify their own strengths and prioritise future planning, but also to have a more nuanced understanding of what it feels like to have these conversations through the experience, aiding more layered volunteering and peer-led capacity building. The group conversations demonstrated that everyone has an open-ended entry point into death literacy conversations. Along with gaining "new skills to practice and add to my toolbox," one participant reported, "I know quite a bit about palliative care but recognise that's a starting point not an end point."

23.4 Modular delivery

The workshop has been designed for modular delivery and exists as a whole or as smaller, digestible components that can be delivered as a series or as standalone events. This allows for a range of funding, timeframes, context, and capacities, see Box 23.4 case study for an example. To date, death literacy workshops have been run with community members, palliative care volunteers, aged care workers, culturally diverse groups and health professionals, and primarily facilitated by the authors. However, anyone can host a death literacy workshop or event, in any setting. A volunteer or GP can use a deck of cards to discuss end-of-life with their patients or clients. A community development worker may host an event, for example, and screen the film, followed by a series of shorter bite-sized workshops. An aged care lifestyle worker might choose to introduce, sort, and discuss the cards with residents and family members on a family day morning tea. Learning can be facilitated in a group setting or via one-on-one reflection using any of the modules or resources and strengths-based questions such as those outlined in Box 23.3.

Modular delivery options include:

1. Complete modular package (four-hour workshop)
2. Short explainer video screening (Figure 23.5) followed by strengths-based questions for reflection
3. A series of shorter workshops facilitating one component at a time
4. Small group sorting and discussion of either card decks, or both
5. One-on-one sorting and discussion of either card decks, or both
6. One-on-one informal discussions using either of the card decks, or the video
7. Working with the modules in another way that suits your intervention

BOX 23.4 STRENGTHS-BASED CONVERSATIONS FOR SMALL GROUP VIDEO SCREENINGS

- What are your experiences, and what difference have they made?
- What have you offered (or been offered) to support friends and family caring for someone at the end-of-life?
- What SEAK do we have in this group?
- What would you like to learn more about?

BOX 23.5 CALD CASE STUDY

In one workshop, 22 people from different culturally and linguistically diverse (CALD) settings in Sydney, Australia, came together to do the complete death literacy workshop in the morning, followed by an afternoon workshop to discuss and support the organisations/groups in adapting and delivering workshops in their communities. CALD settings included culturally specific Associations and Aged Care providers, community centre staff and patrons. The training was led by the authors. Discussion included questions like "what needs to be adapted to suit the communities you serve" and "what support groups/education programs/community events etc. are *already* in place at your organisation – could you do death literacy workshops with these groups?" There was some discussion about the desirability and processes of having the workshops and materials translated into specific languages, sensitivity around cultural barriers with discussing death and dying, especially with older people, and a lot of ideas and enthusiasm for groups that could benefit from this work.

Two months after the initial day-long workshop, participants were invited to separate organisation/group follow-up sessions to discuss their progress and how we might further support them. Some groups had already taken elements of their learning and made changes to organisational policy and practice to reflect higher death literacy, some groups wanted support to adapt some of the materials, and one organisation identified the need for smaller, bite-sized sessions to be held, to minimise potential overwhelm in older people with less fluent English language skills, *and* to help their staff members grow their confidence facilitating new content. This organisation also began the process of engaging with another local business, already high in death literacy, to explore the options of delivering workshops together.

23.5 Workshops for health professionals

In addition to volunteers and community members, we have found the SEAK model offers a powerful and structured way to prompt reflection about personal and professional experiences with death, dying, and caregiving. Using the Death Literacy cards as described, health professionals have the opportunity to reflect on how they developed their knowledge and skills and to identify any gaps in their knowledge or understanding. The card sorting process provides a safe and non-judgemental process for health professionals to take time to reflect on their own end-of-life planning.

A skill that is often expected to promote with their patients and the community at large, but health professionals also find advance care planning challenging [9]. In this sense, reflection exercises can broaden awareness about the role of community education, laying the groundwork for public health and community engagement initiatives.

BOX 23.6 CASE STUDY: A WHOLE OF SERVICE WORKSHOP

This one-day workshop aimed to bring together diverse staff from across a health organisation to build a shared understanding of public health approaches to palliative and end-of-life care. The day began by introducing the core concepts that shape contemporary public health palliative care, framed as compassionate communities (the why), the death system (where), community development (how), and death literacy (what). This framework provided a common language for understanding the social, relational, and systemic layers that influence dying, death, loss, and grief and offered participants an opportunity to consider how these concepts align with their everyday practice and the organisation's strategic direction.

Using the sorting methods already described, the Death Literacy cards were used to create a safe and accessible way to explore values, experiences, and assumptions about dying, grief, and caregiving. They helped make complex issues feel grounded and conversational, and many participants reported an intention to take the cards back to their teams to initiate discussions and build confidence around end-of-life topics. Feedback highlighted that the cards translated death literacy from an abstract concept into something concrete, relational, and applicable across diverse roles and contexts. Individual reflection paired conversations and small group discussions provided a strong foundation for a concluding planning session focused on developing a coordinated program of community engagement and future compassionate communities initiatives.

23.6 Workshop evaluation

23.6.1 Using the Death Literacy Index in evaluation

The DLI was developed to enable an evidence-based approach to evaluating public health palliative care and compassionate community initiatives. Furthermore, a benchmarking approach provides an evidence-based framework for project planning, facilitates progress tracking, and effectively measures impact over time [5,10].

We have utilised the DLI in various ways in our workshops. For example, the DLI can be used as an initial benchmarking tool to capture baseline death literacy level and help to identify strengths and gaps to inform tailored interventions, ensuring workshop content directly addresses population needs and we tend to use the following steps:

1 Baseline assessment (pre-workshop):

- Participants complete the DLI survey to identify initial strengths and areas for growth.
- Immediate reflection exercises initiate conversations about personal experiences, values, and expectations.

2 Immediate post-workshop assessment:

- Participants retake the DLI to measure shifts in death literacy and any actions participants wish to take.
- Group reflection sessions explore insights, key learnings, and actionable next steps.

3 Follow-up assessment:

- Conducted six to eight weeks post-workshop to assess longer-term changes, integration of knowledge/other actions.
- Qualitative feedback explores any other changes and follows up on actions.
- Note, depending on the type of study, the short version of the DLI (DLI-9) can be useful to use at follow-up to reduce the time burden on participants [6].

23.7 Discussion

Compassionate communities' programs are interrelated public health approaches that aim to improve how individuals and communities understand, navigate, and support end-of-life care, death, dying, and bereavement. The model encourages the whole community, not just health professionals, to play a role in caring for people at end-of-life and supporting those who are bereaved. It is based on the idea that "care for one another at times of crisis and loss is not simply a task for health and social services but is everyone's responsibility" [11]. Compassionate communities build death literacy by:

1 Creating safe spaces for discussion and storytelling
2 Providing education and training
3 Empowering people to support each other during death, dying, and grief

In turn, increasing death literacy strengthens compassionate communities by:

1 Increasing confidence in caregiving and support roles
2 Reducing anxiety around death
3 Enhancing community resilience and capacity

Evaluations of the SEAK framework and the tools described have been positive. Overall, participants report an appreciation for the program's combination of practical tools, reflective learning, and accessible frameworks.

Many participants reported being surprised by the depth of insight they gained, particularly in terms of creative and reflective thinking about death literacy. One participant commented,

> "I didn't expect to learn as much about creatively thinking through how to be more death literate," highlighting the program's effectiveness in challenging assumptions and encouraging new perspectives. Others valued the practical aspects of the training, stating, "I learned some new skills to practice and add to my toolbox," and praised the balance of activities: "Great resources! Good mix of doing, listening, and reflecting." Even those with existing knowledge in palliative care acknowledged that learning is an ongoing process: "I know quite a bit about palliative care, but I recognise that's a starting point, not an endpoint."

The use of planning cards and the SEAK framework was particularly well received as a means to prompt meaningful conversations. Participants found the cards effective in facilitating discussions about sensitive topics:

> "Using cards as a tool to inquire about issues and concerns regarding death and dying, it's a clever way to promote deeper dialogue." These tools were also seen as helpful in engaging others, with one participant reflecting, "Planning cards are a great way to introduce the topic and create discussion."

Importantly, the program boosted confidence and motivation to share end-of-life information within their communities:

> "I feel more confident discussing and sharing end-of-life information with the community." The SEAK framework was recognised as a valuable guide for

> proactive planning: "I gained a lot of knowledge, especially that planning for end-of-life is essential when using the SEAK framework."

The illustrations in this chapter serve as tools to support comprehension, engagement, and behaviour modelling in a field that can often feel emotionally charged or daunting for everyday people supporting compassionate communities' projects. Their inclusion is not decorative but purposeful, aiding in knowledge transmission, empathy building, and facilitating accessible, inclusive learning environments.

Research in public health and education highlights that visual storytelling enhances understanding, memory retention, and emotional engagement, particularly in adult learning and community education settings [12,13]. Visual methods have been shown to help convey sensitive or complex concepts, making them more relatable and easier to discuss [14].

For example, figures like the card sorting activity (Figure 23.3) or community workshop scenes (Figure 23.4) do more than depict actions, they model behaviour and social norms around talking, sharing, and reflecting on death-related knowledge and practices. The DLI itself emerged from research that used creative visual methodologies like photovoice and social network mapping to bring visibility to hidden care practices and everyday knowledge of dying and bereavement [2,5].

By integrating illustrations that reflect lived experiences and workshop dynamics, this chapter extends that legacy. The illustrations support experiential learning and collective meaning-making, which is central to community development approaches and compassionate communities programs [11,15]. As such, they embody the public health palliative care principle that ordinary people are the most important resource in end-of-life care, and that tools which foster discussion and self-reflection especially when visually inviting can catalyse profound personal and social change.

23.8 Conclusion

This chapter has outlined a practical and research-informed approach to building death literacy through community education, centred around the SEAK model. By incorporating the DLI and employing experiential, creative methods such as card decks, videos, and illustrations, this chapter demonstrates how communities can engage actively with death literacy in an accessible and reflective manner. The SEAK model transforms death literacy from a static concept into a dynamic, participatory practice that empowers individuals to "talk, learn, and act."

The modular workshop design discussed here has proven effective across various community and professional settings, including culturally and linguistically diverse groups, healthcare workers, and palliative care volunteers. These programs align with the broader goals of public health palliative care and encourage the development of compassionate communities through health promotion activities that foster conversation and strengthen social networks.

Ultimately, this work emphasises that death literacy flourishes through social and community practices. By making the invisible visible through storytelling, reflection, and shared learning, individuals and communities become better equipped to care for one another in the face of dying, death, and loss.

References

1. K. Noonan, D. Horsfall, R. Leonard and J. Rosenberg, "Developing death literacy," *Progress in Palliative Care*, vol. 24, no. 1, pp. 31–35, 2016.
2. D. Horsfall, K. Noonan and R. Leonard, "Bringing our dying home: Creating community at end of life," *Health Sociology Review*, vol. 22, no. 4, pp. 373–383, 2013.
3. J. P. Rosenberg, D. Horsfall, R. Leonard and K. Noonan, "Informal caring networks for people at end of life: Building social capital in Australian communities," *Health Sociology Review*, vol. 24, no. 1, pp. 29–37, 2015.
4. R. Leonard, D. Horsfall and K. Noonan, "Identifying changes in the support networks of end of life carers using social network analysis," *BMJ Supportive and Palliative Care*, Vol. 5, no. 2, pp. 153–159, 2015.
5. R. Leonard, K. Noonan, D. Horsfall and J. Rosenberg, "Death literacy index: A report on its development and use," *Palliative Care and Social Practice*, vol. 14, pp. 1–11, 2020.
6. K. Noonan, A. Grindrod, S. Shrestha, S. Lee, R. Leonard and T. Johansson, "Progressing the Death Literacy Index: The development of a revised version (DLI-R) and a short format (DLI-9)," *Palliative Care and Social Practice*, Vol. 18, pp. 1–10, 2024.
7. P. Leavy, *Methods meets art: Arts-based research practice*, 2nd ed., Guilford Press, 2015.
8. G. Rose, *Visual methodologies: An introduction to researching with visual materials*, 4th ed., Sage Publications, 2016.
9. L. Gomes Souza, D. A. Bouba, R. C. Coroa, S. G. Dofara, V. Robitaille, V. Blanchette, K. Kastner, F. Bergeron, S. Guay-Belanger, S. S. Izumi, A. M. Totten, P. Archambault and F. Legare, "The impact of advance care planning on healthcare professionals' well-being: A systematic review," *Journal of Pain and Symptom Management*, vol. 67, no. 2, pp. 173–187, 2024.
10. K. Noonan, A. Grindrod, S. Shrestha, S. Lee, R. Leonard and T. Johannson, "Progressing the Death Literacy Index: The development of a revised version (DLI-R) and a short format (DLI-9)," *Palliative Care and Social Practice*, Vol. 18, 2024.
11. A. Kellehear, *Compassionate cities: Public health and end of life care*, Routledge, 2005.
12. H. Joffe, "The power of visual material: Persuasion, emotion and identification," *Diogenes*, vol. 55, no. 1, pp. 84–93, 2008.
13. M. J. Green and K. R. Myers, "Graphic medicine: Use of comics in medical education and patient care," *BMJ*, Vol. 340, p. 340, 2010.
14. M. Guillemin, "Understanding illness: Using drawings as a research method," *Qualitative Health Research*, vol. 12, no. 2, pp. 272–289, 2004.
15. J. Abel, J. Bowra, T. Walter and G. Howarth, "Compassionate community networks: Supporting home dying," *BMJ Supportive & Palliative Care*, vol. 1, no. 2, pp. 129–133, 2013.

24

DEATH LITERACY IN PRACTICE – CASE STUDIES FROM THE UK

Emma Hodges and James Byron

Abstract

The Death Literacy Index (DLI) can be used in a variety of ways as a survey and using more creative conversational approaches as outlined in Chapter 23. This chapter outlines the use of the DLI in practice firstly as part of Compassionate Birmingham one of the United Kingdom's largest and most diverse cities. This is followed using the DLI in Brereton, a village in Staffordshire and then as part of a Compassionate Organisations approach and finally by Dorothy House Hospice as part of their work to understand their community. The chapter outlines some of the benefits, challenges and outcomes from using the DLI alongside other compassionate community and public health palliative care approaches.

24.1 Introduction

The DLI is an exciting development and can be a bridge between community development and health system partners [1]. It is a series of questions that cover six areas pertinent to all areas of death, dying, loss and caregiving that allows for communities to better understand their confidence, knowledge and areas of development. The DLI can be used as a survey or via question cards in a community setting (see Chapter 23). So far in the UK the main use has been via a survey; however, using the cards will be a key part of a project in Birmingham going forward.

24.2 Birmingham

As detailed in Chapter 1, the Compassionate Birmingham network, in partnership with Compassionate Communities UK (CCUK), tested the DLI across the city.

DOI: 10.4324/9781003621348-25

TABLE 24.1 Experience in End-of-Life Care [2]

Experience in End-of-Life Care	*Percentage*
Experienced professional in end-of-life care/palliative care	5
Work in end-of-life care/death related profession	7
Have significant lived experience in caring for someone who is dying	40
Have little lived experience in caring for someone who is dying	48

The aim was to obtain a statistically significant response. In total, we collected 391 responses from community members.

It was important whilst testing the DLI that demographics were collected as well because there was concern that respondents working in healthcare might influence the scores. As shown in Table 24.1, most people who completed the survey were not members of the end-of-life or palliative care workforce.

The age range of respondents was broad; most respondents were aged 55–59, followed by 60–64 and 50–54; however, adult age ranges from 18 to 89 were reflected in the results 78% of respondents were female [2].

Ethnic diversity of respondents was of particular interest due to the multicultural nature of Birmingham (see Chapter 1 for further information). However, most people who completed the DLI identified as white English, Welsh, Scottish, Northern Irish or British (65.08%), followed by Caribbean (9.52%) and then Indian (5.56%). There is a large Bangladeshi community in Birmingham, who are not represented in the results.

Like other approaches [1,3], to achieve statistically significant results, convenience sampling was utilised to test the usefulness of the DLI in Birmingham and to compare this community against the UK sample. To really understand death literacy in Birmingham, a deep dive into individual communities, working alongside citizens is required.

Each question of the DLI was summarised individually and respondents were also asked about their experiences. This additional information was important in providing a deeper picture of death literacy, areas of priority for the healthcare system and community experiences. For example, it is highlighted how emotionally and physically draining caring for someone can be when amplified by additional barriers:

> I co cared for my father during his dying and death. I currently provide care for my mother, who is disabled and is very elderly. I understand the emotional and physical drain regarding the above, whilst trying to hold down a full-time job. The guilt and emotional struggle is significant.

For many people, it can be difficult to find support when caring for someone at the end of their life:

> Have cared for someone in their last week of life at home. Despite continually asking, very minimal care support was given. We had to call rapid response

> multiple times, and I took over care as only 6 visits were received in the week. We were not advised of what to expect, how to support, how the person may die. Lost my mother and grandmother within 6 months, established people in general do not know how to discuss death or grief.

This is particularly for marginalised communities:

> I feel Hindus don't raise their voice like other communities; therefore, their needs are not met, maybe it would help to meet with religious leaders what's required under these circumstances.

People commented on how difficult it can be to navigate the systems around death:

> navigating all the paperwork – I don't even know where to look.
>
> If it wasn't for my brothers, my mum wouldn't know what to do. I still don't know the process that needs to take place. I have not been able to share with anyone how I felt after my dad passed away as I took on a caring role in my family so everyone else was ok. It changes you and people don't realise the brain fog, confusion and who do you talk to.
>
> *[2]*

24.2.1 Results

It quickly became obvious from reviewing the individual questions as well as the totals, that respondents had a higher death literacy when relying on personal experience, however that when relying on knowledge of local systems and services, death literacy was significantly reduced. This demonstrates the need to understand the gap between communication of available support and services and community understanding. This is reflected in the first three scales of practice and experience being higher than the next three scales of community and knowledge as seen in Figure 24.1. Birmingham's overall initial score was broadly like the UK average.

Birmingham Public Health Department funded a community development worker to use DLI and engage with some specific community groups including those from ethnically diverse communities. The difference in these smaller community group samples in comparison to broad population results demonstrates the importance of the DLI being utilised as a community development tool. Population-level data can create a broad baseline but those community members who are currently underrepresented and unlikely to complete a survey, may remain unheard. Given the diversity of the city and the results of convenience sampling, this phase two data set made up of smaller samples shown in Figure 24.2 is more likely to be representative of death literacy in Birmingham.

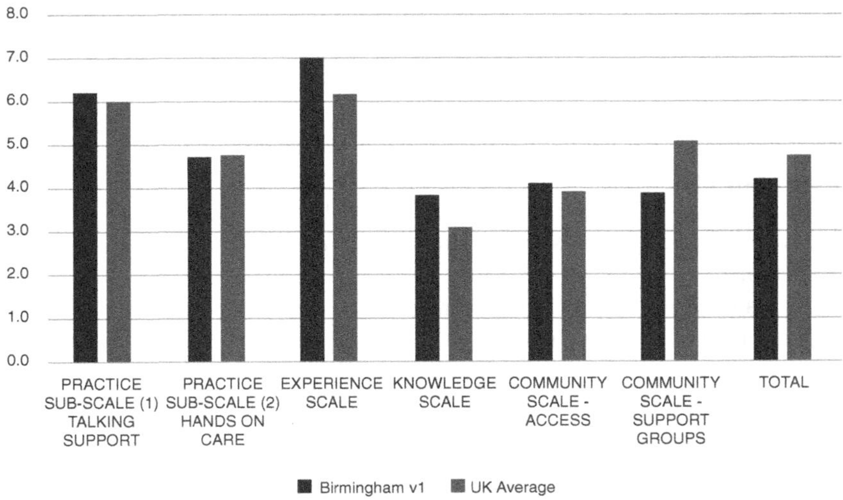

FIGURE 24.1 Birmingham's Initial DLI Results

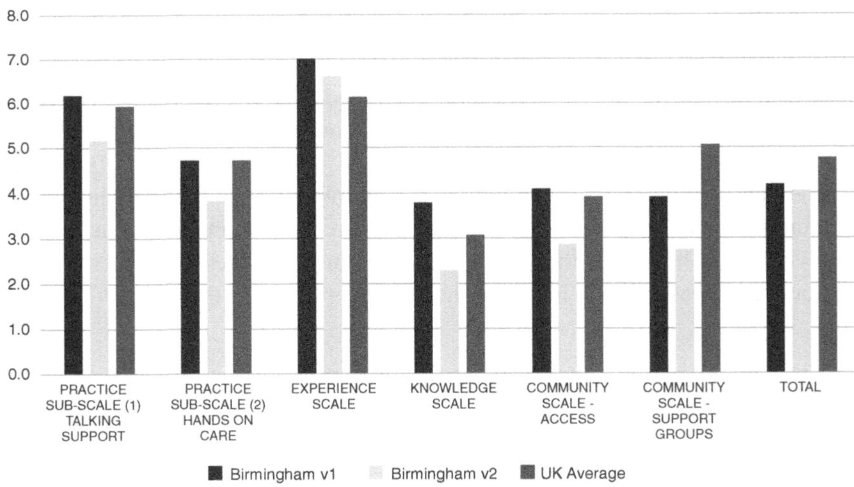

FIGURE 24.2 Birmingham Phase 2 DLI Results Alongside Phase 1 and the UK Average

24.2.2 Application and next steps

Feedback from the initial DLI survey was broadly positive in that it provided some useful information, although it raised more questions than answers. It demonstrated that on areas such as knowledge, community access and community support more awareness needed to be developed. In parallel to this project, the Birmingham and

Solihull Integrated Care Board published a portal that aims to bring together information for healthcare professionals and residents [4]. The hope is that monitoring use of this portal may indicate if it is helping increase death literacy.

Feedback on the DLI was that some of the questions were complex, particularly for people with neurodivergence such as attention deficit disorder and for non-native English speakers. As such, the Compassionate Birmingham network decided to simplify the questions to meet Plain English standards [5] and future work with ethnically diverse communities regarding accessibility of the DLI is also planned.

The Fairer Futures Fund programme, referred to in Chapter 1, will use the DLI as a community development tool, sharing information with residents and exploring together how they, with the support from Compassionate Birmingham, if needed, will develop their death literacy. Of course, the programme may determine that death literacy is not a priority for the residents who form part of the Fairer Futures Fund, but time will tell!

24.3 Brereton

The village of Brereton decided to use DLI to inform their future plans for the compassionate community's initiative. Rather than a digital-only platform for promoting and completing the survey, the team organised a range of conversation, paper surveys alongside an online survey and social media. Due to the work of Brereton Million (see Chapter 2), there was a good understanding of many of the challenges relating to death literacy in the village.

Brereton Million had worked with a start-up organisation that helped simplify the administration required after a death and trained volunteers in the community who could help with this. They had also put on a week of events aimed at supporting increasing knowledge and helping people to 'get their affairs in order'.

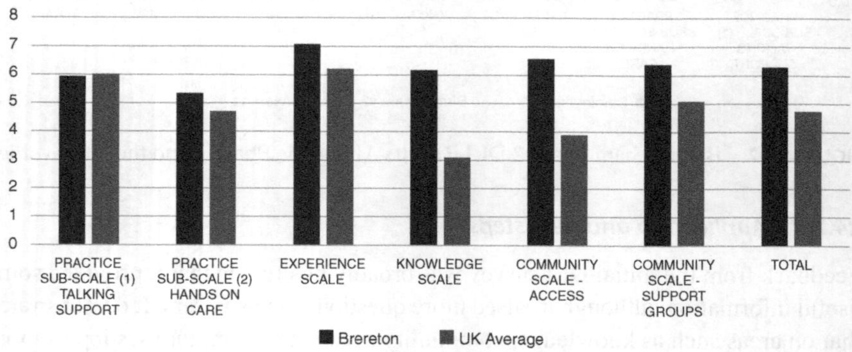

FIGURE 24.3 Brereton's DLI Results Compared to the UK Average [6]

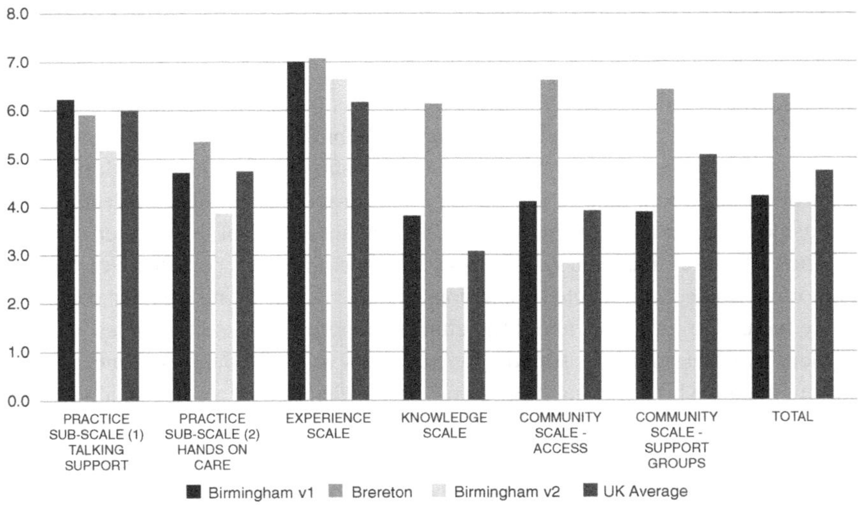

FIGURE 24.4 DLI Brereton, Birmingham and UK Average

These activities were not implemented to increase death literacy for an indicator but due to the knowledge, locally of the experiences of residents. In fact, at the time of running the activities to support the community on death, dying, loss and caregiving, the team at Brereton Million didn't know the DLI existed (Figure 24.3).

Brereton's death literacy results are significantly higher than the UK average [6].

What Brereton has is a central hub and a population of only 6,000 people [7] along with a community leader that everybody knows either in person or via the various social media groups. If a resident does not know how to access support – they usually know who to ask and this made it easier to work on death literacy within the community. There is growing evidence to suggest that death literacy is higher in community with increased social connections and in this case study we saw evidence of that.

Comparing a village with a city is interesting when discussing compassionate communities and optimum size of place for impact (Figure 24.4).

The people of Brereton are continuing their work as a compassionate community and at some stage in the future will repeat the DLI. There are also conversations about an indicator for young adults who are a key focus for their work locally.

24.4 Compassionate organisations

CCUK operates a compassionate organisation and workplace programme. The difference between the two being that a workplace programme and endorsement focus on the 'internal' audience whereas an 'organisation' includes the external community in which the business or school operates.

To become an endorsed workplace or organisation, there are a series of steps. One of which includes using the DLI-9 question tool [8] which is embedded into a wider survey. The use of the DLI-9 was introduced at an employer's event, led by a UK hospice, and was very well received. The business leaders understood the benefit to their workforce of not only having support available during times relating to serious illness, death, dying and loss but also to the benefits of raising the death literacy of the workforce. Being able to use the DLI-9 to provide a snapshot of death literacy alongside the other assessment methods is a real advantage of this shorter survey.

The full survey included questions about the employee's personal experience of supporting someone impacted by serious illness, death, dying, loss or caregiving. There were also questions about the cultural appropriateness of policies, equity of support, available training, support for managers or staff whose role includes supporting people who are dying or grieving. These elements of a compassionate workplace or organisation then form part of a wider assessment of health and well-being factors such as mental health, a sense of belonging, movement and environment.

The use of DLI-9 is emerging, and at the time of writing, there are two organisations whose results we can share. These have been recorded alongside the equivalent indicators in place-based initiatives. The organisations' names have been anonymised.

The comparison is for purposes of interest, rather than a correlation between organisational and place-based results.

Employer B is slightly under in comparison to the other areas, whereas School P is ahead. It is too early in the use of the DLI-9 to draw any conclusions. For both organisations using DLI-9 provided some interesting insights and informed their action plans, particularly around potential partnerships and connections within their local community, and it will be interesting to see how their results change over time (Figure 24.5).

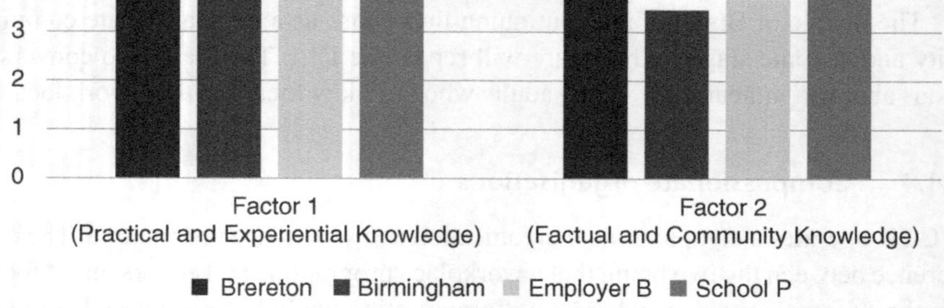

FIGURE 24.5 Use of DLI-9

24.5 Case study – Dorothy House hospice care

In 2022, reflecting both an internal desire to empower communities through strength-based local approaches and an increased sector focus on localised provision of healthcare, Dorothy House created ten Community Palliative Care Teams (CPCT), mirroring the structure of UK primary care networks in our region. In parallel to this change, they used the DLI to benchmark these neighbourhoods through demographically representative samples, seeking to understand where different community strengths and approaches in relationship to them might vary from place to place.

The total sample was 796 responses comprising 526 solicited through hospice communications, 250 sourced from a commercial panel and 20 face-to-face completions to ensure a minimum threshold of 50 responses per neighbourhood and address demographic imbalances (e.g. a shortage of young male responders). While samples were representative in terms of age groups and gender 23% indicated that they 'work or have worked with people at end-of-life' and 51% that they had 'been involved in caring for a person while they were dying at home'. The high number of people with caring experience can be attributed to respondents being sourced through hospice mail lists.

Overall, Death Literacy scored at 5.2 in the sample as a whole compared to 4.8 in the responses from the commercial panel and 4.8 seen in a UK DLI validation study [3] meaning the wider results need to be treated with caution and applied as indicative guides to delivery. This does however evidence the potential impact of the wider supporters and communities that are in relationship to health care institutions and charities, like UK hospices, by evidencing their strength in Death Literacy (Table 24.2).

Due to smaller sample sizes, analysis at the neighbourhood level needed to be treated with caution due to the thresholds needed to attribute statistical significance. However, some metrics and areas stood out. For example the Frome and Mendip Primary Care Network (PCN) area, which is has seen the development of the Frome Model [9] of

TABLE 24.2 Dorothy House Data Compared with Graham-Wisener et al.

DLI Scales and Subscales	*DH Data 2022*	*Graham-Wisener et al. (2022)*
Practical knowledge	5.7	5.4
Talking support	6.2	6.0
Hands on care	5.2	4.7
Experiential knowledge	6.5	6.2
Factual knowledge	4.0	3.1
Community knowledge	5.0	4.5
Accessing help	4.8	3.9
Community groups	5.3	5.1
DLI overall	5.2	4.8

compassionate community delivery had the highest overall level of death literacy (5.6 compared to an area baseline of 5.2), with Community Knowledge (5.6 in Frome versus 5 in the local area) and Community Groups (6 in Frome versus 5.3 in the local area) metrics were found to be statistically higher.

At the other end of the spectrum, the Three Valleys Health PCN, which comprises smaller towns and villages including a former mining community with higher-than-average scores on the Index of Multiple Deprivation, had an overall DLI score of 4.8. The highest scores compared to the UK benchmark were Practical Knowledge (6.3 in Three Valleys PCN versus the UK benchmark of 5.7) and Hands on care (5.9 Three Valleys PCN versus the UK benchmark of 5.2), whilst Factual Knowledge was the lowest (3.0 Three Valleys PCN versus the UK benchmark of 4.0). Like other community projects, Three Valleys Health area is perceived to have a higher number of intergenerational communities where more people were activity involved in caring for friends and relatives. While the lower educational attainment associated with the socio-economic disadvantage was perceived as a potential barrier to the absorption of factual knowledge in the way, it has traditionally been transmitted.

Findings from the community survey were presented to CPCT in order that they could be reflected in their approach to community engagement. Community provision reflects 90% of those cared for by the charity so is hugely significant to the overall experience of end-of-life care in the area.

At a broader level Dorothy House was able to see the impact of the informal community engagement, such as community art and cultural projects, as death literacy tended to be higher in communities where these had historically occurred. This created an increased sense of confidence in the efficacy of creative and informal social events and interventions and an increased willingness to prioritise organisation resources towards their future delivery.

One example of this strengths-based approach is the Firefly Woods at the Dorothy House Winsley site. In response to the pandemic restrictions, Dorothy House collaborated with a local light artist, Bruce Munro. He donated a small installation of Firefly fibre optic lights, into a wooded area to provide a place of reflection. The installation was well received by the community members who engaged with it. An evidence base for the therapeutic benefits of connection to nature was established [10]. Partially inspired by the DLI findings Bruce donated a further installation of lights in 2023 and Wiltshire Wildlife Trust partnered with Dorothy House to support the development of a nature trail focused on facilitating conversations about death and dying with children and young people in 2024. Once access restrictions were removed, the community were encouraged to access the site when a 'place where death is part of life' was relevant to them. Since 2021 thousands of people have chosen to visit the site. An online live stream has also logged hundreds of people attending online each year.

Further, a small group of individual volunteers have stepped forward to help maintain the woods containing the lights. The mentality shift facilitated through the

DLI feedback process encouraged the organisation so support this group and there are now 13 volunteers who help to maintain the Fireflies as an asset to support the wider community. This group also offer peer support and met for a Christmas meal, providing additional social and grief support within the volunteer group.

In 2025, Dorothy House conducted another DLI survey for a sample of 600 sourced via a commercial panel. This group reflected a wider geography than the original sample area. Death literacy had improved slightly overall and across all subscales; however, at the time of writing, the analysis was still underway. It might however be an initial indication that the community engagement by Dorothy House appears to be having an impact on the overall death literacy.

24.6 Summary

This chapter provides some practice-based uses of the DLI. The use of the DLI is emergent and as a community development tool, there is flexibility to test it and use it in creative ways. CCUK has created a DLI Peer Support Group to discuss some of the opportunities and challenges relating to the DLI tools as well as comparing the findings from different communities and considering how to ensure all community voices are heard.

There is an ongoing need to consider the results of national representative studies, and that over time they need to be updated. Additional research is needed to ensure greater representation in national studies. This data will be valuable for both grassroots organisations and health and care system to better co-create target and measure activities that improve death literacy.

The size of communities or neighbourhoods also appears to matter. The Compassionate Birmingham network team, for example, believe that Brereton's results indicate something important about the 'centre of a community' and the practicality of social connectedness at scale. Like with many elements of compassionate city and compassionate community programmes, the usefulness of DLI data is at different levels. At a grassroots level, it can inform the community who completed the DLI as to what strengths and challenges residents are facing and provide opportunities for conversations and action.

At the middle level of organisations and service providers working in the place, it provides useful insight into the effectiveness of interventions and opens the opportunity for additional conversations, community-focused service redesign and co-design of solutions. At strategy and policy level, it can flag what is working well or where the focus of developments needs to be.

In previous years, attempting to demonstrate the impact and importance of compassionate communities to people focused on measurable health outcomes was challenging and relied on tools that were not fit for purpose. As the number of initiatives using the DLI grows, it will strengthen our understanding of the links between compassionate communities, death literacy and health outcomes.

References

1. R. Leonard, K. Noonan, D. Horsfall and J. Rosenberg, "Death literacy index: a report on its development and use," *Palliative Care and Social Practice*, vol. 14, pp. 1–11, 2020.
2. The Compassionate Birmingham Network, *Death Literacy Index*, Compassionate Communities UK, 2023.
3. L. Graham-Wisener, P. Toner, R. Leonard and J. M. Groarke, "Psychometric validation of the Death Literacy Index and benchmarking of death literacy level in a representative UK population sample," *BMC Palliative Care*, vol. 21, no. 1, pp. 1–15, 2022.
4. Birmingham and Solihull Integrated Care Board, "End of Life," [Online]. Available: https://www.birminghamsolihull.icb.nhs.uk/health-information/end-of-life. [Accessed 23 September 2025].
5. Plain English Campaign, "Plain English Campaign," [Online]. Available: https://www.plainenglish.co.uk/. [Accessed 19 September 2025].
6. Brereton Million, *Death Literacy Index*, Brereton Million, 2024.
7. Cannock Chase Council, "Brereton and Ravenhill, 2023," 2023. [Online]. Available: https://www.cannockchasedc.gov.uk/sites/default/files/site-old/brereton_and_ravenhill_2023.pdf. [Accessed 2 September 2025].
8. K. Noonan, A. Grindrod, S. Shrestha, S. Lee, R. Leonard and T. Johansson, "Progressing the death literacy index: the development of a revised version (DLI-R) and a short formal (DLI-9)," *Palliat Care Soc Practice*, vol. 2024. doi: 10.1177/26323524241274806. eCollection, 2024.
9. K. Withers, "A long way from Frome: improving connections between patients, local services and communities to reduce emergency admissions," *BMC Primary Care*, vol. 25, no. 1, p. 307, 2024.
10. R. Lumber, "Beyond knowing nature: contact, emotion, compassion, meaning and beauty are pathways to nature connection," *PLoS One*, vol. 12, no. 5, 2017. https://doi.org/10.1371/journal.pone.0177186

CONCLUSION

Manjula Patel and Emma Hodges

Abstract

This conclusion aims to draw together many of the themes from places featured in this book, starting by outlining areas of shared practice then discussing similar challenges and finally commenting on three practice-based tools, that are utilised in compassionate city and compassionate community initiatives.

Whilst each community is unique, there are similarities in approaches, challenges and lessons learnt that can be helpful to places looking to develop or start a compassionate city or community initiative. The most common approaches within the chapters are practical ingredients needed in developing compassionate cities/communities.

C.1 Introduction

At the beginning of this book, we outlined the aims of drawing together practical examples of compassionate communities/cities activities from around the world.

The cases have captured the journey of how individuals, organisations and communities started out on developing public health approaches to death, dying, loss and caregiving. Underpinning all the cases is the nuance of integrating a new approach within diverse cultural norms. Along the way we learn about the practical steps and barriers they encountered and how they worked through them.

In this conclusion chapter we draw on these diverse cases, and summarise the shared experiences that were the common practical ingredients between them required in developing compassionate communities/cities.

DOI: 10.4324/9781003621348-26

C.2 Common practice ingredients

C.2.1 Social capital

Some initiatives capitalised on the social capital of existing assets, such as Brereton, galvanising the myriads of community assets such as the social club, youth group and much more. Mid and East Antrim started conversations about death, dying and loss with a small charity already supporting older people. In Kerala, the medical students volunteered to befriend people dying. Taipei chose a neighbourhood with historical and cultural significance for their first compassionate communities initiative. While Getxo, initiated a compassionate communities programme to stimulate social capital, where individuals came to appreciate people supporting each other. Many of the chapters included the social capital of volunteers or community members, as well as some forms of education or raising awareness to support the development of compassionate cities/communities spreading the message amongst their own social networks. Building on existing and growing more social capital is a key element of developing a compassionate community initiative.

C.2.2 Partnerships

Aspects of partnerships and relationships with other organisations and stakeholders are featured in all the chapters. The range of partnerships across the areas of civic life listed in the compassionate city charter [1] were clearly key in the achievements of all areas featured. These connections with schools, businesses, workplaces, places of worship, neighbourhoods, community groups and health and care services for example were common. For Kenya, the partnership with a trusted organisation was at the heart of engaging with the community. Partnerships with healthcare organisations and others enabled Taipei, Singapore, Uganda, and Inverclyde to be a bridge into the community and reach more people. For Queensland, as a children hospice partnership was key. The longevity of the partnership or scale of activity varied and of course many of these reflected the social and cultural context.

C.2.3 Diversity & cultural appropriateness

An important feature highlighted in many of the case studies is the how compassionate community initiatives were adapted to be culturally acceptable. For example, in Taiwan they combined the initiative with Madeleine Leininger's cultural care theory, to re-frame discussions about end-of-life to be appropriate with Chinese beliefs. Mid and East Antrim in Northern Ireland, organised cultural exchange through stories, building cohesive communities who discovered their cultures had similar traditions. In some cases, there were no easy translation of the word 'compassion' for example, in Japan or, in Koln where they adapted the word to 'care' as it was more appealing to Germans. Uganda and Kenya both referenced the importance of recognising varied cultural traditions in both challenging taboos and generating community support.

C.2.4 *Young people*

Working with schools is a key area of action within the compassionate city charter [1] and a natural area of focus for compassionate communities. There are some wonderful examples in the chapters of areas doing innovative work with young people. For example, the Hackathon in Singapore, the Palliative Care Clubs in Uganda, and in Kenya they involved the youth to be part of the home visiting team, with the hope of building a resilient future. Often the engagement of young people purely relates to bereavement or education and in Kenya they also focused on supporting young carers.

This book also acknowledges that the engagement of children's palliative care services in the field of public health palliative care is essential. The chapter from Hummingbird House and the case study on service redesign at Acorns Children's Hospice offer emerging new ideas for the application of public health palliative care and compassionate communities for young people with a life limiting condition.

C.2.5 *Arts, culture, and festivals*

The creative arts feature in many of the chapters, for example, in Scotland, a festival to Absent Friends creates opportunities for storytelling and remembrance. In Birmingham, Brum YODO organises annual festival themed 'A Matter of Life and Death' with music and events. The East Suffolk coast initiative installed a 'Before I Die' wall and invited passers-by to write down something they hoped for before they died. They also, worked with libraries to stock bookcases with titles exploring grief, resilience, and hope. In Uganda, school students sang songs of celebration, recited poems reflecting on kindness and compassion, and performed plays at the launch of the palliative care club. In Singapore they hold an annual festival themed 'Live Well, Leave Well.' Mid and East Antrim facilitated art activities such as storytelling, music, movement and visual arts. As well as, holding the first funeral festival in Northern Ireland.

C.2.6 *Training and workshops*

The provision of training or workshops is mentioned in many of the chapters. Most of them such as: Scotland, Brereton, Singapore, Taipei, Japan, Colombia, Koln and Suffolk delivered training or workshops to community members and residents. Training for volunteers was cited by Uganda, Taipei, South West Australia, Queensland, and Ottawa. Getxo provided training for the migrant community. Training or workshops for other audiences included: caregivers, students, children, teachers, staff, healthcare professionals, end-of-life doulas, communities, people with learning disabilities, prison population, and employers. The training and workshops content included: issues about death, dying, loss, grief, bereavement support, compassion, community development, compassionate communities, public health palliative care, end-of-life care, advanced care planning, cultural training, peer support, and community resources.

C.2.7 *Public participation and engagement*

Central to developing compassionate communities, is community participation, so it is not surprising that all the case studies included public engagement in one form or another with a wide group of people. This included for example, community leaders, local businesses, religious representatives in Taipei. In Suffolk this included conversations about death, dying and loss at pubs cafes, prisons, schools, creative hubs, community centres, sporting locations, and hospitals. Koln organised death cafes and in Taipei a cafe with a similar function but called a life cafe and Inverclyde had a bereavement cafe. Bruges had a community neighbourhood programme, and there are many more example of community engagement with community groups, delivering workshops, organising events such as festivals, online resources, school project, encouraging champions and the recruitment of volunteers.

C.2.8 *Volunteering*

Volunteers, feature in many different forms. Volunteers were involved: with being member of a management group, providing practical support to people in the community, undergoing training, and taking part in community conversations. Inverclyde described the intangible benefits of volunteers' experience of making a difference. Volunteers in Getxo were trained to be connectors, their role was like Suffolk's volunteers as community and cultural connectors. Mid and East Antrim's asset-based approach involved older members of the community harnessing their lived experience in the co-produced activities of end-of-life discussions. In Ottawa, volunteers facilitated advance care planning, grief, and bereavement workshops. Volunteers in Colombia thought it was important to support caregivers.

C.3 Challenges

C.3.1 *Definitions*

The first challenge is with the definition is the word compassion itself. Compassion does not directly translate in some languages, e.g. Japanese or German. Or the term is understood as 'empathy' or 'being kind.' Ironically, there are many different dictionary definitions too. The Oxford English Dictionary definitions include "the feeling or emotion, when a person is moved by the suffering or distress of another, and by the desire to relieve it" [2]. Kellehear defines compassion as 'the sharing of suffering' [3].

In practice the exploration of the meaning of the word compassion creates shared learning and deepens understanding of diverse cultural contexts. This can be a valuable exchange that promotes learning.

The terms compassionate city and compassionate community are used interchangeably and there is confusion about the concept of a compassionate city applying to communities that are not cities.

Compassionate communities is a term used to describe community development in the context of public health palliative care; it is a practice method. A compassionate community is likely to be focusing on grass roots activities for example: Brereton, where one community leader during the Covid-19 pandemic mobilised a team of volunteers to be a source of support to members of the community where there was a need. They set out to bring people together, neighbours supporting each other, the foundation of supporting people at the end-of-life. In Kato the journey started from the transforming experience of care and loss an asset borne out of adversity, to support others from the grassroots.

The compassionate city charter [1] requires a wider range of public health methodologies including system redesign, reorientation of resources and policy change across civic life. This may be a city in the traditional sense, e.g. Birmingham in the UK or it might be a different configuration of administrative authority, e.g. Kericho County in Kenya or Matsuzaki Town in Japan. Any administrative authority will have a level they can directly influence and then also would need to influence greater regional or national policy. A compassionate city initiative will of course, also have several examples of compassionate community initiatives active, as they do in Birmingham, Scotland, Singapore and in Japan to enable system change, they are strategically implementing a compassionate city plan and compassionate communities locally.

In many cases local (bottom-up) compassionate community initiatives have found it challenging to impact system change, such as in Ottawa. While a compassionate city (top-down) approach can impact system change but may not have sufficient traction without grass roots engagement. A combined approach of compassionate city and community approaches are needed to have the greatest impact at all levels.

The other important reflection here is that the compassionate city charter [1], is not and was never meant to be prescriptive. Many places create their own charter or adapt the existing template into something that makes sense for their area of focus for example Kato Towns, Western Australia and Birmingham all reference how they created or modified the charter.

C.3.2 Resources and funding

All initiatives featured in this book had some form of resource and funding. These are incredibly varied across the areas. Some initiatives grew from outside of health and care structures, e.g. Ottawa and Brereton. Compassionate Ottawa was formed as an idea with a group of local people and later became more structured and was able to secure funding. Brereton had funding for a community development programme and due to the experience of the village during the pandemic, engaged in compassionate communities to strengthen and recognise the skills they had and work on areas of development.

A compassionate city approach can utilise a wider range of local government/authority resources over a longer period compared to short-term funded local community initiative outside of the system such as Ottawa. In Bruges the community development worker was placed within a healthcare service, in retrospect they reflected a community organisation would have been more suitable. Learning from Scotland's experience, a sustainability plan is needed to prevent the negative impact that short-term funded initiatives can have on a community. When the aim of a compassionate community initiative is increasing agency and control, the power dynamic associated to resources cannot be under-estimated. Compassionate communities are integral to a compassionate city movement to maintain momentum; to influence system change and build community capacity. Both city and community approaches are interdependent.

To create sustainability, appropriate allocation of resources will naturally vary. All the examples shared in this book have some sort of key role of either an individual or a team who are taking the work forward. Who this is, and how it is funded varies significantly from volunteers to funded community leaders, to funded professionals. In Kericho County, Kenya the lead is a nurse and community pastor. In Kerala, India a palliative medicine doctor, in Kato, USA a community member, in Birmingham, UK the public health department, in Scotland, a palliative care team, and in South West Australia a network led by a Professor in Palliative Care.

In many ways, who leads or starts the work is not important. However, the idea that there is a grass roots movement without leadership or resources is not seen in practice. Networks and partnerships are essential as can be seen across all the areas featured.

There is a responsibility of these early adopters to ensure that there is succession planning in place, making the case for a public health palliative care approach and embedding it within communities and systems so that a change of personnel does not bring the movement to a halt. Examples from Kato Towns and Birmingham reference the impact of key personnel changes.

C.3.3 Relationships with health partners and palliative care

There is wide variety in the examples shared relating to the engagement with formal palliative care services or other parts of the healthcare system. These can be loosely categorised as: -

1 For some their compassionate communities and compassionate cities programmes are a natural extension of palliative care, e.g. Singapore, Uganda, Kericho, East Suffolk, Kerala, Kenya, Getxo, East Suffolk, Scotland and Inverclyde

2 For others, the initiatives are separate or loosely connected to formal palliative care services, e.g. Brereton, Birmingham, Bruges, Ottawa and Mid and East Antrim.
3 Others are alongside elements of palliative care, e.g. Japan, Kato Towns, Taiwan, Southwest Australia, Queensland Australia, Koln and Keralty.

As described in the chapter on Kato Towns, co-developing an initiative alongside care provision, where there are different visions or different understandings of a public health movement can create significant challenges for maintaining partnerships.

For a compassionate community it is possible to grow community participation, social connectedness and increase death and grief literacy without too much engagement with formal health services. However, for a compassionate city, this is more problematic. All health and care systems need the three strands of; public health; primary/community health; and secondary/specialist health or as described by Abel et al, the New Essentials of Palliative Care [4] (specialist, generalist, community development, and civic sector) all working together.

This balance of community grown v healthcare-led needs careful navigation and a key area of influence for practitioners and leaders in public health palliative care.

C.3.4 Size

There is a theme about the size of the ideal community or city programme. Singapore for example has a country wide approach with excellent integration and partnership a national government level and across health providers. Constituencies can then get involved at a local level and in October 2025 Singapore launched Compassionate Communities SG with Mountbatten constituency being the first to launch its local initiative. There is no doubt that the combination of integration, partnership, and size of the area of focus provides some benefits to being able to generate ground up, organisational and policy change.

Colombia is also a country wide approach as is Uganda, although working within four regions as a starting point. Scotland also has a national approach alongside areas working at local areas such as the council area of Inverclyde.

Other initiatives are focused on a city or town, e.g. Koln, Bruges, Birmingham, Taipei, Ottawa, and Matsuzaki. For others it is whatever area makes sense to the origin of the compassionate community or city programme, e.g. Kato Towns, Brereton, Oasis of Hope in Kerachi County.

The question is perhaps less one of size and more about aspiration, sphere of influence and structures. For example, in Uganda specific areas have been selected to start growing with others to follow. Singapore has an integrated health and care system, and the Singapore Hospice Council has a unifying voice for their compassionate community programme, they will have a national structure with constituencies focused on areas of practice.

Therefore, a compassionate community needs to be a naturally occurring community that might be placed based, that has the aspiration and capacity to connect and improve issues relating to death, dying, loss and caregiving utilising the many ingredients summarised in this chapter and detailed across the book. A compassionate city needs to be an administrative authority that has the commitment, influence and structure to reorientate policies, redesign systems and support many emerging compassionate communities.

C.3.5 Summary

These challenges whilst similar thematically, vary based on cultural context. Each compassionate city or compassionate community will need to consider how to navigate some of these issues, e.g. where is the community of focus, how big is it, where does the administrative authority lie, who are the key partners and how to facilitate change in often deeply embedded institutional partners. In most of these chapters there is a key person who has social and emotional capital, and therefore sustainability (in the context of ongoing adaptation and change) is a key concern. The demographic changes being experienced, and the pressure this will be putting on both healthcare systems and communities will no doubt create added challenges in how to resource compassionate city and community initiatives at a time when the new essentials of palliative care has never been needed more.

C.4 Tools

As practice develops in compassionate cities and compassionate communities, new methodologies and tools emerge. This book gives three examples of practice methods that support a compassionate city or compassionate community initiative based on themes outlined in the chapters.

C.4.1 Community connectors

The development of key roles in the community was mentioned in many chapters for example in South West Australia and Columbia. The advantages of these roles are set out in Chapter 22 and are critical in supporting compassionate communities.

In some examples a community connector may be a member of the public who has had a bit of training to enable them to have the confidence and knowledge to chat to people and where necessary signpost them to clubs and groups that might be helpful, e.g. the case study from Princes Alice Hospice in Chapter 22. In other examples the roles are more formalised and are part of a healthcare system providing 'social prescribing', e.g. Colombia. Having both is perfectly acceptable, the key is understanding the difference, that one is naturally occurring communities supporting each other and the other is a form of service provision.

C.4.2 Death and grief literacy

Increasing death and grief literacy was one of the aims of all areas featured in this book. Whether these specific terms were used, understanding different attitudes, cultural challenges and barriers relating to death, dying, loss and caregiving was a common theme. Some areas, e.g. Ottawa, Birmingham and Brereton, have used the death literacy index [5] to help understand the community or to provide some baseline information.

Chapters 23 and 24 were dedicated to the use of the death literacy index, how it can be used to prompt community discussions and how it is being used in parts of England as part of a compassionate city or compassionate community programme.

For people who need a more quantifiable method of showing change, the death literacy index is a significant development.

C.4.3 Service redesign

There is a challenge in aligning service providers' interests and a community development approach. For some healthcare professionals the focus of the job is so intense that it is difficult to imagine a new normal and some of the possible changes can threaten role identity and legitimacy [6]. Institutional change is challenging and as the chapter on Kato Towns shows sometimes decoupling key elements for them to survive and grow is essential.

Supporting teams to learn about the possibilities for a service redesign focused on community assets can help the relationship between healthcare professionals and communities. This was shown in the case studies in Chapter 22 with for example Acorns Children's Hospice where the process of using a community-focused service redesign approach enabled new thinking, learning and acceptance of new models of working.

If one of the aims of public health palliative care is the reorientation of health care services and resources to community, then new practice methods that supports institutional change is essential.

C.5 Conclusion

The aim of this book was to offer a range of diverse practice examples from across the globe that would help current and future practitioners involved in compassionate city and compassionate community initiatives. The chapters provide common experiences, challenges, lessons, and many creative ideas. These many shared approaches provide a new and comprehensive framework of practice ingredients that can help in the planning, development and growth of compassionate cities and communities. The hope is that the fantastic examples featured in this book will inspire and help continue to grow the compassionate city and community movement to improve the lives of people affected by death, dying, loss and caregiving.

References

1. A. Kellehear, "Compassionate City Charter," 2020. [Online]. Available: https://compassionate-communitiesuk.com/the-compassionate-city-charter-3/. [Accessed 18 August 2025].
2. Oxford English Dictionary, "Compassion," [Online]. Available: https://www.oed.com/dictionary/compassion_n?tl=true#8806014. [Accessed 26 October 2025].
3. A. Kellehear, "*Discussions in Singapore*." [Interview] *Singapore Hospice Council*, Singapore. 2025. [Online]. Available: https://www.singaporehospice.org.sg/an-interview-with-professor-allan-kellehear/#. [Accessed 18 August 2025].
4. J. Abel, A. Kellehear and A. Karapliagou, "Palliative care – The new essentials," *Annals Palliative Medicine*, Vol 7, Supplement 2, pp. S3-S14, 2018. [Online] Available: https://apm.amegroups.org/article/view/19026/html. [Accessed 18 August 2025].
5. R. Leonard, K. Noonan, D. Horsfall and J. Rosenberg, "Death literacy index: A report on its development and use," *Palliative Care and Social Practice*, vol. 14, pp. 1–11, 2020.
6. E. Hodges and S. Read, "How might organisational institutionalism support the challenges of the modern hospice," *The International Journal of Health Planning and Management*, vol. 33, no. 4, pp. 768–774, 2018.

INDEX

Note: **Bold** page numbers refer to tables and *italic* page numbers refer to figures.